CLINICAL COMPANION FOR

P9-DMB-219

WONG'S

ESSENTIALS *of* PEDIATRIC NURSING

CLINICAL COMPANION FOR

WONG'S
ESSENTIALS
of PEDIATRIC
NURSING

Marilyn J. Hockenberry,
PHD, RN-CS, PNP, FAAN

Director, Center for Research and Evidence-Based Practice
Nurse Scientist, Texas Children's Hospital;
Director of Nurse Practitioners
Texas Children's Cancer Center;
Professor, Department of Pediatrics
Baylor College of Medicine
Houston, Texas

David Wilson,
MS, RNC

Professor, Langston University School of Nursing;
Staff, Pediatric Emergency Center
Saint Francis Hospital
Tulsa, Oklahoma

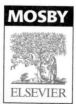

MOSBY

ELSEVIER

11830 Westline Industrial Drive
St. Louis, Missouri 63146

CLINICAL COMPANION FOR WONG'S ESSENTIALS   978-0-323-05354-9
OF PEDIATRIC NURSING, FIRST EDITION

Notice

Knowledge and best practice in this field are constantly changing. As new research and experience
broaden our knowledge, changes in practice, treatment and drug therapy may become necessary
or appropriate. Readers are advised to check the most current information provided (i) on procedures featured or (ii) by the manufacturer of each product to be administered, to verify the recommended dose or formula, the method and duration of administration, and contraindications. It is
the responsibility of the practitioner, relying on their own experience and knowledge of the patient, to make diagnoses, to determine dosages and the best treatment for each individual patient,
and to take all appropriate safety precautions. To the fullest extent of the law, neither the Publisher
nor the Authors assumes any liability for any injury and/or damage to persons or property arising
out of or related to any use of the material contained in this book.

The Publisher

Library of Congress Cataloging-in-Publication Data
Hockenberry, Marilyn J. Clinical companion for Wong's essentials of pediatric nursing /
Marilyn J. Hockenberry, David Wilson. — 1st ed. p. ; cm. Companion v. to: Wong's essentials of pediat-
ric nursing. 8th ed. c2009. Includes bibliographical references and index. ISBN 978-0-323-05354-9
(pbk. : alk. paper) 1. Pediatric nursing—Handbooks, manuals, etc. I. Wilson, David, 1950 Aug. 25- II.
Hockenberry, Marilyn J. Wong's essentials of pediatric nursing. III. Title. [DNLM: 1. Pediatric Nursing—
Handbooks. WY 49 H685c 2009] RJ245.H58 2009 618.92'00231—dc22

                                                                                    2008034172

Managing Editor: Michele D. Hayden
Developmental Editor: Amanda Politte
Publishing Services Manager: Deborah Vogel
Project Manager: Brandilyn Tidwell
Designer: Renee Duenow

Printed in the United States of America
Last digit is the print number: 9   8   7   6   5   4   3   2   1

CONTRIBUTING EDITOR

Patrick Barrera, BS
Assistant Director
Evidence-Based Clinical Decision Support
Center for Research and Evidence-Based Practice
Texas Children's Hospital
Houston, Texas

CONTRIBUTOR

Kathleen E. Carberry, RN, BSN
Research Nurse
Congenital Heart Surgery Service
Texas Children's Hospital
Houston, Texas

REVIEWERS

Pamela Bachmeyer, PhD, RN, CPNP
Associate Professor
Nursing Department
Chicago State University
Chicago, Illinois

Robin Gallagher, DNSc, MS, CRNP
Department of Nursing and Public Administration
Marywood University
Scranton, Pennsylvania

Carrie Huntsman-Jones, MSN, RN, CPN
Faculty
Department of Nursing
Davis Applied Technology College
Kaysville, Utah

Denise Nebel, MSN, RNC
Instructor
Iowa Wesleyan College
Division of Nursing
Mt. Pleasant, Iowa

Preface

This first edition of the *Clinical Companion for Wong's Essentials of Pediatric Nursing, 8th Edition,* provides a compact, user-friendly state-of-the-art resource for clinicians. The *Clinical Companion* is designed to ensure that specific information can be located quickly and easily when needed in a busy clinical setting. **Part 1** focuses on essential components of the history and physical assessment. Important aspects of the family and cultural assessment are included as well as special considerations for the newborn history and physical examination. **Part 2** provides a summary of pain assessment and management including nonpharmacologic interventions. **Part 3** presents a summary of 131 common childhood illnesses or disorders. Each illness/disorder summary includes a concise description of the problem, pathophysiology, clinical signs and symptoms, diagnostic evaluation, treatment, nursing care management and patient and family teaching. **Part 4** reviews common diagnostic tests or tools frequently used in the care of infants, children and adolescents. **Part 5** presents a summary of common nursing care procedures. Information in this book parallels the detailed description of pediatric nursing care found in the textbook.

With this new book we remember Donna Wong, whose knowledge and expertise of pediatric nursing have made us all better nurses. We greatly miss her.

Marilyn J. Hockenberry and David Wilson

Contents

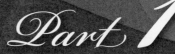

Part 1

History and Physical Assessment

HEALTH HISTORY
Information
Identifying Information
1. Name
2. Address
3. Telephone number
4. Age
5. Birth date
6. Race/ethnic group
7. Gender
8. Religion/spiritual beliefs
9. Nationality
10. Date of interview
11. Informant

    Chief Complaint (CC). To establish the specific reason for the individual seeking professional health attention

Present Illness (PI)
To obtain all details related to the chief complaint
1. Onset
   a. Date of onset
   b. Manner of onset (gradual or sudden)
   c. Precipitating and predisposing factors related to onset (emotional disturbance, physical exertion, fatigue, bodily function, pregnancy, environment, injury, infection, toxins and allergens, therapeutic agents)

2. Characteristics
    a. Character (quality, quantity, consistency, or other)
    b. Location and radiation (e.g., pain)
    c. Intensity or severity
    d. Timing (continuous or intermittent, duration of each, temporal relationship to other events)
    e. Aggravating and relieving factors
    f. Associated symptoms
3. Course since onset
    a. Incidence
        1. Single acute attack
        2. Recurrent acute attacks
        3. Daily occurrences
        4. Periodic occurrences
        5. Continuous chronic episode
        6. Recent travel outside the U. S.
    b. Progress (better, worse, unchanged)
    c. Effect of therapy

Past history (PH)
To elicit a profile of the individual's previous illnesses, injuries, or operations
1. Pregnancy (maternal)
    a. Number (gravida)
        1. Dates of delivery
    b. Outcome (parity)
        1. Gestation (full-term, near-term, preterm, postterm)
        2. Stillbirths, abortions
    c. Health during pregnancy
    d. Medications taken
2. Labor and delivery
    a. Duration of labor
    b. Type of delivery
    c. Place of delivery
    d. Medications
3. Perinatal period
    a. Weight and length at birth
    b. Time of regaining birth weight
    c. Condition of health immediately after birth
    d. Apgar score

    e. Presence of problems including congenital anomalies

    f. Date of discharge from nursery or NICU

4. Previous illnesses, operations, or injuries

    a. Onset, symptoms, course, termination

    b. Occurrence of complications

    c. Incidence of disease in other family members or in community

    d. Emotional response to previous hospitalization

    e. Circumstances and nature of injuries

5. Allergies

    a. Hay fever, asthma, or eczema

    b. Unusual reactions to foods, drugs, animals, plants, latex products, or household products

6. Current medications

    a. Name, dose, schedule, duration, and reason for administration

7. Alternative remedies

    a. Herbs, natural products, special foods, drinks

8. Pain

    a. Previous experiences

    b. Reactions

    c. Effective management

    d. Cultural influences

9. Immunizations

    a. Name, number of doses, age when given

    b. Occurrence of reaction

    c. Administration of horse or other foreign serum, gamma-globulin, or blood transfusion

10. Growth and development

    a. Weight at birth, 6 months, 1 year, and present

    b. Dentition

        1. Age of eruption/shedding

        2. Number

        3. Problems with teething

    c. Age of head control, sitting unsupported, walking, first words

    d. Present grade in school, scholastic achievement

    e. Interaction with peers and adults

    f. Participation in organized activities, such as scouting, sports

11. Habits
    a. Behavior patterns
        1. Nail biting
        2. Thumb sucking
        3. Pica
        4. Rituals, such as security blanket
        5. Unusual movements (head banging, rocking)
        6. Temper tantrums
    b. Activities of daily living
        1. Hour of sleep and arising
        2. Duration of nighttime sleep/naps
        3. Age of toilet training
        4. Pattern of stools and urination; occurrence of enuresis or encopresis
        5. Type of exercise
    c. Use/abuse of drugs, alcohol, coffee (caffeine), tobacco, vitamins/supplements, or alternative therapies
    d. Usual disposition; response to frustration
12. Nutrition
    a. Infant
        1. Breast fed or bottle fed
        2. Frequency and amount
        3. Duration
        4. Supplements
    b. Preschool and older
        1. 24-hour diet recall

Family Medical History
To identify the presence of genetic traits or diseases that have familial tendencies; to assess family habits and exposure to a communicable disease that may affect family members
Familial diseases, such as heart disease, hypertension, cancer, diabetes mellitus, obesity, congenital anomalies, allergy, asthma, tuberculosis, seizures, sickle cell disease, depression, mental retardation, mental illness or other emotional problems, syphilis, or rheumatic fever; indicate symptoms, treatment, and sequelae.

REVIEW OF SYSTEMS

General—Overall state of health, fatigue, recent and/or unexplained weight gain or loss (period of time for either), contributing factors (change of diet, illness, altered appetite), exercise tolerance, fevers (time of day), chills, night sweats (unrelated to climatic conditions), frequent infections, general ability to carry out activities of daily living, behavior

Integument—Pruritus, pigment or other color changes, acne, moles, birthmarks, discoloration, eruptions, rashes (location), tendency toward bruising, petechiae, excessive dryness, general texture, disorders or deformities of nails, hair growth or loss, hair color change (for adolescent, use of hair dyes or other potentially toxic substances such as hair straighteners)

Head—Headaches, dizziness, injury (specific details)

Eyes—Visual problems (ask about behaviors indicative of blurred vision, such as bumping into objects, clumsiness, sitting very close to the television, holding a book close to the face, writing with head near desk, squinting, rubbing the eyes, bending the head in an awkward position), cross-eye (strabismus), nystagmus, eye infections, edema of lids, excessive tearing, use of glasses or contact lenses, date of last optic examination

Nose—Nosebleeds (epistaxis), constant or frequent running or stuffy nose, nasal obstruction (difficulty in breathing), alteration or loss of sense of smell

Ears—Earaches, discharge, evidence of hearing loss (ask about behaviors such as need to repeat requests, loud speech, inattentive behavior), results of any previous auditory testing, pulling or rubbing ear

Mouth—Mouth breathing, gum bleeding, toothaches, toothbrushing, use of fluoride, difficulty with teething (symptoms), last visit to dentist (especially if temporary dentition is complete), response to dentist

Throat—Sore throats, difficulty in swallowing, choking (especially when chewing food—may be from poor chewing habits), hoarseness or other voice irregularities

Neck—Pain, limitation of movement, stiffness, difficulty in holding head straight (torticollis), thyroid enlargement, enlarged nodes or other masses

Chest—Breast enlargement, discharge, masses, enlarged axillary nodes (for adolescent female, ask about breast self-examination)

Respiratory—Chronic cough, frequent colds (number per year), wheezing, shortness of breath at rest or on exertion, difficulty in breathing, sputum production, infections (pneumonia, tuberculosis), date of last chest x-ray examination, and skin reaction from tuberculin testing

Cardiovascular—Cyanosis or fatigue on exertion, cold extremities, history of heart murmur or rheumatic fever, anemia, date of last blood count, blood type, recent transfusion

Gastrointestinal—nausea, vomiting (not associated with eating, may be indicative of brain tumor or increased intracranial pressure), jaundice or yellowing skin or sclera, belching, flatulence, recent change in bowel habits (blood in stools, change in color, diarrhea, and constipation)

Genitourinary—Pain on urination, frequency, hesitancy, urgency, hematuria, nocturia, polyuria, unpleasant odor to urine, force of stream, discharge, change in size of scrotum, date of last urinalysis (for adolescent, sexually transmitted disease, type of treatment; for male adolescent, ask about testicular self-examination)

Gynecologic—Menarche, date of last menstrual period, regularity or problems with menstruation, vaginal discharge, pruritus, date and result of last Pap smear (include obstetric history as discussed under birth history when applicable); if sexually active, type of contraception

Musculoskeletal—Weakness, clumsiness, lack of coordination, unusual movements, back or joint stiffness, muscle pains or cramps, abnormal gait, deformity, fractures, serious sprains, activity level, redness, swelling, tenderness

Neurologic—Seizures, tremors, dizziness, loss of memory, general affect, fears, nightmares, speech problems, any unusual habit

Endocrine—Intolerance to weather changes, excessive thirst and urination, excessive sweating, salty taste to skin, signs of early puberty

Lymphatic—History of frequent infections, enlarged lymph nodes in any region, swelling, tenderness, red streaks

CULTURAL ASSESSMENT

1. Communication
   a. What language is spoken at home?
   b. How does the family demonstrate respect or disrespect?
   c. How well does the family understand English (spoken and written)?
   d. Is an interpreter needed?

2. Health beliefs
   a. How are health and illness defined by the family?
   b. How are feelings expressed regarding illness or death?
   c. What are the attitudes toward sickness?
   d. Who makes the decisions regarding health practices in the family?
   e. Are there cultural practices that would restrict the type of care needed?
   f. Is a health professional of a specific gender or ethnic background an issue for the family?
3. Religious practices and rituals
   a. What is the family's religious preference?
   b. To whom does the family turn for support and counseling?
   c. Are there special practices or rituals that may affect care?
   d. Are there special rituals or ceremonies when a patient is ill or dying?
   e. Are special rituals or ceremonies attached to birth, baptism, puberty, or death?
4. Diet practices
   a. Are some foods restricted by the family's culture?
   b. Are there cultural practices in observance of certain occasions or events?
   c. How is food prepared?
   d. Who is responsible for food preparation?
   e. Do certain foods have special meaning to the family or child?
   f. Are special foods believed to cause or cure an illness or disease?
   g. Are there times of required food fasting?
   h. How are the periods of fasting defined, and who fasts in the family?
5. Family characteristics
   a. Who makes the decisions in the family?
   b. How many generations are thought to be a single family?
   c. Which relatives compose the family unit?
   d. When are children disciplined or punished?
   e. How is affection demonstrated in the family?
   f. How are emotions exhibited in the family?
   g. What is the attitude toward children?

6. Sources of support
   a. What ethnic or cultural organizations does the family belong to?
   b. How do the organizations influence the family's approach to health care?
   c. Who is most responsible for influencing the family's health beliefs?
   d. Is there a specific cultural group with which the family identifies?
   e. Is the specific cultural group identified by where the child was born and has lived?

SUMMARY OF PHYSICAL ASSESSMENT OF THE NEWBORN
Usual Findings
1. General measurements
   a. *Head circumference*—33-35 cm (13-14 inches); about 2-3 cm (1 inch) larger than chest circumference
   b. *Chest circumference*—30.5-33 cm (12-13 inches)
   c. *Crown-to-rump length*—31-35 cm (12.5-14 inches); approximately equal to head circumference
   d. *Head-to-heel length*—48-53 cm (19-21 inches)
   e. *Birth weight*—2700-4000 g (6-9 pounds)
2. Vital signs
   a. *Temperature*
   b. Axillary—36.5°-37° C (97.9°-98.6° F)
   c. *Heart rate*
   d. Apical—110-160 beats/min
   e. *Respirations*
   f. 30-60 breaths/min
   g. *Blood pressure (BP)*
   h. Oscillometric—65/41 mm Hg (average) in arm and calf
3. General appearance
   a. *Posture*—Flexion of head and extremities, which rest on chest and abdomen
4. Skin
   a. At birth, puffy, smooth
   b. Second to third day, pink, flaky, dry
   c. Vernix caseosa
   d. Lanugo

e. Edema around eyes, face, legs, dorsa of hands, feet, and scrotum or labia
f. *Acrocyanosis*—Cyanosis of hands and feet
g. *Cutis marmorata*—Transient mottling when infant is exposed to stress, decreased temperature, or overstimulation

5. Head
   a. *Anterior fontanel*—Diamond-shaped, 2.5-4 cm (1-1.75 inches)
   b. *Posterior fontanel*—Triangular, 0.5-1 cm (0.2-0.4 inch)
   c. Fontanels should be flat and firm.
   d. Widest part of fontanel measured from bone to bone, not suture to suture

6. Eyes
   a. Lids usually edematous
   b. Iris color—slate gray, dark blue, brown; absence of tears
   c. Presence of red reflex
   d. Corneal reflex in response to touch
   e. Pupillary reflex in response to light
   f. Blink reflex in response to light or touch
   g. Rudimentary fixation on objects and ability to follow to midline

7. Ears
   a. Position—Top of pinna on horizontal line with outer canthus of eye
   b. Startle reflex elicited by a loud, sudden noise
   c. Pinna flexible, cartilage present

8. Nose
   a. Nasal patency
   b. Nasal discharge—Thin, white mucus
   c. Sneezing
   d. Milia

9. Mouth and throat
   a. Intact, high-arched palate
   b. Uvula in midline
   c. Frenulum of tongue
   d. Frenulum of upper lip
   e. Sucking reflex—Strong and coordinated
   f. Rooting reflex
   g. Gag reflex
   h. Extrusion reflex

    i. Absent or minimal salivation

    j. Vigorous cry

10. Neck
    a. Short, thick, usually surrounded by skin folds
    b. Tonic neck reflex
11. Chest
    a. Anteroposterior and lateral diameters equal
    b. Slight sternal retractions evident during inspiration
    c. Xiphoid process evident
    d. Breast enlargement
12. Back and rectum
    a. Spine intact; no openings, masses, or prominent curves
    b. Trunk incurvation reflex
    c. Anal reflex
    d. Patent anal opening
    e. Passage of meconium within 48 hours
13. Extremities
    a. Ten fingers and ten toes
    b. Full range of motion
    c. Nail beds pink, with transient cyanosis immediately after birth
    d. Creases on anterior two thirds of sole
    e. Sole usually flat
    f. Symmetry of extremities
    g. Equal muscle tone bilaterally, especially resistance to opposing flexion
    h. Equal bilateral brachial and femoral pulses
14. Neuromuscular system
    a. Extremities usually maintain some degree of flexion.
    b. Extension of an extremity followed by previous position of flexion
    c. Head lag while sitting, but momentary ability to hold head erect
    d. Able to turn head from side to side when prone
    e. Able to hold head in horizontal line with back when held prone

PHYSICAL ASSESSMENT SUMMARY

1. Growth measurements
   a. Measure weight and height/length, chest and head circumference (see Tables 1-3 and 1-6).

2. Physiologic measurements
   a. Obtain vital sign measurements.
3. General appearance
   a. Observe the following during the assessment:
      1. Face
      2. Posture
      3. Body movement
      4. Hygiene
      5. Nutrition
      6. Behavior
      7. Development
      8. State of awareness
4. Skin
   a. Observe skin in natural daylight or neutral artificial light.
   b. *Color*—Most reliably assessed in sclera, conjunctiva, nail beds, tongue, buccal mucosa, palms, and soles
   c. *Texture*—Note moisture, smoothness, roughness, integrity of skin, and temperature.
   d. *Temperature*—Compare each part of body for even temperature.
   e. *Turgor*—Grasp skin on abdomen between thumb and index finger, pull taut, and release quickly; indent skin with finger.
5. Accessory structures
   a. *Hair*—Inspect color, texture, quality, distribution, elasticity, and hygiene.
   b. *Nails*—Inspect color, shape, texture, quality, distribution, elasticity, and hygiene.
   c. *Dermatoglyphics*—Observe flexion creases of palm.
6. Lymph nodes
   a. Palpate using distal portion of fingers.
   b. Press gently but firmly in a circular motion.
   c. Note size, mobility, temperature, tenderness, and any change in enlarged nodes.
7. Head
   a. Note shape and symmetry.
   b. Note head control (especially in infants) and head posture.
   c. Evaluate range of motion (ROM).
   d. Palpate skull for fontanels, nodes, or obvious swellings.
   e. Examine scalp for hygiene, lesions, infestation, signs of trauma, loss of hair, discoloration.
   f. Percuss frontal sinuses in children over 7 years.

8. Neck
   a. *Trachea*—Palpate for deviation; place thumb and index finger on each side and slide fingers back and forth.
   b. *Thyroid*—Palpate, noting size, shape, symmetry, tenderness, nodules; place pads of index and middle fingers below cricoid cartilage; feel for isthmus (tissue connecting lobes) rising during swallowing; feel each lobe laterally and posteriorly.
   c. *Carotid arteries*—Palpate on both sides.
   d. Note any deviation, masses, or nodules when palpating neck structures.
   e. Note unequal pulses and protruding neck veins.
9. Eyes
   a. Inspect placement and alignment; if abnormality is suspected, measure inner canthal distance.
   b. *Palpebral slant*—Draw imaginary line through two points of medial (inner) canthal.
   c. *Epicanthal fold*—Observe for excess fold from roof of nose to inner termination of eyebrow.
   d. *Lids*—Observe placement, movement, and color.
   e. *Bulbar conjunctiva*—Observe color.
   f. *Eyelashes* and *eyebrows*—Observe distribution and direction of growth.
   g. *Sclera*—Observe color.
   h. *Cornea*—Check for opacities by shining light toward eye.
   i. *Pupils*
      1. Compare size, shape, and movement.
      2. Test reaction to light; shine light source toward and away from eye.
      3. Test accommodation; have child focus on object from distance and bring object close to face.
   j. *Iris*—Observe shape, color, size, and clarity.
   k. *Lens*—Inspect.
   l. *Fundus*
   m. Examine with ophthalmoscope set at 0; approach the child from a 15° angle; change to plus or minus diopters to produce clear focus.
10. Ears
   a. *Pinnae*—Inspect placement and alignment.
   b. Observe the usual landmarks of the pinna.

    c. Note presence of any abnormal openings, tags of skin, or sinuses.

    d. Inspect hygiene (odor, discharge, color).

    e. Examine external canal and middle ear structures with otoscope.

11. Nose

    a. Inspect size, placement, and alignment.

    b. *Mucosal lining*—Redder than oral membranes, moist, but no discharge

    c. *Turbinate and meatus*—Same color as mucosal lining

    d. *Septum*—In midline

12. Mouth and throat

    Internal structures

    Ask cooperative child to open mouth wide and say "Ahh"; usually not necessary to use tongue blade.

    a. *Lips*—Note color, texture, any obvious lesions.

    b. *Mucous membranes*—Bright pink, glistening, smooth, uniform, and moist

    c. *Gingiva*—Firm, coral pink, and stippled; margins are "knife-edged"

    d. *Teeth*—Number appropriate for age, white, good occlusion of upper/lower jaws

      1. General rule for estimating number of teeth in children under 2 years: age (in months) minus 6 (e.g., 8 months minus 6 5 2 teeth)

13. Chest

    a. Inspect size, shape, symmetry, movement, and breast development.

    b. Describe findings according to geographic and imaginary landmarks.

14. Lungs

    a. Evaluate respiratory movements for rate, rhythm, depth, quality, and character (see Table 1-1).

    b. With child sitting, place each hand flat against back or chest with thumbs in midline along lower costal margins.

    c. *Vocal fremitus*—Palpate as above, and have child say "99," "eee".

    d. Percuss each side of chest in sequence from apex to base.

  e. Lobes are resonant except for:
     1. Dullness at fifth interspace right midclavicular line (liver)
     2. Dullness from second to fifth interspace over left sternal border to midclavicular line (heart)
     3. Tympany below left fifth interspace (stomach)
  f. Auscultate breath and voice sounds for intensity, pitch, quality, and relative duration of inspiration and expiration.
     1. Vesicular breath sounds
     2. Bronchovesicular breath sounds
     3. Bronchial breath sounds
  g. Note adventitious sounds.
     1. *Crackles*—Discrete, noncontinuous crackling sound
     2. *Wheezes*—Continuous musical sounds
     3. *Audible inspiratory wheeze (stridor)*—Sonorous, musical wheeze heard without a stethoscope
     4. *Audible expiratory wheeze*—Whistling, sighing wheeze heard without a stethoscope
     5. *Pleural friction rub*—Crackling, grating sound during inspiration and expiration

TABLE 1-1	
Various Patterns of Respiration	
Tachypnea	Increased rate
Bradypnea	Decreased rate
Dyspnea	Distress during breathing
Apnea	Cessation of breathing
Hyperpnea	Increased depth
Hypoventilation	Decreased depth (shallow) and irregular rhythm
Hyperventilation	Increased rate and depth
Kussmaul respiration	Deep and labored respiration, usually seen in respiratory acidosis (e.g., diabetic ketoacidosis)
Cheyne-Stokes respiration	Gradually increasing rate and depth with periods of apnea
Biot respiration	Periods of hyperpnea alternating with apnea (similar to Cheyne-Stokes except that the depth remains constant)
Seesaw (paradoxic) respiration	Chest falls on inspiration and rises on expiration
Agonal respiration	Last gasping breaths before death

15. Heart
    a. Begin with inspection, followed by palpation, then auscultation.
    b. Palpate to determine the location of the apical impulse (AI).
    c. Palpate skin for capillary filling time.
    d. Auscultate for heart sounds.
    e. Listen with child in sitting and reclining positions.
    f. Use both diaphragm and bell chest pieces.
    h. Evaluate sounds for quality, intensity, rate, and rhythm.
    i. Follow sequence:
        1. *Aortic area*—Second right intercostal space close to sternum
        2. *Pulmonic area*—Second left intercostal space close to sternum
        3. *Erb point*—Second and third left intercostal spaces close to sternum
        4. *Tricuspid area*—Fifth left intercostal spaces close to sternum
        5. *Mitral or apical are*a—Fifth intercostal space, left mid-clavicular line (third to fourth intercostal space and lateral to left midclavicular line [MCL] in infants)
    j. Listen in the following areas for these findings (see Box 1-1)
        1. *S_1-S_2*—Clear, distinct, rate equal to radial pulse; rhythm regular and even
        2. *Aortic area*—S_2 heard louder than S_1
        3. *Pulmonic area*—Splitting of S_2 heard best (normally widens on inspiration)
        4. *Erb point*—Frequent site of innocent murmurs
        5. *Tricuspid area*—S_1 louder sound preceding S_2
        6. *Mitral or apical area*—S_1 heard loudest; splitting of S_1 may be audible
        7. *Quality*—Clear and distinct
        8. *Intensity*—Strong, but not pounding
        9. *Rate*—Same as radial pulse
        10. *Rhythm*—Regular and even
    k. Usual findings of innocent murmurs
        1. *Timing within S_1-S_2 cycle*—Systolic, that is, they occur with or after S_1
        2. *Quality*—Usually of a low-pitched, musical, or groaning quality

      3. *Loudness*—Grade III or less in intensity and do not increase over time

      4. *Area best heard*—Usually loudest in the pulmonic area with no transmission to other areas of the heart

      5. *Change with position*—Audible in the supine position but absent in the sitting position

      6. *Other physical signs*—Not associated with any physical signs of cardiac disease

16. Abdomen

    a. Inspection is followed by auscultation, percussion, and palpation, which may distort the normal abdominal sounds.

    b. Inspect contour, size, and tone.

    c. Note condition of skin.

    d. Note movement.

    e. Inspect umbilicus for herniation, fistulas, hygiene, and discharge.

    f. Observe for hernias.

      1. *Inguinal*—Slide little finger into external inguinal ring at base of scrotum; ask child to cough.

      2. *Femoral*—Place finger over femoral canal (located by placing index finger over femoral pulse and middle finger against skin toward midline).

    g. Auscultate for bowel sounds and aortic pulsations.

      1. *Bowel sounds*—Short, metallic, tinkling sounds like gurgles, clicks, or growls heard every 10-30 seconds

      2. *Aortic pulsations*—Heard in epigastrium, slightly left of midline

---

▌ BOX 1-1

Grading of the Intensity of a Heart Murmur

I—Very faint, frequently not heard if child sits up

II—Usually readily heard, slightly louder than grade I, audible in all positions

III—Loud but not accompanied by a thrill

IV—Loud, accompanied by a thrill

V—Loud enough to be heard with the stethoscope barely on the chest, accompanied by a thrill

VI—Loud enough to be heard with the stethoscope not touching the chest, often heard with the human ear close to the chest, accompanied by a thrill

    l. Percuss the abdomen.
       1. Tympany over stomach on left side and most of abdomen, except for dullness or flatness just below right costal margin (liver)
   m. Palpate abdominal organs.
      1. **Liver**—May be palpated 1-2 cm below right costal margin in infants and young children
      2. **Spleen**—Sometimes palpated 1-2 cm below left costal margin in infants and young children
   n. Elicit abdominal reflex—Scratch skin from side to midline in each quadrant.
17. Genitalia
   a. Proceed in same manner as examination of other areas; explain procedure and its significance before doing it, such as palpating for testes.
   b. Respect privacy at all times.
   c. Use opportunity to discuss concerns about sexual development with older child and adolescent.
   d. Use opportunity to discuss sexual safety with young children.
   e. If in contact with bodily substances, wear gloves.
   f. Assess Tanner Stage.
18. Penis
   a. Inspect size.
   b. *Glans* and *shaft*—Inspect for signs of swelling, skin lesions, inflammation.
   c. *Prepuce*—Inspect in uncircumcised male.
   d. *Urethral meatus*—Inspect location, and note any discharge.
   e. *Scrotum*—Inspect size, location, skin, and hair distribution.
   f. *Testes*—Palpate each scrotal sac using thumb and index finger.
19. Female
   a. *External genitalia*—Inspect structures; place young child in semireclining position in parent's lap with knees bent and soles of feet in apposition.
   b. *Labia*—Palpate for any masses.
   c. *Urethral meatus*—Inspect for location; identified as V-shaped slit by wiping downward from clitoris to perineum.

  d. *Skene glands*—Palpate or inspect.
  e. *Vaginal orifice*—Internal examination usually not performed; inspect for obvious opening.
  f. *Bartholin glands*—Palpate or inspect.
20. Anus
  a. *Anal area*—Inspect for general firmness, condition of skin.
  b. *Anal reflex*—Elicit by gently pricking or scratching perianal area.
21. Back and extremities
  a. Inspect curvature and symmetry of spine.
  b. Test for scoliosis.
    1. Have child stand erect; observe from behind, and note asymmetry of shoulders and hips.
    2. Have child bend forward at the waist until back is parallel to floor; observe from side and note asymmetry.
    3. Note mobility of spine.
  c. Inspect each extremity joint for symmetry, size, temperature, color, tenderness, and mobility.
  d. Assess shape of bones.
  e. Measure distance between the knees when child stands with malleoli in apposition.
  f. Measure distance between the malleoli when the child stands with knees together.
  g. Inspect position of feet.
  h. Inspect gait.
  i. Have child walk in straight line.
  j. Estimate angle of gait by drawing imaginary line through center of foot and line of progression.
22. Neurologic assessment (see Table 1-2)
  a. Mental status
    1. Observe behavior, mood, affect, general orientation to surroundings, level of consciousness.
  b. Motor functioning (see Tables 1-4 and 1-5)
    1. Test muscle strength, tone, and development.
    2. Test coordination.
      ■ *Finger-to-nose test*—With the child's arm extended, have child touch nose with the index finger.
      ■ *Heel-to-shin test*—With child standing, have child run the heel of one foot down the shin of the other leg.

- ▪ *Romberg test*—Have child stand erect with feet together and eyes closed.
- ▪ Have child touch tip of each finger to thumb in rapid succession.
- ▪ Have child pat leg with first one side, then the other side of hand in rapid sequence.
- ▪ Have child tap your hand with ball of foot as quickly as possible.

  c. Sensory functioning
    1. Test vision and hearing.
    2. *Sensory intactness*—Touch skin lightly with a pin, and have child point to stimulated area while keeping eyes closed.
    3. *Sensory discrimination:*
- ▪ Touch skin with pin and cotton; have child describe it as sharp or dull.
- ▪ Touch skin with cold and warm object (e.g., metal and rubber heads of reflex hammer); have child differentiate between temperatures.
- ▪ Using two pins, touch skin simultaneously with both or only one pin; have child discriminate when one or two pins are used.

  d. Reflexes (deep tendon)
    1. *Biceps*—Hold child's arm by placing the partially flexed elbow in your hand with the thumb over the antecubital space; strike your thumbnail with the hammer.
    2. *Triceps*—Bend the arm at the elbow, and rest the palm in your hand; strike the triceps tendon. *Alternate procedure*—If the child is supine, rest arm over chest and strike the triceps tendon.
    3. *Brachioradialis*—Rest the forearm on the lap or abdomen, with the arm flexed at the elbow and palm down; strike the radius about 1 inch (depending on child's size) above the wrist.
    4. *Knee jerk or patellar reflex*—Sit child on the edge of the examining table or on parent's lap with the lower legs flexed at the knee and dangling freely; tap the patellar tendon just below the knee cap.
    5. *Achilles*—Use the same position as for the knee jerk; support the foot lightly in your hand and strike the Achilles tendon.

6. *Ankle clonus*— Dorsiflex child's foot and assess for rhythmical contraction of the calf muscles.
7. *Kernig sign*—Flex child's leg at hip and knee while supine; note pain or resistance.
8. *Brudzinski sign*—With child supine, flex the head; note pain and involuntary flexion of hip and knees.
9. Usual grading of reflexes:

Grade 0	0	Absent
Grade 1	+	Diminished
Grade 2	+ +	Normal, average
Grade 3	+ + +	Brisker than normal
Grade 4	+ + + +	Hyperactive (clonus)

TABLE 1-2

Assessment of Cranial Nerves

CRANIAL NERVE	DISTRIBUTION/FUNCTION	TEST
I—Olfactory (S)*	Olfactory mucosa of nasal cavity	With eyes closed, have child identify odors such as coffee, alcohol, or other smells from a swab; test each nostril separately.
II—Optic (S)	Rods and cones of retina, optic nerve	Check for perception of light, visual acuity, peripheral vision, color vision, and normal optic disc.
III—Oculomotor (M)*	Extraocular muscles (EOM) of eye: Superior rectus (SR)—Moves eyeball up and in Inferior rectus (IR)—Moves eyeball down and in Medial rectus (MR)—Moves eyeball nasally Inferior oblique (IO)—Moves eyeball up and out Pupil constriction and accommodation Eyelid closing	Have child follow an object (toy) or light in the six cardinal positions of gaze. Perform PERRLA (see p. 12). Check for proper placement of lid (see p. 12).
IV—Trochlear (M)	Superior oblique (SO) muscle—Moves eye down and out	Have child look down and in.

*S, Sensory; M, motor.

Continued

TABLE 1-2—cont'd

Assessment of Cranial Nerves

CRANIAL NERVE	DISTRIBUTION/FUNCTION	TEST
V—Trigeminal (M, S)	Muscles of mastication	Have child bite down hard and open jaw; test symmetry and strength.
	Sensory: Face, scalp, nasal and buccal mucosa	With child's eyes closed, see if child can detect light touch in the mandibular and maxillary regions. Test corneal and blink reflex by touching cornea lightly (approach child from the side so that child does not blink before cornea is touched).
VI—Abducens (M)	Lateral rectus (LR) muscle—Moves eye temporally	Have child look toward temporal side.
VII—Facial (M, S)	Muscles for facial expression	Have child smile, make funny face, or show teeth to see symmetry of expression.
	Anterior two thirds of tongue (sensory)	Have child identify a sweet or salty solution; place each taste on anterior section and sides of protruding tongue; if child retracts tongue, solution will dissolve toward posterior part of tongue.
VIII—Auditory, Acoustic, or Vestibulocochlear (S)	Internal ear Hearing, balance	Test hearing; note any loss of equilibrium or presence of vertigo (dizziness).

IX—Glossopharyngeal (M, S)	Pharynx, tongue	Stimulate the posterior pharynx with a tongue blade; the child should gag.
	Posterior one third of tongue (sensory)	Test sense of sour or bitter taste on posterior segment of tongue.
X—Vagus (M, S)	Muscles of larynx, pharynx, some organs of gastrointestinal system, sensory fibers of root of tongue, heart, lung, and some organs of gastrointestinal system	Note hoarseness of the voice, gag reflex, and ability to swallow. Check that uvula is in midline; when stimulated with a tongue blade, should deviate upward and to the stimulated side.
XI—Accessory (M)	Sternocleidomastoid and trapezius muscles of shoulder	Have child shrug shoulders while applying mild pressure; with the hands placed on shoulders, have child turn head against opposing pressure on either side; note symmetry and strength.
XII—Hypoglossal (M)	Muscles of tongue	Have child move tongue in all directions; have child protrude tongue as far as possible; note any midline deviation.
		Test strength by placing tongue blade on one side of tongue and having child move it away.

TABLE 1-3

General Trends in Height and Weight Gain During Childhood

AGE GROUP	WEIGHT	HEIGHT
Birth-6 months	Weekly gain: 140-200 g (5-7 oz) Birth weight doubles by end of first 4-7 months	Monthly gain: 2.5 cm (1 inch)
6-12 months	Weight gain: 85-140 g (3-5 oz) Birth weight triples by end of first year	Monthly gain: 1.25 cm (0.5 inch) Birth length increases by approximately 50% by end of first year
Toddlers	Birth weight quadruples by age 2.5	Height at age 2 is approximately 50% of eventual adult height Gain during second year: about 12 cm (4.75 inches) Gain during third year: about 6-8 cm (2.375-3.25 inches)
Preschoolers	Yearly gain: 2-3 kg (4.5-6.5 lb)	Birth length doubles by age 4 Yearly gain: 5-7.5 cm (2-3 inches)
School-age children	Yearly gain: 2-3 kg (4.5-6.5 lb)	Yearly gain after age 7: 5 cm (2 inches) Birth length triples by about age 13
PUBERTAL GROWTH SPURT		
Females— 10-14 years	Weight gain: 7-25 kg (15-55 lb) Mean: 17.5 kg (38.125 lb)	Height gain: 5-25 cm (2-10 inches); approximately 95% of mature height achieved by onset of menarche or skeletal age of 13 years Mean: 20.5 cm (8.25 inches)

TABLE 1-3—cont'd		
General Trends in Height and Weight Gain During Childhood		
AGE GROUP	**WEIGHT**	**HEIGHT**
Males— 11-16 years	Weight gain: 7-30 kg (15-65 lb) Mean: 23.7 kg (52.125 lb)	Height gain: 10-30 cm (4-12 inches); approximately 95% of mature height achieved by skeletal age of 15 years Mean: 27.5 cm (11 inches)

TABLE 1-4

Motor Development During Infancy

AGE (MONTHS)	GROSS MOTOR	FINE MOTOR
1	Assumes flexed position with pelvis high but knees not under abdomen when prone (at birth, knees flexed under abdomen)* Can turn head from side to side when prone; lifts head momentarily from bed* Has marked head lag, especially when pulled from lying to sitting position Holds head momentarily parallel and in midline when suspended in prone position Assumes asymmetric tonic neck reflex position when supine When infant is held in standing position, body limp at knees and hips In sitting position back is uniformly rounded, head control is absent	Hands predominantly closed Grasp reflex strong Hand clenches on contact with rattle
2	Assumes less flexed position when prone—hips flat, legs extended, arms flexed, head to side* Less head lag when pulled to sitting position Can maintain head in same plane as rest of body when held in ventral suspension When infant is prone, can lift head almost 45° off table When infant is held in sitting position, head is held up but bobs forward Assumes asymmetric tonic neck reflex position intermittently	Hands frequently open Grasp reflex fading

3	Able to hold head more erect when sitting but still bobs forward Has only slight head lag when pulled to sitting position Assumes symmetric body positioning Able to raise head and shoulders from prone position to a 45° to 90° angle from table; bears weight on forearms When infant is held in standing position, able to bear slight fraction of weight on legs Regards own hand	Actively holds rattle but will not reach for it* Grasp reflex absent Hands kept loosely open Clutches own hand; pulls at blankets and clothes
4	Has almost no head lag when pulled to sitting position* Balances head well in sitting position* Back less rounded, curved only in lumbar area Able to sit erect if propped up Able to raise head and chest off surface to angle of 90° Assumes predominant symmetric position Rolls from back to side*	Inspects and plays with hands; pulls clothing or blanket over face in play* Tries to reach object with hand but overshoots Grasps object with both hands Plays with rattle placed in hand, shakes it, but cannot pick it up if dropped Can carry objects to mouth
5	No head lag when pulled to sitting position When infant is sitting, able to hold head erect and steady Able to sit for longer periods when back is well supported Back straight When infant is prone, assumes symmetric positioning with arms extended Can turn over from abdomen to back* When infant is supine, puts feet to mouth	Able to grasp objects voluntarily* Uses palmar grasp, bidextrous approach Plays with toes Takes objects directly to mouth Holds one cube while regarding a second one

Continued

TABLE 1-4—cont'd

Motor Development During Infancy

AGE (MONTHS)	GROSS MOTOR	FINE MOTOR
6	When infant is prone, can lift chest and upper abdomen off table, bearing weight on hands When infant is about to be pulled to a sitting position, lifts head Sits in highchair with back straight Rolls from back to abdomen When infant is held in standing position, bears almost all of weight Hand regard absent	Resecures a dropped object Drops one cube when another is given Grasps and manipulates small objects Holds bottle Grasps feet and pulls to mouth
7	When infant is supine, spontaneously lifts head off table Sits, leaning forward on hands* When infant is prone, bears weight on one hand Sits erect momentarily Bears full weight on feet When infant is held in standing position, bounces actively	Transfers objects from one hand to the other* Has unidextrous approach and grasp Holds two cubes more than momentarily Bangs cube on table Rakes at a small object

8	Sits steadily unsupported* Readily bears weight on legs when supported; may stand holding on to furniture Adjusts posture to reach an object	Has beginning pincer grasp using index, fourth, and fifth fingers against lower part of thumb Releases objects at will Rings bell purposely Retains two cubes while regarding third cube Secures an object by pulling on a string Reaches persistently for toys out of reach
9	Creeps on hands and knees Sits steadily on floor for prolonged time (10 minutes) Recovers balance when leans forward but cannot do so when leaning sideways Pulls self to standing position and stands holding on to furniture*	Uses thumb and index finger in crude pincer grasp* Preference for use of dominant hand now evident Grasps third cube Compares two cubes by bringing them to-gether
10	Can change from prone to sitting position Stands while holding on to furniture, sits by falling down Recovers balance easily while sitting While child is standing, lifts one foot to take a step	Crude release of an object beginning Grasps bell by handle

Continued

TABLE 1-4—cont'd

Motor Development During Infancy

AGE (MONTHS)	GROSS MOTOR	FINE MOTOR
11	When child is sitting, pivots to reach toward back to pick up an object Cruises or walks holding on to furniture or with both hands held*	Explores objects more thoroughly (e.g., clapper inside bell) Has neat pincer grasp Drops object deliberately for it to be picked up Puts one object after another into a container (sequential play) Able to manipulate an object to remove it from tight-fitting enclosure
12	Walks with one hand held* Cruises well May attempt to stand alone momentarily; may attempt first step alone* Can sit down from standing position without help	Releases cube in cup Attempts to build two-block tower but fails Tries to insert a pellet into a narrow-necked bottle but fails Can turn pages in a book, many at a time

*Milestones that represent essential integrative aspects of development that lay the foundation for the achievement of more advanced skills.

TABLE 1-5

Motor Development During Toddler Years

AGE (MONTHS)	GROSS MOTOR	FINE MOTOR
15	Walks without help (usually since age 13 months) Creeps up stairs Kneels without support Cannot walk around corners or stop suddenly without losing balance Assumes standing position without support Cannot throw ball without falling	Constantly casting objects to floor Builds tower of two cubes Holds two cubes in one hand Releases a pellet into a narrow-necked bottle Scribbles spontaneously Uses cup with lid well but rotates spoon
18	Runs clumsily, falls often Walks up stairs with one hand held Pulls and pushes toys Jumps in place with both feet Seats self on chair Throws ball overhand without falling	Builds tower of three or four cubes Release, prehension, and reach well developed Turns pages in a book two or three at a time In drawing, makes stroke imitatively Manages spoon without rotation

Continued

TABLE 1-5—cont'd

Motor Development During Toddler Years

AGE (MONTHS)	GROSS MOTOR	FINE MOTOR
24	Goes up and down stairs alone with two feet on each step Runs fairly well, with wide stance Picks up object without falling Kicks ball forward without overbalancing	Builds tower of six or seven cubes Aligns two or more cubes like a train Turns pages of book one at a time In drawing, imitates vertical and circular strokes Turns doorknob, unscrews lid
30	Jumps with both feet Jumps from chair or step Stands on one foot momentarily Takes a few steps on tiptoe	Builds tower of eight cubes Adds chimney to train of cubes Good hand-finger coordination; holds crayon with fingers rather than fist Moves fingers independently In drawing, imitates vertical and horizontal strokes, makes two or more strokes for cross

Motor Development: Preschool Years

AGE (YEARS)	GROSS MOTOR	FINE MOTOR
3	Rides tricycle Jumps off bottom step	Builds tower of nine or 10 cubes Builds bridge with three cubes

	Gross Motor	Fine Motor
	Stands on one foot for a few seconds Goes up stairs using alternate feet, may still come down using both feet on step Broad jumps May try to dance, but balance may not be adequate	Adeptly places small pellets in narrow-necked bottle In drawing, copies a circle, imitates a cross, names what has been drawn, cannot draw stick figure but may make circle with facial features
4	Skips and hops on one foot Catches ball reliably Throws ball overhand Walks down stairs using alternate footing	Uses scissors successfully to cut out picture following outline Can lace shoes but may not be able to tie bow In drawing, copies a square, traces a cross and diamond, adds three parts to stick figure
5	Skips and hops on alternate feet Throws and catches ball well Jumps rope Skates with good balance Walks backward with heel to toe Balances on alternate feet with eyes closed	Ties shoelaces Uses scissors, simple tools, or pencil very well In drawing, copies a diamond and triangle; adds seven to nine parts to stick figure; prints a few letters, numbers, or words, such as first name

TABLE 1-6

Growth and Development During School-Age Years

AGE (YEARS)	PHYSICAL AND MOTOR	MENTAL	PERSONAL AND SOCIAL
6	Height and weight gain continues slowly Weight: 16-23.6 kg (35.5-58 pounds); height: 106.6-123.5 cm (42-48 inches) Central mandibular incisors erupt Loses first tooth Gradual increase in dexterity Active age; constant activity Often returns to finger feeding More aware of hand as a tool Likes to draw, print, color Vision reaches maturity	Develops concept of numbers Can count 13 pennies Knows whether it is morning or afternoon Defines common objects such as fork and chair in terms of their use Obeys triple commands in succession Knows right and left hands Says which is pretty and which is ugly of a series of drawings of faces Describes the objects in a picture rather than simply enumerating them Attends first grade	Can share and cooperate better Has great need for children of own age Will cheat to win Often engages in rough play Often jealous of younger brother or sister Does what adults are seen doing May have occasional temper tantrums Is a boaster Is more independent, probably influence of school Has own way of doing things Increases socialization

7	Begins to grow at least 5 cm (2 inches) in height per year	Notices that certain items are missing from pictures	Is becoming a real member of the family group
	Weight: 17.7-30 kg (39-66.5 pounds); height: 111.8-129.7 cm (44-51 inches)	Can copy a diamond	Takes part in group play
	Maxillary central incisors and lateral mandibular incisors erupt	Repeats three numbers backward	Boys prefer playing with boys; girls prefer playing with girls
	More cautious in approaches to new performances	Develops concept of time; reads ordinary clock or watch correctly to nearest quarter hour; uses clock for practical purposes	Spends a lot of time alone; does not require a lot of companionship
	Repeats performances to master them	Attends second grade	
	Jaw begins to expand to accommodate permanent teeth	More mechanical in reading; often does not stop at the end of a sentence, skips words such as "it," "the," and "he"	
8-9	Continues to gain 5 cm (2 inches) in height per year	Gives similarities and differences between two things from memory	Is easy to get along with at home
	Weight: 19.6-39.6 kg (43-87 pounds); height: 117-141.8 cm (46-56 inches)	Counts backward from 20 to 1; understands concept of reversibility	Likes the reward system
	Lateral incisors (maxillary) and mandibular cuspids erupt	Repeats days of the week and months in order; knows the date	Dramatizes
	Movement fluid; often graceful and poised	Describes common objects in detail, not merely their use	Is more sociable

Continued

TABLE 1-6—cont'd

Growth and Development During School-Age Years

AGE (YEARS)	PHYSICAL AND MOTOR	MENTAL	PERSONAL AND SOCIAL
	Always on the go; jumps, chases, skips	Makes change out of a quarter	Is better behaved
	Increased smoothness and speed in fine motor control; uses cursive writing	Attends third and fourth grades	Is interested in boy-girl relationships but will not admit it
	Dresses self completely	Reads more; may plan to wake up early just to read	Goes about home and community freely, alone or with friends
	Likely to overdo; hard to quiet down after recess	Reads classic books, but also enjoys comics	Likes to compete and play games
	More limber; bones grow faster than ligaments	More aware of time; can be relied on to get to school on time	Shows preference in friends and groups
		Can grasp concepts of parts and whole (fractions)	Plays mostly with groups of own sex but is beginning to mix
		Understands concepts of space, cause and effect, nesting (puzzles), conservation (permanence of mass and volume)	Develops modesty
		Classifies objects by more than one quality; has collections	Compares self with others
		Produces simple paintings or drawings	Enjoys organizations, clubs, and group sports

10-12	Boys: Slow growth in height and rapid weight gain; may become obese in this period	Writes brief stories	Loves friends; talks about them constantly
	Weight: 24.3-58 kg (54-128 pounds); height: 127.5-162.3 cm (50-64 inches)	Attends fifth to seventh grades	Chooses friends more selectively; may have a "best friend"
	Posture is more similar to an adult's; will overcome lordosis	Writes occasional short letters to friends or relatives on own initiat ve	Enjoys conversation
	Girls: Pubescent changes may begin to appear; body lines soften and round out	Uses telephone for practical purposes	Develops beginning interest in opposite sex
	Remainder of teeth will erupt and tend toward full development (except wisdom teeth)	Responds to magazine, radio, or other advertising	Is more diplomatic
		Reads for practical information or own enjoyment—stories or library books of adventure or romance, animal stories	Likes family; family really has meaning
			Likes mother and wants to please her in many ways
			Demonstrates affection
			Likes father, who is admired and may be idolized

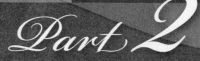

Part 2

Pain Assessment and Management

Children's ability to describe pain changes as they grow older and as they cognitively and linguistically mature. Three types of measures—behavioral, physiologic, and self-report—have been developed to measure children's pain, and their applicability depends on the child's cognitive and linguistic ability.

DEVELOPMENTAL CHARACTERISTICS OF CHILDREN'S RESPONSES TO PAIN

Preterm Infant

1. The preterm infant's response may be behaviorally blunted or absent; however, there is sufficient evidence that preterm infants are neurologically capable of experiencing pain.
2. Use a preterm infant pain scale.
3. Assume that painful procedures in older child and adult are also painful in preterm infant (e.g., venipuncture, lumbar puncture, endotracheal intubation, circumcision, chest tube insertion, heel puncture).

Young Infant

1. Generalized body response of rigidity or thrashing, possibly with local reflex withdrawal of stimulated area
2. Loud crying
3. Facial expression of pain (brows lowered and drawn together, eyes tightly closed, and mouth open and squarish)
4. No association demonstrated between approaching stimulus and subsequent pain

Older Infant
1. Localized body response with deliberate withdrawal of stimulated area
2. Loud crying
3. Facial expression of pain or anger
4. Physical resistance, especially pushing the stimulus away after it is applied

Young Child
1. Loud crying, screaming
2. Verbal expressions such as "Ow," "Ouch," "It hurts"
3. Thrashing of arms and legs
4. Attempts to push stimulus away before it is applied
5. Lack of cooperation; need for physical restraint
6. Requests termination of procedure
7. Clings to parent, nurse, or other significant person
8. Requests emotional support, such as hugs or other forms of physical comfort
9. May become restless and irritable with continuing pain
10. Behaviors occurring in anticipation of actual painful procedure

School-Age Child
1. May see all behaviors of young child, especially during actual painful procedure, but less in anticipatory period
2. Stalling behavior, such as "Wait a minute" or "I'm not ready"
3. Muscular rigidity, such as clenched fists, white knuckles, gritted teeth, contracted limbs, body stiffness, closed eyes, wrinkled forehead

Adolescent
1. Less vocal protest
2. Less motor activity
3. More verbal expressions, such as "It hurts" or "You're hurting me"
4. Increased muscle tension and body control

NONPHARMACOLOGIC STRATEGIES FOR PAIN MANAGEMENT
General Strategies
1. Use nonpharmacologic interventions to supplement, not replace, pharmacologic interventions, and use for mild pain and pain that is reasonably well controlled with analgesics.

TABLE 2-1

Behavioral Pain Assessment Scales for Infants and Young Children

AGES OF USE	INSTRUMENT
4 months to 18 years	Objective Pain Score (OPS) (Hannallah and others, 1987)
1 to 5 years	Children's Hospital of Eastern Ontario Pain Scale (CHEOPS) (McGrath and others, 1985)
Newborn to 16 years	Nurses Assessment of Pain Inventory (NAPI) (Stevens, 1990)
3 to 36 months	Behavioral Pain Score (BPS) (Robieux and others, 1991)
4 to 6 months	Modified Behavioral Pain Scale (MBPS) (Taddio and others, 1995)
<36 months and children with cerebral palsy	Riley Infant Pain Scale (RIPS) (Schade and others, 1996)
2 months to 7 years	FLACC Postoperative Pain Tool (Merkel and others, 1997)
1 to 7 months	Postoperative Pain Score (POPS) (Attia and others, 1987)
Average gestational age 33.5 weeks	Neonatal Infant Pain Scale (NIPS) (Lawrence and others, 1993)
27 weeks gestational age to full term	Pain Assessment Tool (PAT) (Hodgkinson and others, 1994)
1 to 36 months	Pain Rating Scale (PRS) (Joyce and others, 1994)
32 to 60 weeks gestational age	CRIES (Krechel, Bildner, 1995)
28 to 40 weeks gestational age	Premature Infant Pain Profile (PIPP) (Stevens and others, 1996)
0 to 28 days	Scale for Use in Newborns (SUN) (Blauer, Gerstmann, 1998)
Birth (23 weeks gestational age) and full-term newborns up to 100 days	Neonatal Pain, Agitation, and Sedation Scale (NPASS) (Puchalski, Hummel, 2002)

TABLE 2-2
FLACC Scale*

	0	1	2
Face	No particular expression or smile	Occasional grimace or frown, withdrawn, disinterested	Frequent to constant frown, clenched jaw, quivering chin
Legs	Normal position or relaxed	Uneasy, restless, tense	Kicking, or legs drawn up
Activity	Lying quietly, normal position, moves easily	Squirming, shifting back and forth, tense	Arched, rigid, or jerking
Cry	No cry (awake or asleep)	Moans or whimpers, occasional complaint	Crying steadily, screams or sobs, frequent complaints
Consolability	Content, relaxed	Reassured by occasional touching, hugging, or talking to; distractible	Difficult to console or comfort

*From Merkel S and others: The FLACC: a behavioral scale for scoring postoperative pain in young children, *Pediatr Nurs* 23(3):293-297, 1997. Used with permission of Jannetti Publications, Inc., and the University of Michigan Health System. Can be reproduced for clinical and research use.

TABLE 2-3

Pain Rating Scales for Children

PAIN SCALE, DESCRIPTION	RECOMMENDED AGE, COMMENTS
FACES Pain Rating Scale (Wong and Baker, 1988) Uses six cartoon faces ranging from smiling face for "no pain" to tearful face for "worst pain" 0 No hurt 1 or 2 Hurts little bit 2 or 4 Hurts little more 3 or 6 Hurts even more 4 or 8 Hurts whole lot 5 or 10 Hurts worst	Children as young as three years. Use original instructions without affect words, such as *happy* or *sad*, or brief words resulted in same range of pain rating, probably reflecting child's rating of pain intensity. For coding purposes, numbers 0, 2, 4, 6, 8, 10 can be substituted for 0-5 system to accommodate 0-10 system. Provides three scales in one: facial expressions, numbers, and words. Research supports cultural sensitivity of FACES for Caucasian, African-American, Hispanic, Thai, Chinese, and Japanese children.
Oucher (Beyer, Denyes, and Villarruel, 1992) Uses six photographs of Caucasian child's face representing "no hurt" to "biggest hurt you could ever have"; also includes vertical scale with numbers from 0 to 100; scales for African-American and Hispanic children have been developed (Villarruel and Denyes, 1991)	Children 3 to 13 years. Use numeric scale if child can count any 2 numbers, or by tens (Jordan-Marsh and others, 1994). Determine whether child has cognitive ability to use photographic scale; child should be able to rate 6 geometric shapes from largest to smallest.

Continued

TABLE 2-3—cont'd

Pain Rating Scales for Children

PAIN SCALE, DESCRIPTION	RECOMMENDED AGE, COMMENTS
	Determine which ethnic version of Oucher to use. Allow child to select version of Oucher, or use version that most closely matches physical characteristics of child. NOTE: Ethnically similar scale may not be preferred by child when given choice of ethnically neutral cartoon scale (Luffy and Grove, 2003).
Poker Chip Tool† (Hester and others, 1998) Uses four red poker chips placed horizontally in front of child	Children as young as 4 years. Determine whether child has cognitive ability to use numbers by identifying larger of any 2 numbers.
Word-Graphic Rating Scale‡ (Tesler and others, 1991) Uses descriptive words (may vary in other scales) to denote varying intensities of pain	Children 4 to 17 years

No   Little   Medium   Large   Worst
pain   pain   pain   pain   possible pain

Numeric Scale
Uses straight line with end points identified as "no pain" and "worst pain" and sometimes "medium pain" in the middle; divisions along line marked in units from 0-10 (high number may vary)

No pain   Worst pain

| | | | | | | | | | | |
|0|1|2|3|4|5|6|7|8|9|10|

Children as young as 5 years, as long as they can count and have some concept of numbers and their values in relation to other numbers
Scale may be used horizontally or vertically
Number coding should be same as other scales used in facility

Visual AnalogueScale (VAS) (Cline and others, 1992)
A vertical or horizontal line is drawn to a certain length, such as 10 cm (4 in), and anchored by items that represent extremes of the subjective phenomenon, such as pain, which is measured

No pain   Worst pain

Children as young as 4.5 years, preferably 7 years
Vertical or horizontal scale may be used
Research shows that children ages 3 to 18 years least prefer VAS compared with other scales (Luffy and Grove, 2003; Wong and Baker, 1988).

Color Tool (Eland and Banner, 1999)
Uses markers for child to construct own scale that is used with body outline

Children as young as 4 years, provided they know their colors, are not color blind, and are able to construct the scale if in pain

TABLE 2-4

CRIES Neonatal Postoperative Pain Scale (Krechel and Bildner, 1995)

	0	1	2
Crying	No	High pitched	Inconsolable
Requires oxygen for saturation >95%	No	<30%	>30%
Increased vital signs	Heart rate and blood pressure less than or equal to preoperative state	Heart rate and blood pressure increase <20% of preoperative state	Heart rate and blood pressure increase >20% of preoperative state
Expression	None	Grimace	Grimace/grunt
Sleepless	No	Wakes at frequent intervals	Constantly awake

2. Form a trusting relationship with child and family. Express concern regarding their reports of pain, and intervene appropriately.
3. Use general guidelines to prepare child for procedure.
4. Prepare child before potentially painful procedures, but avoid "planting" the idea of pain. For example, instead of saying, "This is going to (or may) hurt," say, "Sometimes this feels like pushing, sticking, or pinching, and sometimes it doesn't bother people. Tell me what it feels like to you."
5. Use "nonpain" descriptors when possible (e.g., "It feels like heat" rather than "It's a burning pain"). This allows for variation in sensory perception, avoids suggesting pain, and gives the child control in describing reactions.
6. Avoid evaluative statements or descriptions (e.g., "This is a terrible procedure" or "It really will hurt a lot").
7. Stay with child during a painful procedure.
8. Allow parents to stay with child if child and parent desire; encourage parent to talk softly to child and to remain near child's head.

9. Involve parents in learning specific nonpharmacologic strategies and in assisting child with their use.
10. Educate child about the pain, especially when explanation may lessen anxiety (e.g., that pain may occur after surgery and does not indicate something is wrong); reassure the child that he or she is not responsible for the pain.
11. For long-term pain control, give child a doll, which represents "the patient," and allow child to do everything to the doll that is done to the child; pain control can be emphasized through the doll by stating, "Dolly feels better after the medicine."
12. Teach procedures to child and family for later use.

Specific Strategies

1. Distraction
   a. Involve parent and child in identifying strong distracters.
   b. Involve child in play; use radio, tape recorder, CD player, or computer game; have child sing or use rhythmic breathing.
   c. Have child take a deep breath and blow it out until told to stop.
   d. Have child blow bubbles to "blow the hurt away."
   e. Have child concentrate on yelling or saying "ouch," with instructions to "yell as loud or soft as you feel it hurt; that way I know what's happening."
   f. Have child look through kaleidoscope (type with glitter suspended in fluid-filled tube) and encourage him or her to concentrate by asking, "Do you see the different designs?"
   g. Use humor, such as watching cartoons, telling jokes or funny stories, or acting silly with child.
   h. Have child read, play games, or visit with friends.
2. Relaxation
   a. With an infant or young child:
      1. Hold in a comfortable, well-supported position, such as vertically against the chest and shoulder.
      2. Rock in a wide, rhythmic arc in a rocking chair or sway back and forth, rather than bouncing child.
   b. With a slightly older child:
      1. Ask child to take a deep breath and "go limp as a rag doll" while exhaling slowly; then ask child to yawn (demonstrate if needed).

    2. Help child assume a comfortable position (e.g., pillow under neck and knees).

    3. Begin progressive relaxation: starting with the toes, systematically instruct child to let each body part "go limp" or "feel heavy"; if child has difficulty relaxing, instruct child to tense or tighten each body part and then relax it.

    4. Allow child to keep eyes open, since children may respond better if eyes are open rather than closed during relaxation.

3. Guided Imagery
   a. Have child identify a highly pleasurable real or imaginary experience.
   b. Have child describe details of the event, including as many senses as possible (e.g., "feel the cool breezes," "see the beautiful colors," "hear the pleasant music").
   c. Have child write down or tape-record script.
   d. Encourage child to concentrate only on the pleasurable event during the painful time; enhance the image by recalling specific details through reading the script or playing the tape.
   e. Combine with relaxation and rhythmic breathing.

4. Positive Self-Talk
   a. Teach child positive statements to say when in pain (e.g., "I will be feeling better soon," "When I go home, I will feel better, and we will eat ice cream").

5. Thought Stopping
   a. Identify positive facts about the painful event (e.g., "It does not last long").
   b. Identify reassuring information (e.g., "If I think about something else, it does not hurt as much").
   c. Condense positive and reassuring facts into a set of brief statements, and have child memorize them (e.g., "Short procedure, good veins, little hurt, nice nurse, go home").
   d. Have child repeat the memorized statements whenever thinking about or experiencing the painful event.

6. Behavioral Contracting
   a. **Informal**—May be used with children as young as four or five years of age:
      1. Use stars, tokens, or cartoon character stickers as rewards.
      2. Give a child who is uncooperative or procrastinating during a procedure a limited time (measured by a visible timer) to complete the procedure.

3. Proceed as needed if child is unable to comply.
4. Reinforce cooperation with a reward if the procedure is accomplished within specified time.

b. **Formal**—Use written contract, which includes:
  1. Realistic (seems possible) goal or desired behavior
  2. Measurable behavior (e.g., agrees not to hit anyone during procedures)
  3. Contract written, dated, and signed by all persons involved in any of the agreements
  4. Identified rewards or consequences that are reinforcing
  5. Goals that can be evaluated
  6. Commitment and compromise requirements for both parties (e.g., while timer is used, nurse will not nag or prod child to complete procedure)

ROUTES AND METHODS OF ANALGESIC DRUG ADMINISTRATION
Oral
1. Oral route preferred because of convenience, cost, and relatively steady blood levels
2. Higher dosages of oral form of opioids required for equivalent parenteral analgesia
3. Peak drug effect occurs after 1 to 2 hours for most analgesics
4. Delay in onset a disadvantage when rapid control of severe pain or of fluctuating pain is desired

Sublingual, Buccal, or Transmucosal
1. Tablet or liquid placed between cheek and gum (buccal) or under tongue (sublingual)
2. Highly desirable because more rapid onset than oral route
3. Produces less first-pass effect through liver than oral route, which normally reduces analgesia from oral opioids (unless sublingual or buccal form is swallowed, which occurs often in children)
4. Few drugs commercially available in this form
5. Many drugs can be compounded into sublingual troche or lozenge.
  a. **Actiq**—Oral transmucosal fentanyl citrate in hard confection base on a plastic holder; indicated only for management of breakthrough cancer pain in patients with malignancies who

are already receiving and are tolerant to opioid therapy, but can be used for preoperative or preprocedural sedation and analgesia

Intravenous (IV) (Bolus)
1. Preferred for rapid control of severe pain
2. Provides most rapid onset of effect, usually in about 5 minutes
3. Advantage for acute pain, procedural pain, and breakthrough pain
4. Needs to be repeated hourly for continuous pain control
5. Drugs with short half-life (morphine, fentanyl, hydromorphone) preferable to avoid toxic accumulation of drug

IV (Continuous)
1. Preferred over bolus and intramuscular injection for maintaining control of pain
2. Provides steady blood levels
3. Easy to titrate dosage

Subcutaneous (SC) (Continuous)
1. Used when oral and IV routes not available
2. Provides equivalent blood levels to continuous IV infusion
3. Suggested initial bolus dose to equal 2-hour IV dose; total 24-hour dose usually requires concentrated opioid solution to minimize infused volume; use smallest gauge needle that accommodates infusion rate

Patient-Controlled Analgesia (PCA)
1. Generally refers to self-administration of drugs, regardless of route
2. Typically uses programmable infusion pump (IV, epidural, SC) that permits self-administration of boluses of medication at preset dose and time interval (lockout interval is time between doses)
3. PCA bolus administration often combined with initial bolus and continuous (basal or background) infusion of opioid
4. Optimum lockout interval not known but must be at least as long as time needed for onset of drug
5. Should effectively control pain during movement or procedures
6. Longer lockout provides larger dose.

Family-Controlled Analgesia
1. One family member (usually a parent) or other caregiver designated as child's primary pain manager with responsibility for pressing PCA button
2. Guidelines for selecting a primary pain manager for family-controlled analgesia:
   a. Spends a significant amount of time with the patient
   b. Is willing to assume responsibility of being primary pain manager
   c. Is willing to accept and respect patient's reports of pain (if able to provide) as best indicator of how much pain the patient is experiencing; knows how to use and interpret a pain rating scale
   d. Understands the purpose and goals of patient's pain management plan
   e. Understands concept of maintaining a steady analgesic blood level
   f. Recognizes signs of pain and side effects and adverse reactions to opioid

Nurse-Activated Analgesia
1. Child's primary nurse designated as primary pain manager and is only person who presses PCA button during that nurse's shift
2. Guidelines for selecting primary pain manager for family-controlled analgesia also applicable to nurse-activated analgesia
3. May be used in addition to a basal rate to treat breakthrough pain with bolus doses; patients assessed every 30 minutes for the need for a bolus dose
4. May be used without a basal rate as a means of maintaining analgesia with around-the-clock bolus doses

Intramuscular
NOTE: **Not recommended for pediatric pain control; not current standard of care**
1. Painful administration (hated by children)
2. Some drugs can cause tissue and nerve damage.
3. Wide fluctuation in absorption of drug from muscle
4. Faster absorption from deltoid than from gluteal sites

5. Shorter duration and more expensive than oral drugs
6. Time consuming for staff, and unnecessary delay for child

Intranasal
1. Available commercially as butorphanol (Stadol NS); approved for those older than 18 years of age
2. Should not be used in patient receiving morphine-like drugs because butorphanol is partial antagonist that will reduce analgesia and may cause withdrawal

Intradermal
1. Used primarily for skin anesthesia (e.g., before lumbar puncture, bone marrow aspiration, arterial puncture, skin biopsy)
2. Local anesthetics (e.g., lidocaine) cause stinging, burning sensation.
3. Duration of stinging dependent on type of "caine" used
4. To avoid stinging sensation associated with lidocaine:
   a. Buffer the solution by adding 1 part sodium bicarbonate (1 mEq/ml) to 9 to 10 parts 1% or 2% lidocaine with or without epinephrine.

Topical or Transdermal
1. EMLA (eutectic mixture of local anesthetics [lidocaine and prilocaine]) cream and anesthetic disk or LMX4 (4% lidocaine cream)
   a. Eliminates or reduces pain from most procedures involving skin puncture
   b. Must be placed on intact skin over puncture site and covered by occlusive dressing or applied as anesthetic disc for 1 hour or more before procedure
2. LAT (lidocaine-adrenaline-tetracaine) or tetracaine-phenylephrine (tetraphen)
   a. Provides skin anesthesia about 15 minutes after application on nonintact skin
   b. Gel (preferable) or liquid placed on wounds for suturing
   c. Adrenaline not for use on end arterioles (fingers, toes, tip of nose, penis, earlobes) because of vasoconstriction
3. Numby Stuff
   a. Uses iontophoresis to transport lidocaine 2% and epinephrine 1:100,000 (Iontocaine) into the skin

     b. Current delivered by small battery-powered device that has an electrode with Iontocaine and a ground electrode

     c. Produces local dermal anesthesia in about 10 minutes to a depth of approximately 10 mm at maximum setting

     d. May be frightening to young children when they see the device and feel the current

     e. Child should be observed during iontophoresis, and all metal, such as jewelry, should be removed from application site to prevent burns.

4. Transdermal fentanyl (Duragesic)
     a. Available as patch for continuous pain control
     b. Safety and efficacy not established in children younger than 12 years of age
     c. Not appropriate for initial relief of acute pain because of long interval to peak effect (12 to 24 hours); for rapid onset of pain relief, give an immediate-release opioid
     d. Orders for "rescue doses" of an immediate-release opioid recommended for breakthrough pain, a flare of severe pain that breaks through the medication being administered at regular intervals for persistent pain
     e. Has duration of up to 72 hours for prolonged pain relief
     f. If respiratory depression occurs, possible need for several doses of naloxone

5. Vapocoolant
     a. Use of prescription spray coolant, such as Fluori-Methane or ethyl chloride (Pain-Ease); applied to the skin for 10 to 15 seconds immediately before the needle puncture; anesthesia lasts about 15 seconds
     b. Cold disliked by some children; may be less uncomfortable to spray coolant on a cotton ball and then apply this to the skin
     c. Application of ice to the skin for 30 seconds found to be ineffective

Rectal
1. Alternative to oral or parenteral routes
2. Variable absorption rate
3. Generally disliked by children

4. Many drugs able to be compounded into rectal suppositories*

Regional Nerve Block
1. Use of long-acting local anesthetic (bupivacaine or ropivacaine) injected into nerves to block pain at site
2. Provides prolonged analgesia postoperatively, such as after inguinal herniorrhaphy
3. May be used to provide local anesthesia for surgery, such as dorsal penile nerve block for circumcision or for reduction of fractures

Inhalation
1. Use of anesthetics, such as nitrous oxide, to produce partial or complete analgesia for painful procedures
2. Side effects (e.g., headache) possible from occupational exposure to high levels of nitrous oxide

Epidural or Intrathecal
1. Involves catheter placed into epidural, caudal, or intrathecal space for continuous infusion or single or intermittent administration of opioid with or without a long-acting local anesthetic (e.g., bupivacaine, ropivacaine)
2. Analgesia primarily from drug's direct effect on opioid receptors in spinal cord
3. Respiratory depression rare but may have slow and delayed onset; can be prevented by checking level of sedation and respiratory rate and depth hourly for initial 24 hours and decreasing dose when excessive sedation is detected
4. Nausea, itching, and urinary retention are common dose-related side effects from the epidural opioid.
5. Mild hypotension, urinary retention, and temporary motor or sensory deficits are common unwanted effects of epidural local anesthetic.

Data primarily from American Pain Society: *Principles of analgesic use in the treatment of acute pain and chronic cancer pain,* ed 4, Skokie, Ill, 1999, The Society; and McCaffery M, Pasero C: *Pain: a clinical manual,* ed 2, St Louis, 1999, Mosby.

*For further information about compounding drugs in troche or suppository form, contact **Professional Compounding Centers of America (PCCA),** 9901 S. Wilcrest Drive, Houston, TX 77009; (800) 331-2498; www.pccarx.com.

6. Catheter for urinary retention inserted during surgery to decrease trauma to child; if inserted when child is awake, anesthetize urethra with lidocaine.

SIDE EFFECTS OF OPIOIDS
General
1. Constipation (possibly severe)
2. Respiratory depression
3. Sedation
4. Nausea and vomiting
5. Agitation, euphoria
6. Mental clouding
7. Hallucinations
8. Orthostatic hypotension
9. Pruritus
10. Urticaria
11. Sweating
12. Miosis (may be sign of toxicity)
13. Anaphylaxis (rare)

Signs of Tolerance
1. Decreasing pain relief
2. Decreasing duration of pain relief

Signs of Withdrawal Syndrome in Patients with Physical Dependence
1. Initial signs of withdrawal
   a. Lacrimation
   b. Rhinorrhea
   c. Yawning
   d. Sweating
2. Later signs of withdrawal
   a. Restlessness
   b. Irritability
   c. Tremors
   d. Anorexia
   e. Dilated pupils
   f. Gooseflesh
   g. Nausea, vomiting

TABLE 2-5
Nonsteroidal Antiinflammatory Drugs (NSAIDs) Approved for Children*

DRUG	DOSAGE	COMMENTS
Acetaminophen (Tylenol)	10-15 mg/kg/dose every 4-6 hours, not to exceed 5 doses in 24 hours or 75 mg/kg/day, orally	Available in numerous preparations Nonprescription Higher dosage range may provide increased analgesia
Choline magnesium trisalicylate (Trilisate)	Children <37 kg (81.5 lb): 50 mg/kg/day divided into 2 doses Children >37 kg (81.5 lb): 2250 mg/day divided into 2 doses	Available in suspension, 500 mg/5 ml Prescription
Ibuprofen† (Children's Motrin, Children's Advil)	Children <6 months: 5-10 mg/kg/dose every 6-8 hours, not to exceed 40 mg/kg/day	Available in numerous preparations Available in suspension, 100 mg/5 ml, and drops, Nonprescription 100 mg/2.5 ml
Naproxen (Naprosyn)	Children >2 years: 10 mg/kg/day divided into 2 doses	Available in suspension, 125 mg/5 ml, and several different dosages for tablets Prescription
Tolmetin (Tolectin)	Children >2 yr: 20 g/kg/day divided into 3-4 doses	Available in 200-mg, 400-mg, and 600-mg tablets Prescription

Data from Olin BR and others: *Drug facts and comparisons*, St Louis, 2002, Facts and Comparisons.
NOTE: Newer formulations of NSAIDs selectively inhibit one of the enzymes of cycloxygenase (COX-2, which is responsible for pain transmission) but do not inhibit the other (COX-1). Inhibition of COX-1 decreases prostaglandin production, which is necessary for normal organ function. For example, prostaglandins help maintain gastric

mucosal blood flow and barrier protection, regulate blood flow to the liver and kidneys, and facilitate platelet aggregation and clot formation. Theoretically, the COX-2 NSAIDs provide similar analgesic and antiinflammatory benefits with fewer gastric and platelet side effects than the nonselective agents. COX-2 NSAIDs are approved for use in patients older than 18 years of age.

*All NSAIDs in this table (except acetaminophen) have significant antiinflammatory, antipyretic, and analgesic actions. Acetaminophen has a weak antiinflammatory action, and its classification as an NSAID is controversial. Patients respond differently to various NSAIDs; therefore changing from one drug to another may be necessary for maximum benefit.

Acetylsalicylic acid (aspirin) is also an NSAID but is not recommended for children because of its possible association with Reye's syndrome. The NSAIDs in this table have no known association with Reye's syndrome. However, caution should be exercised in prescribing any salicylate-containing drug (e.g., Trilisate) for children with known or suspected viral infection.

Side effects of ibuprofen, naproxen, and tolmetin include nausea, vomiting, diarrhea, constipation, gastric ulceration, bleeding nephritis, and fluid retention. Acetaminophen and choline magnesium trisalicylate are well tolerated in the gastrointestinal tract and do not interfere with platelet function. NSAIDs (except acetaminophen) should not be given to patients with allergic reactions to salicylates. All NSAIDs should be used cautiously in patients with renal impairment.

TABLE 2-6

Dosage of Selected Opioids for Children

DRUG	APPROPRIATE EQUIANALGESIC	APPROXIMATE EQUIANALGESIC PARENTERAL DOSE	Recommended Starting Dose (Children <50 kg (110 lb) Body Weight)*	
			ORAL	PARENTERAL*
Morphine	30 mg every 3-4 hr	10 mg every 3-4 hr	0.2-0.4 mg/kg every 3-4 hr	0.1-0.2 mg/kg IM every 3-4 hr
			0.3-0.6 mg/kg time released every 12 hr	0.02-0.1 mg/kg IV bolus every 2 hr
				0.015 mg/kg every 8 min PCA
				0.01-0.02 mg/kg/hr IV infusion (neonates)
				0.01-0.06 mg/kg/hr IV infusion (child)
Fentanyl (Sublimaze) (oral mucosal form [Actiq])†	Not available	0.1 mg IV	5-15 mcg/kg; maximum dose 400 mcg	0.5-1.5 mcg/kg IV bolus every 30 min
				1-2 mcg/hr IV infusion
Codeine‡	200 mg every 3-4 hr	130 mg every 3-4 hr	1 mg/kg every 3-4 hr	Not recommended
Hydromorphone§ (Dilaudid)	7.5 mg every 3-4 hr	1.5 mg every 3-4 hr	0.04-0.1 mg/kg every 3-4 hr	0.02-0.1 mg/kg every 3-4 hr
				0.005-0.2 mg/kg IV bolus every 2 hr

Hydrocodone and acetaminophen (Lorcet, Lortab, Vicodin, others)	30 mg every 3-4 hr	Not available	0.2 mg/kg every 3-4 hr	Not available
Levorphanol (Levo-Dromoran)	4 mg every 6-8 hr	2 mg every 6-8 hr	0.04 mg/kg every 6-8 hr	0.02 mg/kg every 6-8 hr
Methadone (Dolophine, others¶)	20 mg every 6-8 hr	10 mg every 6-8 hr	0.2 mg/kg every 6-8 hr	0.1 mg/kg every 6-8 hr
Oxycodone (Roxicodone, OxyContin; also in Percocet, Percodan, Tylox, others)	20 mg every 3-4 hr	Not available	2 mg/kg every 3-4 hr#	Not available

Data from Acute Pain Management Guideline Panel: *Acute pain management: operative or medical procedures and trauma: clinical practice guideline*, AHCPR Pub No 92-0032, Rockville, Md, 1992, Agency for Health Care Policy and Research, Public Health Service, U. S. Department of Health and Human Services; Berde C and others: Report of the subcommittee on disease-related pain in childhood cancer, *Pediatrics* 86(5 pt 2):820, 1990.

IM, Intramuscular; *IV*, intravenous; *PCA*, patient-controlled analgesia.

Note: Published tables vary in suggested doses that are equianalgesic to morphine. Clinical response is criterion that must be applied for each patient; titration to clinical response is necessary. Because there is no complete cross-tolerance among these drugs, it is usually necessary to use a lower than equianalgesic dose when changing drugs and to retitrate to response.

Caution: Recommended doses do not apply to patients with renal or hepatic insufficiency or other conditions affecting drug metabolism and kinetics.

***Caution:** Doses listed for patients with body weight less than 50 kg (110 lb) cannot be used as initial starting doses in infants less than 6 months of age. For nonventilated infants younger than 6 months, the initial opioid dose should be about ¼ to ⅓ of the dose recommended for older infants and children. For example, morphine could be used at a dose of 0.03 mg/kg instead of the traditional 0.1 mg/kg.

¶Actiq is indicated only for management of breakthrough cancer pain in patients with malignancies who are already receiving and are tolerant to opioid therapy, but it can be used for preoperative or preprocedural sedation/analgesia.

Continued

*Caution: Codeine doses above 65 mg often are not appropriate because of diminishing incremental analgesia with increasing doses but continually increasing constipation and other side effects. Dosages are from McCaffery M, Pasero C: *Pain: a clinical manual*, ed 2, St Louis, 1999, Mosby.

§For morphine, hydromorphone, and oxymorphone, rectal administration is an alternate route for patients unable to take oral medications, but equianalgesic doses may differ from oral and parenteral doses because of pharmacokinetic differences.

¶Initial dose is 10%-25% of equianalgesic morphine dose. Parenteral Dolophine is no longer available in the United States.

#Caution: Doses of aspirin and acetaminophen in combination with opioid or nonsteroidal antiinflammatory drug preparations must also be adjusted to patient's body weight. Daily dose of acetaminophen should not exceed 75 mg/kg, or 4000 mg.

TABLE 2-7

Management of Opioid Side Effects

SIDE EFFECT	ADJUVANT DRUGS	NONPHARMACOLOGIC TECHNIQUES
Constipation	**Senna and docusate sodium**	Increase water intake
	Tablet:	Prune juice, bran cereal, vegetables
	2 to 6 years: Start with ½ tablet once a day; maximum: 1 tablet twice a day	
	6 to 12 years: Start with 1 tablet once a day; maximum: 2 tablets twice a day	
	>12 yr: Start with 2 tablets once a day; maximum: 4 tablets twice a day	
	Liquid:	
	1 month to 1 year: 1.25-5 ml q hs	
	1 to 5 years: 2.5-5 ml q hs	
	5 to 15 years: 5-10 ml q hs	
	>15 years: 10-25 ml q hs	
	Casanthranol and docusate sodium	
	Liquid: 5-15 ml q hs	
	Capsules: 1 cap PO q hs	
	Bisacodyl: PO or PR	
	3 to 12 years: 5 mg/dose/day	
	>12 years: 10-15 mg/dose/day	
	Lactulose	
	7.5 ml/day after breakfast	
	Adult: 15-30 ml/day PO	

Continued

TABLE 2-7—cont'd

Management of Opioid Side Effects

SIDE EFFECT	ADJUVANT DRUGS	NONPHARMACOLOGIC TECHNIQUES
	Mineral oil: 1-2 tsp/day PO **Magnesium citrate** <6 years: 2-4 ml/kg PO once 6 to 12 years: 100-150 ml PO once >12 years: 150-300 ml PO once **Milk of Magnesia** <2 years: 0.5 ml/kg/dose PO once 2 to 5 years: 5-15 ml/day PO 6 to 12 years: 15-30 ml PO once >12 years: 30-60 ml PO once	
Sedation	**Caffeine:** single dose of 1-1.5 mg PO **Dextroamphetamine:** 2.5-5 mg PO in AM and early afternoon **Methylphenidate:** 2.5-5 mg PO in AM and early afternoon Consider opioid switch if sedation is persistent	Caffeinated drinks (e.g., Mountain Dew, cola drinks)
Nausea, vomiting	**Promethazine:** 0.5 mg/kg q 4-6 hr; maximum: 25 mg/dose **Ondansetron:** 0.1-0.15 mg/kg IV or PO q 4 hr; maximum: 8 mg/dose **Granisetron:** 10-40 mcg/kg q 2-4 hr; maximum: 1 mg/dose **Droperidol:** 0.05-0.06 mg/kg IV q 4-6 hr; can be very sedating	Imagery, relaxation Deep, slow breathing

Pruritus	**Diphenhydramine:** 1 mg/kg IV or PO q 4-6 hr prn; max: 25 mg/dose	Oatmeal baths, good hygiene
	Hydroxyzine: 0.6 mg/kg/dose PO q 6 hr; maximum: 50 mg/dose	Exclude other causes of itching
	Naloxone: 0.5 mcg/kg q 2 min until pruritus improves (diluted in solution of	Change opioids
	0.1 mg of naloxone per 10 ml of saline)	
	Butorphanol: 0.3-0.5 mg/kg IV (use cautiously in opioid-tolerant children; may	
	cause withdrawal symptoms); maximum: 2 mg/dose because mixed	
	agonist-antagonist	
Respiratory depression: mild to moderate	Hold dose of opioid	Arouse gently, give oxygen,
	Reduce subsequent doses by 25%	encourage to deep breathe
Respiratory depression: severe	**Naloxone**	Oxygen, bag and mask if indicated
	During disease pain management:	
	0.5 mcg/kg in 2-min increments until breathing improves (American Pain	
	Society, 1999; McCaffery and Pasero, 1999)	
	Reduce opioid dose if possible	
	Consider opioid switch	
	During sedation for procedures:	
	5-10 mcg/kg until breathing improves (Yaster, 1997)	
	Reduce opioid dose if possible	
	Consider opioid switch	

Continued

TABLE 2-7—cont'd
Management of Opioid Side Effects

SIDE EFFECT	ADJUVANT DRUGS	NONPHARMACOLOGIC TECHNIQUES
Dysphoria, confusion, hallucinations	Evaluate medications, eliminate adjuvant medications with central nervous system effects as symptoms allow Consider opioid switch if possible **Haloperidol** (Haldol): 0.05-0.15 mg/kg/day divided in 2-3 doses; maximum: 2-4 mg/day	Rule out other physiologic causes
Urinary retention	Evaluate medications, eliminate adjuvant medications with anticholinergic effects (e.g., antihistamines, tricyclic antidepressants) Occurs with spinal analgesia more frequently than with systemic opioid use **Oxybutynin** 1 year: 1 mg tid 1 to 2 years: 2 mg tid 2 to 3 years: 3 mg tid 4 to 5 years: 4 mg tid >5 years: 5 mg tid	Rule out other physiologic causes In/out or indwelling urinary catheter

hs, At bedtime; *IV*, intravenous; *PO*, by mouth; *PR*, by rectum; *prn*, as needed; *q*, every; *tid*, three times a day.

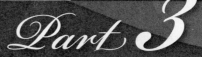

Part 3

Common Childhood Illnesses/Disorders

ACUTE RESPIRATORY DISTRESS SYNDROME

Description

Acute respiratory distress syndrome (ARDS) is a complex respiratory illness characterized by respiratory distress and hypoxemia that occur within 72 hours of a serious injury or surgery in a person with previously normal lungs. ARDS may occur as a result of clinical conditions and injuries such as sepsis, trauma, viral pneumonia, fat emboli, drug overdose, reperfusion injury after lung transplantation, smoke inhalation, and near-drowning.

Pathophysiology

The hallmark of ARDS is increased permeability of the alveolar-capillary membrane that results in pulmonary edema. During the acute phase of ARDS, the alveolocapillary membrane is damaged, with an increasing pulmonary capillary permeability and resulting interstitial edema. When fibrosis occurs, the child may demonstrate respiratory distress and the need for mechanical ventilation. The lungs become stiff as a result of surfactant inactivation, gas diffusion is impaired, and eventually bronchiolar mucosal swelling and congestive atelectasis occur. The net effect is decreased functional residual capacity, pulmonary hypertension, and increased intrapulmonary right-to-left shunting of pulmonary blood flow. Surfactant secretion is reduced, and the atelectasis and fluid-filled alveoli provide an excellent medium for bacterial growth. Hypoxemia is expressed as the partial pressure of oxygen (PaO_2) to fraction of inspired oxygen (FiO_2) ratio, or P/F ratio; the P/F ratio for ARDS is 200.

Clinical Signs and Symptoms

The child with ARDS may first demonstrate only symptoms caused by an injury or infection, but, as the condition deteriorates, hyperventilation, tachypnea, increasing respiratory effort, cyanosis, and decreasing oxygen saturation occur. At times the developing hypoxemia is not responsive to oxygen administration.

Diagnostic Evaluation

The criteria for diagnosis of ARDS in children are an acute antecedent illness or injury, acute respiratory distress or failure, no evidence of prior cardiopulmonary disease, and diffuse bilateral infiltrates evidenced on chest radiography.

Treatment

Treatment involves supportive measures, such as:

- Maintenance of adequate oxygenation and pulmonary perfusion
- Treatment of infection (or the precipitating cause)
- Maintenance of adequate cardiac output and vascular volume, hydration, adequate nutritional support, comfort measures, prevention of complications, such as GI ulceration and aspiration, and psychologic support
- Prone positioning may be used to improve oxygenation. The use of endotracheal intubation, positive end-expiratory pressure, and low tidal volume may be required to ensure maximum oxygen delivery by increasing functional residual capacity, reducing intrapulmonary shunting, and reducing pulmonary fluid.
- Additional supportive strategies in the treatment of ARDS in children include the use of lung-protective ventilator strategies, permissive hypercapnia, inhaled nitric oxide, exogenous surfactant administration, high-frequency ventilation, partial liquid ventilation, and extracorporeal life support (extracorporeal membrane oxygenation, or ECMO).

Nursing Care Management

- Respiratory assessment; oxygenation and respiratory status; arterial blood gas monitoring
- Management of mechanical ventilation; oral care; prevention of accidental extubation

- Monitoring of cardiac output, perfusion, fluid and electrolyte balance, and renal function (urinary output)
- Pain management and comfort needs
- Sedation may be required in acute phase.
- Family support and information on child's status
- Hemodynamic monitoring and care of central lines
- Medications: diuretics, vasopressors
- Managing the effects of immobilization: skin care, hydration, positioning, passive range of motion
- Nutritional management: enteral and parenteral nutrition

Patient and Family Teaching
- Information about child's status
- Communication techniques with intubated and mechanically ventilated child
- Involvement in care of child during acute phase
- Safety prevention: avoidance of conditions that may cause severe respiratory illness such as house fire; reduce exposure to noxious chemicals.

ADRENAL HYPERPLASIA, CONGENITAL
Description
Congenital adrenal hyperplasia (CAH) is a family of disorders caused by decreased enzyme activity required for cortisol production in the adrenal cortex. The most common defect is 21-hydroxylase deficiency, which constitutes more than 90% of all cases of CAH.

Pathophysiology
Interference in the biosynthesis of cortisol during fetal life results in an increased production of ACTH, which stimulates hyperplasia of the adrenal gland. Depending on the enzymatic defect, increased quantities of cortisol precursors and androgens are secreted. There are six major types of biochemical defects. The most common is partial or complete 21-hydroxylase deficiency. With partial deficiency, enough aldosterone is produced to preserve sodium, and adequate cortisol is produced to prevent signs of adrenocortical insufficiency.

Clinical Signs and Symptoms
- Masculinization of external female genitalia causes the clitoris to enlarge so that it appears as a small phallus. Fusion of the

labia produces a sac-like structure resembling the scrotum without testes. However, no abnormal changes occur in the internal sexual organs, although the vaginal orifice is usually closed by the fused labia.

▪ In males, *ambiguous genitalia* should be considered in any male infant with hypospadias or micropenis and no palpable gonads, and a diagnostic evaluation for CAH should be contemplated. Males do not display genital abnormalities at birth.

▪ Increased pigmentation of skin creases and genitalia caused by increased ACTH may be a subtle sign of adrenal insufficiency.

▪ A salt-wasting crisis frequently occurs, usually within the first few weeks of life.

▪ Infants fail to gain weight, and hyponatremia and hyperkalemia may be significant.

▪ Untreated CAH results in early sexual maturation, with enlargement of the external sexual organs; development of axillary, pubic, and facial hair; deepening of the voice; acne; and marked increase in musculature.

Diagnostic Evaluation

Clinical diagnosis is initially based on congenital abnormalities that lead to difficulty in assigning gender to the newborn and on signs and symptoms of adrenal insufficiency or hypertension.

▪ Evidence of increased 17-ketosteroid levels is found in most types of CAH.

▪ In complete 21-hydroxylase deficiency, blood electrolytes demonstrate loss of sodium and chloride and elevation of potassium.

▪ Chromosome typing for positive sex determination and to rule out any other genetic abnormality (e.g., Turner syndrome) is always done in any case of ambiguous genitalia.

▪ Ultrasound to identify the absence or presence of female reproductive organs in a newborn or child with ambiguous genitalia

▪ In older children bone age is advanced, and linear growth is increased.

Treatment

▪ The initial medical objective is to confirm the diagnosis and assign a gender to the child, usually according to the genotype.

- In both sexes, cortisone is administered to suppress the abnormally high secretion of ACTH.
- Depending on the degree of masculinization in the female, reconstructive surgery may be required to reduce the size of the clitoris, separate the labia, and create a vaginal orifice.

Nursing Care Management
- Early recognition of ambiguous genitalia in newborns is essential
- If there is any question regarding assignment of gender, the parents need to be told immediately to prevent the embarrassing situation of informing family members of the child's gender and then having to change the announcement.

Patient and Family Teaching
- Because infants are especially prone to dehydration and salt-losing crises, parents need to be aware of signs of dehydration and the urgency of immediate medical intervention to stabilize the child's condition.
- Parents should have injectable hydrocortisone available and know how to prepare and administer the intramuscular injection. The parents should be advised that there is no physical harm in treating for suspected adrenal insufficiency that is not present, whereas the consequence of not treating acute adrenal insufficiency can be fatal.

ALLERGIC RHINITIS
Description
Allergic rhinitis affects many children and is associated with numerous airway disorders, including asthma, OME, and chronic sinusitis. Seasonal allergic rhinitis (or hay fever) usually follows a spring-fall pattern and is caused by tree, grass, and weed pollens. Seasonal allergic rhinitis usually does not develop until the individual has been sensitized by two or more pollen seasons. Peak incidence for allergic rhinitis is in the adolescent and postadolescent age groups, but younger children are also affected.

Pathophysiology
Allergic rhinitis requires two conditions: a familial predisposition to develop allergy and exposure of a sensitized person to the allergen. Inhalants in the form of microscopic airborne particles

(e.g., pollens, mold, animal danders, and environmental dusts) enter the upper respiratory tract with inhalation and bind to submucosal mast cells in the respiratory tract epithelium. In the allergic child, symptoms are mediated by immunoglobulin E (IgE), which is produced by the child's B lymphocytes. The IgE molecules on the cell surfaces trigger the rapid release of mast cell mediators (e.g., histamine, prostaglandins, and leukotrienes), as well as cell interactive compounds called cytokines. Histamine, a potent vasodilator, acts directly on local receptors to produce vasodilation, mucosal edema, and increased production of mucus. The cytokines summon cells to the area and are responsible for the slower late-phase allergic reaction of inflammation and destruction of the mucosal surface that progresses to chronic nasal obstruction. Repeated exposure of these sensitized membranes to specific aeroallergens results in clinical allergic disease.

Clinical Signs and Symptoms
- Watery rhinorrhea
- Nasal obstruction
- Sneezing
- Itching of the nose, eyes, palate, pharynx, and conjunctiva
- Mucus secretion with postnasal drainage
- Snoring during sleep
- Fatigue
- Malaise
- Poor school performance
- Associated URI
- Shiners (dark circles under the eyes)
- Anorexia

Diagnostic Evaluation
- Based on a thorough history and physical examination
- Nasal smear to determine the number of eosinophils in the nasal secretions
- Blood examination for total IgE and elevated eosinophils
- Skin allergen tests
- Radioallergosorbent tests (RAST): used to determine the level of specific IgE antibodies to specific allergens

Treatment
- Avoidance of offending allergens (food, drugs, animal dander, chemicals, dust, pollen)
- Medications: antihistamines; nasal corticosteroids; leukotriene modifier; immunotherapy

Nursing Care Management
- Recognition of symptoms and referral for further evaluation
- Preparation for administration of skin (allergen) and immuno-therapy

To distinguish allergies from colds, be aware that:
- Allergies occur repeatedly and are often seasonal.
- Allergies are seldom accompanied by fever.
- Allergies often involve itching in the eyes and nose.
- Allergies usually trigger constant and consistent bouts of sneezing.
- Allergies are often accompanied by ear and eye problems.

Patient and Family Teaching
- Medication administration
- Allergen avoidance
- Symptom management
- Skin testing

ANEMIA, IRON-DEFICIENCY
Description
Anemia caused by an inadequate supply of dietary iron is the most prevalent nutritional disorder in the United States and the most common mineral disturbance. Children 12 to 36 months of age are at risk for anemia as a result of cow's milk being a major staple of many infants' diet. Preterm infants are especially at risk because of their reduced fetal iron supply. Adolescents are also at risk because of their rapid growth rate combined with poor eating habits.

Pathophysiology
Iron-deficiency anemia can be caused by any number of factors that decrease the supply of iron, impair its absorption, increase the body's need for iron, or affect the synthesis of Hgb.

Clinical Signs and Symptoms
■ Pallor, fatigue, irritability, loss of appetite, decreased physical activity
■ In severe cases, congestive heart failure may develop.

Diagnostic Evaluation
■ CBC, MCV, RDW, reticulocyte count
■ Transferrin saturation, FEP, ferritin

Treatment
■ In formula-fed infants the most convenient and best sources of supplemental iron are iron-fortified commercial formula and iron-fortified infant cereal.
■ Dietary addition of iron-rich foods is usually inadequate as the sole treatment of iron-deficiency anemia, because the iron is poorly absorbed and thus provides insufficient supplemental quantities of iron.
■ Oral iron supplements at a dose of 4-6mg/kg of elemental iron are prescribed for approximately 3 months. Ferrous sulfate, more readily absorbed than ferric iron, results in higher Hgb levels. Ascorbic acid (vitamin C) appears to facilitate absorption of iron and may be given as vitamin C–enriched foods and juices with the iron preparation.
■ If the Hgb level fails to rise after 1 month of oral therapy, it is important to assess for persistent bleeding, iron malabsorption, noncompliance, improper iron administration, or other causes for the anemia.

Nursing Care Management
■ An essential nursing responsibility is instructing parents in the administration of iron.
■ Oral iron should be given as prescribed in three divided doses between meals, when the presence of free hydrochloric acid is greatest, because more iron is absorbed in the acidic environment of the upper GI tract.
■ A citrus fruit or juice taken with the medication aids in absorption.

Patient and Family Teaching
■ A primary nursing objective is to prevent nutritional anemia through family education. Because breast milk is a poor iron

source after 5 months of lactation, reinforce the importance of administering iron supplementation in the exclusively breast-fed infant by 6 months of age.

■ In the formula-fed infant, discuss with parents the importance of using iron-fortified formula and the introduction of solid foods at the appropriate age during the first year of life. Cereals are one of the first semisolid foods to be introduced into the infant's diet at approximately 6 months of age.

■ Diet education of teenagers is especially difficult, especially because teenage girls are particularly prone to following weight-reduction diets. Emphasizing the effect of anemia on appearance (pallor) and energy level (difficulty maintaining popular activities) may be useful.

■ Discuss side-effects of iron therapy:
  ■ An adequate dosage of oral iron turns the stools a tarry green color.
  ■ Vomiting or diarrhea can occur with iron therapy. If the parents report these symptoms, the iron can be given with meals and the dosage reduced and then gradually increased until tolerated.
  ■ Liquid preparations of iron may temporarily stain the teeth. If possible, the medication should be taken through a straw or given through a syringe or medicine dropper placed toward the back of the mouth. Brushing the teeth after administration of the drug lessens the discoloration.

ANOREXIA NERVOSA
Description
Anorexia nervosa (AN) is an eating disorder characterized by a refusal to maintain a minimally normal body weight and by severe weight loss in the absence of obvious physical causes.

Pathophysiology
The disorder appears to be caused by a combination of genetic, neurochemical, psychodevelopmental, and sociocultural factors. The dominant aspects of AN are a relentless pursuit of thinness and a fear of fatness, usually preceded by a period of mood disturbances and behavior changes.

Clinical Signs and Symptoms
- Severe and profound weight loss
- Secondary amenorrhea (if menarche attained)
- Primary amenorrhea (if menarche not attained)
- Sinus bradycardia
- Lowered body temperature
- Hypotension
- Intolerance to cold
- Dry skin and brittle nails
- Appearance of lanugo hair
- Thinning hair
- Abdominal pain
- Bloating
- Constipation
- Fatigue
- Lightheadedness
- Evidence of muscle wasting (cachectic appearance)
- Bone pain with exercise

Diagnostic Evaluation
Diagnosis is made on the basis of criteria established by the American Psychiatric Association (see Box 17-16 in text book).

Treatment
- Immediate medical care for person with life-threatening medical (fluid and electrolyte imbalance); or psychiatric disturbance such as suicide attempt
- Restore a healthy weight.
- Establish healthy eating patterns.
- Psychotherapy to correct deficits and distortions in psychologic functioning
- Resolve disturbed family interaction patterns.

Nursing Care Management
- Monitor nutritional status.
- Enforce healthy eating habits.
- Help adolescent set limits and avoid destructive behaviors/habits.
- Assist with treatment of life-threatening conditions such as electrolyte imbalance.

- Reinforce behavioral contract and plan of care with adolescent.
- Participate in individual and family therapy.

Patient and Family Teaching
- Nutritional counseling
- Behavioral modification techniques
- Individual and family coping skills that are not disruptive to family functioning
- Teach family how to support adolescent and how to help adolescent set realistic goals.

AORTIC STENOSIS
Description
Narrowing or stricture of the aortic valve, causing resistance to blood flow from the left ventricle, decreased cardiac output, left ventricular hypertrophy, and pulmonary vascular congestion. The prominent anatomic consequence of aortic stenosis (AS) is the hypertrophy of the left ventricular wall, which eventually leads to increased end-diastolic pressure resulting in pulmonary venous and pulmonary arterial hypertension. Left ventricular hypertrophy also interferes with coronary artery perfusion and may result in myocardial infarction or scarring of the papillary muscles of the left ventricle, which causes mitral insufficiency. Valvular stenosis, the most common type, is usually caused by malformed cusps that result in a bicuspid rather than tricuspid valve or fusion of the cusps. Subvalvular stenosis is a stricture caused by a fibrous ring below a normal valve; supravalvular stenosis occurs infrequently. Valvular AS is a serious defect for the following reasons: (1) the obstruction tends to be progressive; (2) sudden episodes of myocardial ischemia, or low cardiac output, can result in sudden death; and (3) surgical repair rarely results in a normal valve. This is one of the rare instances in which strenuous physical activity may be curtailed because of the cardiac condition.

Pathophysiology
A stricture in the aortic outflow tract causes resistance to ejection of blood from the left ventricle. The extra workload on the left ventricle causes hypertrophy. If left ventricular failure develops, left

atrial pressure will increase; this causes increased pressure in the pulmonary veins, which results in pulmonary vascular congestion (pulmonary edema).

Clinical Signs and Symptoms

Newborns with critical AS demonstrate signs of decreased cardiac output with faint pulses, hypotension, tachycardia, and poor feeding (see Box 3-1, Common Signs and Symptoms of Congestive Heart Failure). Children show signs of exercise intolerance, chest pain, and dizziness when standing for a long period. There is a characteristic murmur that is low-pitched, harsh, and rasping, heard loudest at the base in the second intercostal space. Patients are at risk for bacterial endocarditis, coronary insufficiency, and ventricular dysfunction.

BOX 3-1

Common Signs and Symptoms of Congestive Heart Failure

Impaired Myocardial Function	Pulmonary Congestion
Tachycardia	Tachypnea
Sweating (inappropriate)	Dyspnea
Decreased urinary output	Retractions (infants)
Fatigue	Flaring nares
Weakness	Exercise intolerance
Restlessness	Orthopnea
Anorexia	Cough, hoarseness
Nausea	Cyanosis
Vomiting	Wheezing
Pale, cool extremities	Grunting
Weak peripheral pulses	
Decreased blood pressure	**SYSTEMIC VENOUS CONGESTION**
Chest pain	Weight gain
Palpitations	Hepatomegaly
Gallop rhythm	Peripheral edema, especially periorbital
Cardiomegaly	Ascites
Duskiness	Neck vein distention (children)
Change in level of consciousness	

Diagnostic Evaluation

See Table 3-1, Procedures for Cardiac Diagnosis; and Table 3-2, Current Interventional Cardiac Catheterization Procedures in Children.

TABLE 3-1	
Procedures for Cardiac Diagnosis	
PROCEDURE	**DESCRIPTIVE**
Chest radiograph (X-ray)	Provides information on heart size and pulmonary blood flow patterns
Electrocardiography (ECG)	Graphic measure of electrical activity of heart
Holter monitor	24-hour continuous ECG recording used to assess dysrhythmias
Echocardiography	Use of high-frequency sound waves obtained by a transducer to produce an image of cardiac structures
Transthoracic	Done with transducer on chest
M-mode	One-dimensional graphic view used to estimate ventricular size and function
Two-dimensional (2-D)	Real-time, cross-sectional views of heart used to identify cardiac structures and cardiac anatomy
Doppler	Identifies blood flow patterns and pressure gradients across structures
Fetal	Imaging fetal heart in utero
Transesophageal (TEE)	Transducer placed in esophagus behind heart to obtain images of posterior heart structures or in patients with poor images from chest approach
Cardiac catheterization	Imaging study using radiopaque catheter placed in a peripheral blood vessel and advanced into heart to measure pressures and oxygen levels in heart chambers and visualize heart structures and blood flow patterns
Hemodynamics	Measures pressures and oxygen saturations in heart chambers
Angiography	Use of contrast material to illuminate heart structures and blood flow patterns

Continued

TABLE 3-1—cont'd
Procedures for Cardiac Diagnosis

PROCEDURE	DESCRIPTIVE
Biopsy	Use of special catheter to remove tiny samples of heart muscle for microscopic evaluation; used in assessing infection, inflammation, or muscle dysfunction disorders; also to assess the level of rejection after heart transplant
Electrophysiology (EPS)	Special catheters with electrodes employed to record electrical activity from within heart; used to diagnose rhythm disturbances
Exercise stress test	Monitoring of heart rate, blood pressure, electrocardiogram (ECG), and oxygen consumption at rest and during progressive exercise on a treadmill or bicycle
Cardiac magnetic resonance imaging (MRI)	Noninvasive imaging technique; used in evaluation of cardiac and vascular anatomy of the heart (i.e., coarctation of the aorta, vascular rings), estimates of ventricular mass and volume; uses for MRI are expanding

TABLE 3-2
Current Interventional Cardiac Catheterization Procedures in Children

INTERVENTION	DIAGNOSIS
Balloon atrial septostomy: Use is well established in newborns; may also be done under echocardiographic guidance	Transposition of great arteries (BAS used as an intermediary step to improve cyanosis until surgery) Some complex single-ventricle defects
Balloon dilation: Treatment of choice	Valvular pulmonic stenosis Branch pulmonary artery stenosis Congenital valvular aortic stenosis Rheumatic mitral stenosis Recurrent coarctation of aorta Further follow-up required in native coarctation of aorta in patients >7 mo Congenital mitral stenosis

TABLE 3-2—cont'd	

Current Interventional Cardiac Catheterization Procedures in Children

INTERVENTION	DIAGNOSIS
Coil occlusion: Accepted alternative to surgery	Patent ductus arteriosus (<4 mm) Aortopulmonary collaterals
Transcatheter device closure: Several devices in clinical trials	Atrial septal defect (ASD)
Amplatzer septal occluder: Approved for ASD closure	ASD
Ventricular septal defect devices: In clinical trials	Ventricular septal defects
Stent placement	Pulmonary artery stenosis Coarctation of the aorta in adolescents Use to treat other lesions; investigational
Radiofrequency ablation	Some tachydysrhythmias

Data from Allen HD, Beekman RH 3rd, Garson A Jr, and others: Pediatric therapeutic cardiac catheterization: AHA scientific statement, *Circulation* 97:609-625, 1998; updated from Rome J, Kreutzer J: Pediatric interventional catheterization: reasonable expectations and outcomes, *Pediatr Clin North Am* 51:1589-1610, 2004.

Treatment
Valvular Aortic Stenosis
Surgical Treatment. Aortic valvotomy is performed under inflow occlusion. It is used rarely because balloon dilation in the catheterization laboratory is the first-line procedure. Newborns with critical AS and small left-sided structures may undergo a Stage 1 Norwood procedure.

Nonsurgical Treatment. The narrowed valve is dilated using balloon angioplasty in the catheterization laboratory. This procedure is usually the first intervention.

Subvalvular Aortic Stenosis
Surgical Treatment. Procedure may involve incising a membrane if one exists or cutting the fibromuscular ring. If the obstruction results from narrowing of the left ventricular outflow tract and a small aortic valve annulus, a patch may be required to enlarge the

entire left ventricular outflow tract and annulus and replace the aortic valve, an approach known as the Konno procedure.

Nursing Care Management
Assist in Measures to Assess and Improve Cardiac Function
Monitor Cardiac Function
- Vital signs monitoring
- Respiratory assessment
- Cardiac assessment
  - Cardiac output (color, pulses, perfusion, capillary refill, renal function, and neurologic function)
  - Heart sounds
  - Dysrhythmias
- Keep accurate record of intake and output.
- Weigh child or infant on same scale at same time of day.
Administer Medications
- Review child's history related to cardiac management.
- Administer medications on schedule.
- Assess effectiveness of medications and any side effects noted.
- Be aware of drug-drug and drug-food interactions.
- Follow guidelines for medication administration.

Manage Common Side Effects of Cardiac Defects
- Prevent fatigue during feeding; offer small frequent feedings to infant's or child's tolerance.
- Organize nursing care to allow child/infant uninterrupted rest.
- Promote activities that do not cause fatigue.

Provide Support for the Child and Family
- Communicate with the child and family in an appropriate style.
- Provide the child and family with honest answers.
- Provide emotional support.
- Offer age-appropriate interventions.
- Provide information on available resources for support for the child and family.

Patient and Family Teaching
Prepare the Child and Family for Diagnostic and Operative Procedures
- Provide explanation of diagnostic tests and why each test is performed because many of them are invasive procedures.

- Prepare the child prior to the invasive procedure. Remember discussion is dependent upon the child's age and development.
- Use simple words or pictures to describe procedures and answer all questions the child and family may have.
- Postoperative wound care teaching as needed
- Post-cardiac catheterization wound care teaching as needed
- Assess and record results of teaching and family's participation in care.

Educate the Child and Family
- Assess child's and family's level of knowledge regarding aortic stenosis.
- Assess child's and family's understanding of what they have heard about aortic stenosis.
- Assess child's and family's understanding of the surgery and/or cardiac catheterization.
- Teach the child and/or family at least four characteristics of congestive heart failure that may occur because of the aortic stenosis such as:
    - Fatigue after exertion
    - Fast heart rate
    - Fast breathing, shortness of breath, dyspnea
    - Retractions
    - Nasal flaring
    - Cool extremities
    - Diaphoresis
    - Decreased urinary output
    - Puffiness (edema)
    - Fussiness
    - Decreased appetite
- Educate child and family about care such as medication preparation and administration.
- Assess child's and family's access to appropriate pharmacy for any special preparation medications.
- If the child is on anticoagulation therapy, educate the child and family about:
    - Anticoagulation therapy
    - Dietary restrictions
    - Laboratory testing required
    - The need for close medical follow-up

- ▪ Signs and symptoms of complications from blood clots and bleeding
- ▪ Educate child and family about when to notify their physician of any clinical changes.
- ▪ Provide appropriate educational resources and review materials with them.
- ▪ Clarify information presented by the health care team including appointment for follow-up visit.
- ▪ Discuss SBE (subacute bacterial endocarditis) prophylaxis with the pediatric cardiologist.

APLASTIC ANEMIA
Description
Aplastic anemia (AA) refers to a condition in which the formed elements of the blood are simultaneously depressed. The peripheral blood smear demonstrates pancytopenia or the triad of profound anemia, leukopenia, and thrombocytopenia. Aplastic anemia can be *primary* (*congenital,* or present at birth) or *secondary* (acquired). The best-known congenital disorder of which aplastic anemia is an outstanding feature is *Fanconi syndrome,* a rare hereditary disorder characterized by pancytopenia, hypoplasia of the bone marrow, and patchy brown discoloration of the skin resulting from the deposit of melanin and associated with multiple congenital anomalies of the musculoskeletal and genitourinary systems. The syndrome appears to be inherited as an autosomal recessive trait with varying penetrance; therefore, affected siblings may demonstrate several different combinations of defects.

Pathophysiology
Most of the cases of AA are considered idiopathic where no cause is found. Several etiologic factors contribute to the development of acquired hypoplastic anemia:

- ▪ Human parvovirus infection, hepatitis, or overwhelming infection
- ▪ Irradiation
- ▪ Immune disorders such as eosinophilic fasciitis and hypoimmunoglobulinemia
- ▪ Drugs such as certain chemotherapeutic agents, anticonvulsants, and antibiotics

- Industrial and household chemicals, including benzene and its derivatives, which are found in petroleum products, dyes, paint remover, shellac, and lacquers
- Infiltration and replacement of myeloid elements, such as in leukemia or the lymphomas

Clinical Signs and Symptoms
- Onset of clinical symptoms of anemia, leukopenia, and decreased platelet count are usually insidious.

Diagnostic Evaluation
- Definitive diagnosis is determined from bone marrow aspiration, which demonstrates the conversion of red bone marrow to yellow, fatty bone marrow.
- Severe AA is defined as less than 25% bone marrow cellularity with at least two of the following findings: absolute granulocyte count <500 mm^3, platelet count $<20,000$/mm^3, and absolute reticulocyte count $<40,000$/mm^3.
- Moderate AA is defined as more than 25% bone marrow cellularity with the presence of mild or moderate cytopenias.

Treatment
- Therapy is directed at restoring function to the marrow and involves two main approaches:
  - Immunosuppressive therapy to remove the presumed immunologic functions that prolong aplasia. *Antilymphocyte globulin* (ALG) or *antithymocyte globulin* (ATG) is the principal drug treatment used for aplastic anemia. Cyclosporine may also be used. ATG and cyclosporine suppress T cell–dependent autoimmune responses but do not cause bone marrow suppression.
  - Replacement of the bone marrow through transplantation. Bone marrow transplantation is the treatment of choice for severe aplastic anemia when a suitable donor exists. Hematopoietic stem cell transplantation should be considered early in the course of the disease if a compatible donor can be found.
- Colony-stimulating factor (CSF), and granulocyte-macrophage colony-stimulating factor (GM-CSF) given parenterally, may be used to enhance bone marrow production.

■ Androgens also may be used with ATG to stimulate erythropoiesis if the AA is nonresponsive to initial therapies.

Nursing Care Management
■ The care of the child with aplastic anemia is similar to that of the child with leukemia (see pp. 243–244)—specifically, preparing the child and family for the diagnostic and therapeutic procedures, preventing complications from the severe pancytopenia, and emotionally supporting them in terms of a potentially fatal outcome.

Patient and Family Teaching
■ Provide explanation of diagnostic tests and why each test is performed because many of them, such as bone marrow aspiration and biopsy, are invasive procedures.
■ Prepare the child prior to the invasive procedure. Remember discussion is dependent upon the child's age and development.
■ Use simple words to describe procedures, and answer all questions the child and family may have.
■ Assess child's and family's level of knowledge regarding aplastic anemia and treatment.
■ Assess child's and family's understanding of what they have heard about aplastic anemia and treatment.
■ Educate the family regarding neutropenia, anemia, and thrombocytopenia; the signs and symptoms of infection; and fever precautions.
■ Provide appropriate educational resources and review materials with child and family.
■ Clarify information presented by the health care team.

ACUTE APPENDICITIS
Description
Appendicitis is an inflammation of the *vermiform appendix* (blind sac at the end of the cecum); appendicitis is the most common cause of emergency abdominal surgery in childhood.

Pathophysiology
Appendicitis may be caused by obstruction of the lumen of the appendix by hardened fecal material (fecalith); swollen lymphoid tissue, occurring after a viral infection; or a parasite such as

Enterobius vermicularis or pinworms, that can obstruct the appendiceal lumen.

With acute obstruction, the outflow of mucus secretion is blocked and pressure builds within the lumen, resulting in compression of blood vessels. The resulting ischemia is followed by ulceration of the epithelial lining and bacterial invasion. Subsequent necrosis causes perforation or rupture with fecal and bacterial contamination of the peritoneal cavity. The resulting inflammation spreads rapidly throughout the abdomen *(peritonitis),* especially in young children, who are unable to localize infection.

Clinical Signs and Symptoms
▪ Periumbilical pain followed by nausea, right lower quadrant pain, and later vomiting with fever; anorexia
▪ Localized tenderness at McBurney point: a point midway between the anterior superior iliac crest and the umbilicus
▪ Sudden absence of pain may indicate perforation.

Diagnostic Evaluation
▪ Complete blood count
▪ Urinalysis (to rule out UTI)
▪ Serum hCG (human chorionic gonadotropin) in females to rule out an ectopic pregnancy
▪ White blood cell (WBC) count greater than $10,000/mm^3$ and a C-reactive protein (CRP) are common but are not necessarily specific for appendicitis.
▪ Computed tomography (CT) scan of the abdomen (may show enlarged appendiceal diameter, appendiceal wall thickening, periappendiceal inflammatory changes including fat streaks, phlegmon, fluid collection, and/or extraluminal gas)
▪ Abdomen ultrasound may be helpful.

Treatment
▪ Before perforation: rehydration, antibiotics, and surgical removal of the appendix *(appendectomy)*
▪ Laparoscopic surgery is commonly used to treat nonperforated acute appendicitis.
▪ With perforated (ruptured) appendix: IV hydration, systematic antibiotics; possibly NG suction for bowel decompression

■ Postoperative care—without perforation: pain management; hydration, fluid and electrolyte management

■ Postoperative care—with perforation: pain management; fluid and electrolyte replacement; systemic antibiotics; bowel decompression until return of bowel function

■ Abdominal wound may be closed or remain open with perforation.

Nursing Care Management

■ Preoperative: early detection; assist with diagnostic tests; comfort measures; initiate IV access for hydration; prepare for surgery (emotionally and physically); keep family informed of child's status perioperatively; fever management.

■ Postoperative: pain management; assessment of return of bowel function; assessment of incisions, drains (as applicable); administration of antibiotics, fluids, and electrolytes; in some cases, management of bowel decompression with NG tube (ensure adequate NG tube function); ambulate and encourage oral fluid intake as tolerated to promote return of bowel function; emotional support and care of child and family; fever management.

Patient and Family Teaching

■ Administration of pain medication at home
■ Dietary intake during recovery phase
■ Evaluation of incision(s)
■ Ambulation and fluid intake

ARTHRITIS, JUVENILE (FORMERLY RHEUMATOID)

Description

Juvenile idiopathic arthritis (JIA) is a chronic autoimmune inflammatory disease causing inflammation of joints and other tissue with an unknown cause. JIA starts before age 16 with peak onset between 1 and 3 years of age.

Pathophysiology

A popular causal theory is an infectious or environmental agent, which triggers an abnormal inflammatory response in a genetically predisposed child, resulting in chronic arthritis, but there is no substantiating evidence. The disease process is characterized by chronic inflammation of the synovium with joint effusion and eventual erosion, destruction, and fibrosis of the articular cartilage. Adhesions between joint surfaces and ankylosis of joints occur if the inflammatory process persists.

Clinical Signs and Symptoms
- Joint tenderness and pain, stiffness
- Systemic: fever, rash, lymphadenopathy, hepatosplenomegaly, and serositis
- Psoriasis or an associated dactylitis, nail pitting, or onycholysis
- Enthesitis: inflammation at the tendon insertion site; sacroiliac or lumbarsacral pain
- Inflammatory bowel disease
- Uveitis: inflammation of the uvea, which lies between the sclera and the retina

Diagnostic Evaluation
JIA is a diagnosis of exclusion; there are no definitive tests. Classifications are based on the clinical criteria of age of onset before 16 years, arthritis in one or more joints for 6 weeks or longer, and exclusion of other etiologies. Additional diagnostic tests may include:
- ESR: erythrocyte sedimentation rate may be elevated
- Rheumatoid factor
- CBC: leukocytosis may be present.
- Slit lamp eye exam to detect uveitis
- Radiographs
- Antinuclear antibodies (ANA)

Treatment
There is no cure for JIA. The major goals of therapy are to:
- control pain
- preserve joint range of motion and function
- minimize effects of inflammation such as joint deformity
- promote normal growth and development

Medications
- NSAIDS: Naproxen, ibuprofen, Tolmetin
- Methotrexate
- Corticosteroids: orally, as intraarticular joint injections, as intravenous infusions, or in eye drop form for uveitis

- Etanercept: a tumor necrosis factor alpha receptor blocker
- Slow-acting antirheumatic drugs (SAARDs): sulfasalazine, hydroxychloroquine, gold, and D-penicillamine
- Physical and occupational therapy: focuses on strengthening muscles, mobilizing restricted joint motion, and preventing or correcting deformities

Nursing Care Management
- Assessment of the child's general health, the status of involved joints, and the child's emotional response to all ramifications of the disease
- Teaching medication administration to child and family
- Encouraging child to be involved in school and other age-appropriate activities
- Helping child and family explore options for pain management
- Preventing complications such as muscle contracture for disuse; follow-up medical exams for eye exams (to detect uveitis)
- Encouraging use of heat and exercise to decrease joint pain
- Support child and family: referrals may be necessary for family to cope with financial aspect of care, transportation needs, medications.

Patient and Family Teaching
- Medication administration
- Pain management
- Joint exercises and other therapies
- Importance of medical follow-up examinations

ASTHMA
Description
Asthma is a chronic inflammatory disorder of the airways characterized by recurrent episodes of wheezing, breathlessness, chest tightness, and cough.

Pathophysiology
Inflammation contributes to heightened airway reactivity in asthma. The mechanisms contributing to airway inflammation are multiple and involve a number of different pathways. Another important component of asthma is bronchospasm and obstruction. The

mechanisms responsible for the obstructive symptoms in asthma include: (1) inflammation and edema of the mucous membranes, (2) accumulation of tenacious secretions from mucous glands, and (3) spasm of the smooth muscle of the bronchi and bronchioles, which decreases the caliber of the bronchioles. Bronchial constriction is a normal reaction to foreign stimuli, but in the child with asthma it is abnormally severe, producing impaired respiratory function. The smooth muscle arranged in spiral bundles around the airway causes narrowing and shortening of the airway, which significantly increases airway resistance to airflow. Because the bronchi normally dilate and elongate during inspiration and contract and shorten on expiration, the respiratory difficulty is more pronounced during the expiratory phase of respiration.

Increased resistance in the airway causes forced expiration through the narrowed lumen. The volume of air trapped in the lungs increases as airways are functionally closed at a point between the alveoli and the lobar bronchi. This trapping of gas forces the individual to breathe at higher and higher lung volumes. Consequently, the person with asthma fights to inspire sufficient air. This expenditure of effort for breathing causes fatigue, decreased respiratory effectiveness, and increased oxygen consumption. The inspiration occurring at higher lung volumes hyperinflates the alveoli and reduces the effectiveness of the cough. As the severity of obstruction increases, there is a reduced alveolar ventilation with carbon dioxide retention, hypoxemia, respiratory acidosis, and, eventually, respiratory failure.

Clinical Signs and Symptoms
- Cough: hacking, paroxysmal, irritative, and nonproductive
- Shortness of breath
- Prolonged expiratory phase
- Audible wheeze
- Malar flush and red ears
- Lips, deep, dark red color
- Restlessness
- Apprehension
- Sweating
- Older children may sit upright with shoulders in a hunched-over position, hands on the bed or chair, and arms braced (tripod).
- May speak with short, panting, broken phrases

- ■ Coarse, loud breath sounds
- ■ Crackles

Diagnostic Evaluation

Asthma is classified into four categories based on the symptom indicators of disease severity. These categories are:

- ■ Intermittent—has least number of symptoms
- ■ Mild persistent
- ■ Moderate persistent
- ■ Severe persistent
- ■ Symptoms increase in frequency or intensity until the last category of severe persistent asthma. These categories provide a stepwise approach to the pharmacologic management, environmental control, and educational interventions needed for each category.

Additional diagnostic measures may include:

- ■ Pulmonary function tests (PFTs)
- ■ Peak expiratory flow rate (PEFR) using a peak expiratory flow meter (PEFM) to determine child's personal best value at optimal functioning
- ■ Bronchoprovocation testing
- ■ Exercise challenge
- ■ Skin testing for allergens
- ■ Chest radiograph
- ■ Complete blood count: eosinophilia

Treatment

The overall goals of asthma management are to:

- ■ Maintain normal activity levels.
- ■ Maintain normal pulmonary function.
- ■ Prevent chronic symptoms and recurrent exacerbations.
- ■ Provide optimum drug therapy with minimum or no adverse effects.
- ■ Assist the child in living as normal and happy a life as possible.

These may be accomplished with the following:

- ■ Recognition and avoidance of allergens
- ■ Pharmacotherapy: inhaled corticosteroids (anti-inflammatory); cromolyn sodium and nedocromil; short- and long-acting β_2-agonists (bronchodilator); methylxanthines (bronchodilator);

leukotriene modifiers; anticholinergics (bronchodilator); and systemic corticosteroids (anti-inflammatory)

▪ Methods of drug administration include: MDI inhaler with or without spacer; nebulized inhalation for smaller children; and dry powder inhaler.

Nursing Care Management
▪ Review child's health history, home, school, and play environment.
▪ Perform a comprehensive physical assessment with focus on the respiratory system.
▪ Asthma education (see below)
▪ Assist family and child in management of asthma symptoms by reducing exposure to allergens.
▪ Assist with allergen testing.
▪ Assist with pulmonary function tests.
▪ Provide emotional support child and family.
▪ Referral for financial and social assistance
▪ Monitor child's and family's progress with asthma care and effects on home and school life.
▪ Administration of medications during asthma exacerbation
▪ Emergent care

Patient and Family Teaching
▪ Education related to recognition and management of symptoms
▪ Education about reducing exposure to asthma triggers
▪ Education regarding medication use and PEFM monitoring
▪ Managing asthma exacerbation during illness
▪ Education regarding play activities, nutrition, and involvement in exercise
▪ Community resource education

ATOPIC DERMATITIS (ECZEMA)
Description
Eczema or *eczematous inflammation* of the skin refers to a descriptive category of dermatologic diseases and not to a specific etiology. AD is a type of pruritic eczema that usually begins during infancy and is associated with allergy with a hereditary tendency (atopy). Three forms of AD are recognized: infantile (infantile eczema), childhood, and preadolescent and adolescent. The majority of children with infantile AD have a family history of

eczema, asthma, food allergies, or allergic rhinitis, which strongly supports a genetic predisposition; many children with AD will develop asthma.

Pathophysiology
The cause of AD is unknown but may be related to an immune reaction with abnormal function of the skin, including alterations in perspiration, peripheral vascular function, and heat intolerance. Patients with AD have dry skin and evidence of increased transepidermal water loss; a defect in the ceramide cells, which help retain water and provide a barrier function; and increased colonization of the skin with *Staphylococcus aureus*. House dust mites, certain foods, mold, and animal hair may play a role in the etiology of AD. Many children with AD have elevated toxic-specific IgE levels. IgE food sensitization has been found to be a major risk factor for infantile AD.

Clinical Signs and Symptoms
Distribution of Lesions
■ Infantile form: generalized, especially cheeks, scalp, trunk, and extensor surfaces of extremities
■ Childhood form: flexural areas (antecubital and popliteal fossae, neck), wrists, ankles, and feet
■ Adolescent and preadolescent form: face, sides of neck, hands, feet, and antecubital and popliteal fossae (to a lesser extent)

Appearance of Lesions
■ Infantile form
  ■ Erythema
  ■ Vesicles
  ■ Papules
  ■ Weeping
  ■ Oozing
  ■ Crusting
  ■ Scaling
  ■ Often symmetric
■ Childhood form
  ■ Symmetric involvement
  ■ Clusters of small erythematous or flesh-colored papules or minimally scaling patches

- Dry; may be hyperpigmented
- Lichenification (thickened skin with accentuation of creases)
- Keratosis pilaris (follicular hyperkeratosis) common
- Adolescent and Adult Form
  - Same as childhood manifestations
  - Dry, thick lesions (lichenified plaques) common
  - Confluent papules

Other Manifestations
- Intense itching
- Unaffected skin dry and rough
- African-American children likely to exhibit more papular or follicular lesions than Caucasian children
- May exhibit one or more of the following:
  - Lymphadenopathy, especially near affected sites
  - Increased palmar creases (many cases)
  - Atopic pleats (extra line or groove of lower eyelid)
  - Tendency toward cold hands
  - Pityriasis alba (small, poorly defined areas of hypopigmentation)
  - Facial pallor (especially around nose, mouth, and ears)
  - Bluish discoloration beneath eyes ("allergic shiners")
  - Increased susceptibility to unusual cutaneous infections (especially viral)

Diagnostic Evaluation
Diagnosis is based on a combination of history and morphologic findings (see Clinical Signs and Symptoms on the previous page).

Treatment
The major goals of management are to (1) hydrate the skin, (2) relieve pruritus, (3) reduce flare-ups or inflammation, and (4) prevent and control infection.
- Skin hydration: emollients, colloid baths, avoiding harsh soaps, avoiding overheating
- Relieve pruritis : medications (antipruritic), wear soft cotton clothing.
- Reduce flare-ups: topical corticosteroids, systemic antibiotics may be necessary.
- Prevent infection: cover lesions or prevent scratching in infants to reduce infection.

- Topical immunomodulators: tacrolimus and pimecrolimus (Elidel) are best used at the beginning of a flare-up just as the skin becomes red and begins to itch.
- General prevention: in those who are at high risk (parents may have atopy), reduce exposure to allergens; breastfeed for first six months; avoid whole cow's milk until 15-18 months; avoid highly allergenic foods until 24-30 months.

Nursing Care Management
- Assist in identifying condition.
- Administration of medications.
- Education regarding management of symptoms and prevention of complications (see Patient and Family Teaching).
- Provide family support and referrals as necessary.

Patient and Family Teaching
- Skin hydration with moisturizers and emollients; colloid baths
- Avoidance of allergens
- Medication administration
- Prevention of scratching (infection may occur) by managing pruritis: cotton mittens, cotton clothing, short fingernails, elbow restraints, antipruritic medications

ATRIAL SEPTAL DEFECT
Description
Abnormal opening between the atria, allowing blood from the higher-pressure left atrium to flow into the lower-pressure right atrium. There are three types of atrial septal defect (ASD):

Primum ASD: opening at lower end of septum; may be associated with mitral valve abnormalities

Secundum ASD: opening near center of septum

Sinus venosus defect: opening near junction of superior vena cava and right atrium; may be associated with partial anomalous pulmonary venous connection

Pathophysiology
Because left atrial pressure slightly exceeds right atrial pressure, blood flows from the left to the right atrium, causing an increased flow of oxygenated blood into the right side of the heart. Despite the low pressure difference, a high rate of flow can still occur

because of low pulmonary vascular resistance and the greater distensibility of the right atrium, which further reduces flow resistance. This volume is well tolerated by the right ventricle because it is delivered under much lower pressure than with a ventricular septal defect. Although there is right atrial and ventricular enlargement, cardiac failure is unusual in an uncomplicated ASD. Pulmonary vascular changes usually occur only after several decades if the defect is left unrepaired.

Clinical Signs and Symptoms

Patients are typically asymptomatic, although they may demonstrate mild exercise intolerance or frequent upper respiratory infections. Development of congestive heart failure is rare in the pediatric population with ASD but becomes more prevalent in adults (see Box 3-1). The physical exam is mostly unremarkable. There may be a systolic ejection murmur through the pulmonary valve, but the most significant finding upon auscultation is a fixed splitting of the second heart sound. Patients are at risk for atrial dysrhythmias (probably caused by atrial enlargement and stretching of conduction fibers) and pulmonary vascular obstructive disease and emboli formation later in life from chronically increased pulmonary blood flow.

Diagnostic Evaluation
Procedures for Cardiac Diagnosis
Treatment

Surgical Treatment. Surgical patch closure (pericardial patch or Dacron patch) is done for moderate to large defects. Smaller defects may be repaired by direct suture closure. Open repair with cardiopulmonary bypass is usually performed before school age. A minimally invasive approach may also be employed with a limited median sternotomy. Sinus venosus ASDs can be closed with a pericardial patch, unless there is also anomalous pulmonary venous drainage. In this case, the Warden procedure may be performed that utilizes a patch to baffle pulmonary venous return appropriately to the left atrium. Primum ASDs may require mitral valve repair or, rarely, replacement of the mitral valve.

Nonsurgical Treatment. Secundum ASD closure with a device during cardiac catheterization is becoming commonplace and can be done as an outpatient procedure. The Amplatzer septal occluder is most commonly used. Smaller defects that have a rim around them for attachment of the device can be closed with a device; large, irregular defects without a rim require surgical closure. Successful closure in appropriately selected patients yields results similar to surgery, but involves shorter hospital stays and fewer complications. Surgical closure is still considered the standard therapy as long-term outcomes following device closure are yet to be defined.

Nursing Care Management
Assist in Measures to Assess and Improve Cardiac Function
Monitor Cardiac Function
- Vital signs monitoring
- Respiratory assessment
- Cardiac assessment
    - Cardiac output (color, pulses, perfusion, capillary refill, renal function, and neurologic function)
    - Heart sounds
    - Dysrhythmias
- Keep accurate record of intake and output.
- Weigh child or infant on same scale at same time of day.
- Monitor for signs and symptoms of postpericardiotomy syndrome following surgery:
    - Fever
    - Malaise
    - Nausea
    - Vomiting
    - Abdominal pain
    - Friction rub may be auscultated.

Administer Medications
- Review child's history related to cardiac management.
- Administer medications on schedule.
- Assess effectiveness of medications and any side effects noted.
- Be aware of drug-drug and drug-food interactions.
- Follow guidelines for medication administration.

Manage Common Side Effects of Cardiac Defects
- Prevent fatigue during feeding; offer small frequent feedings to infant's or child's tolerance.
- Organize nursing care to allow child/infant uninterrupted rest.
- Promote activities that do not cause fatigue.

Provide Support for the Child and Family
- Communicate with the child and family in an appropriate style.
- Provide the child and family with honest answers.
- Provide emotional support.
- Offer age-appropriate interventions.
- Provide information on available resources for support for the child and family.

Patient and Family Teaching
Prepare the Child and Family for Diagnostic and Operative Procedures
- Provide explanation of diagnostic tests and why each test is performed because many of them are invasive procedures.
- Prepare the child prior to the invasive procedure. Remember discussion is dependent upon the child's age and development.
- Use simple words or pictures to describe procedures and answer all questions the child and family may have.
- Postoperative wound care teaching as needed.
- Post-cardiac catheterization wound care teaching as needed.
- Assess and record results of teaching and family's participation in care.

Educate the Child and Family
- Assess child's and family's level of knowledge regarding the ASD.
- Assess child's and family's understanding of what they have heard about ASD.
- Assess child's and family's understanding of the surgery and/or cardiac catheterization.
- Teach the child and/or family at least four characteristics of congestive heart failure that may occur because of the ASD such as:
    - Fatigue after exertion
    - Fast heart rate
    - Fast breathing, shortness of breath, dyspnea
    - Retractions
    - Nasal flaring
    - Cool extremities
    - Diaphoresis

- ▪ Decreased urinary output
- ▪ Puffiness (edema)
- ▪ Fussiness
- ▪ Decreased appetite
- ▪ Educate child and family about care such as medication preparation and administration.
- ▪ Assess child's and family's access to appropriate pharmacy for any special preparation medications.
- ▪ Teach the child and family to notify their physician of any clinical changes.
- ▪ Assess and record results and family's participation in care.
- ▪ Provide appropriate educational resources and review materials with them.
- ▪ Clarify information presented by the health care team including appointment for follow-up visit.
- ▪ Discuss SBE (subacute bacterial endocarditis) prophylaxis with pediatric cardiologist.

ATTENTION DEFICIT HYPERACTIVITY DISORDER
Description
Attention deficit hyperactivity disorder (ADHD) refers to developmentally inappropriate degrees of inattention, impulsiveness, and hyperactivity. To be diagnosed as ADHD, the symptoms must have been present before age 7 years and must be present in at least two settings.

Pathophysiology
While the cause of ADHD is unknown, there is some support for a genetic origin. Psychologic adversity and perinatal brain insults are also being considered.

Clinical Signs and Symptoms
- ▪ Inattention
- ▪ Distractibility
- ▪ Impulsivity
- ▪ Hyperactivity

Diagnostic Evaluation
- ▪ Comprehensive history and physical; special emphasis on school problems can assist in the diagnosis.

- Behavioral checklists and adaptive scales are helpful in measuring school adaptive functioning in children with ADHD.
- Psychiatric disorders and medical problems as well as traumatic experiences are ruled out, including lead poisoning, seizures, partial hearing loss, psychosis, and witnessing of sexual activity and/or violence.

Treatment
- Management of the child with ADHD usually involves multiple approaches that include family education and counseling, medication, proper classroom placement, environmental manipulation, and behavioral or psychotherapy for the child.

Nursing Care Management
- Management begins with an explanation to the parents and the child about the diagnosis, including the nature of the problem.
- Evaluation of medication and its effect
- Follow-up on school participation.

Patient and Family Teaching
- To some parents, a diagnosis of ADHD is confirmation of the fear that their child has some irreversible, serious disease; to others it is a relief. All need the opportunity to vent their feelings and suspicions.
- The greater their understanding of the disorder and its effects, the more likely they will be to carry out the recommended program of therapy.

AUTISM SPECTRUM DISORDERS
Description
Autism spectrum disorders (ASD) are complex neurodevelopmental disorders of brain function accompanied by intellectual and social behavioral deficits.

Pathophysiology
ASD is now recognized as a genetic disorder of prenatal and postnatal brain development. Immune and environmental factors (e.g., viral infections) may interact with the genetic susceptibility to increase the development of ASD.

Clinical Signs and Symptoms
- Children with ASD demonstrate several peculiar and often seemingly bizarre characteristics, primarily in social interactions, communication, and behavior.
  - Inability to maintain eye contact with another person
  - Avoidance of body contact, and language delay at a very early age
  - Limited functional play; may interact with toys in an unusual or odd manner
- ASD children may have significant gastrointestinal symptoms. Constipation is a common symptom and can be associated with acquired megarectum in children with ASD.

Diagnostic Evaluation
- Early recognition of behaviors associated with ASD is critical to implement appropriate interventions and family involvement.
- Developmental history is essential.
- Physical examination for genetic syndromes or neurologic findings
- Often young children present with behavior difficulties.

Treatment
- The most promising results have been through highly structured and intensive behavior modification programs.
- In general, the objective in treatment is to promote positive reinforcement, increase social awareness of others, teach verbal communication skills, and decrease unacceptable behavior.
- Providing a structured routine for the child to follow is a key in the management of ASD.

Nursing Care Management
- Because physical contact often upsets these children, minimum holding and eye contact may be necessary to avoid behavioral outbursts.
- Care must be taken when performing procedures on, administering medicine to, or feeding these children.
- Children with ASD need to be introduced slowly to new situations.

■ Communication should be at the child's developmental level, brief, and concrete.

Patient and Family Teaching
■ Parents need expert counseling early in the course of the disorder.
■ Support groups and experts in ASD provide needed education and support for parents.

BILIARY ATRESIA
Description
Biliary atresia (BA) is a destructive, idiopathic, inflammatory process that leads to fibrosis and obliteration of the biliary tree. Untreated biliary atresia results in progressive cirrhosis and death in most children by 2 years of age.

Pathophysiology
The exact cause of BA is unknown. BA has two distinct forms, postnatal and fetal/embryonic, and different pathogenic mechanisms are suggested for each. Postnatal BA is probably the result of infection or an immune-mediated mechanism. An abnormal direct bilirubin has been designated as ≥ 1.0 mg/dL if the total bilirubin is ≤ 5 mg/dL or a value of direct bilirubin that represents more than 20% of the total bilirubin if it is ≥ 5 mg/dL. Direct hyperbilirubinemia first appears after the resolution of physiologic jaundice of the newborn. Histology demonstrates bile duct remnants and a progressive inflammatory process. In the fetal embryonic form of BA, there is a congenital absence of biliary ductal patency and an absence of bile duct remnants; many infants have associated congenital anomalies. Varying degrees of cholestasis occur, resulting in retention of irritants and toxins. Cholestasis is the accumulation of compounds that cannot be excreted because of occlusion or obstruction of the biliary tree. Injury to the liver occurs as the result of the inflammation caused by the cholestasis.

Clinical Signs and Symptoms
■ Jaundice
■ Dark urine
■ Pale stool (*acholic* stool, indicative of an absence of bile)

- Pruritis with advanced disease process
- Growth failure (failure to thrive)

Diagnostic Evaluation
- Blood tests should include a CBC, electrolytes, bilirubin, and liver enzymes.
- Alpha$_1$-antitrypsin level, TORCH titers, hepatitis serology, alpha-fetoprotein, urine cytomegalovirus, and a sweat test to rule out other conditions that cause persistent cholestasis and jaundice
- Abdominal ultrasonography to inspect liver and biliary system
- Hepatobiliary scintigraphy demonstrates biliary patency.
- Endoscopic retrograde cholangiopancreatography (ERCP) is performed in very young infants.
- Percutaneous liver biopsy is highly reliable when the biopsy contains specimens from a number of portal areas.
- Definitive diagnosis during surgical laparotomy and an intra-operative cholangiogram

Treatment
- ***Hepatic portoenterostomy (Kasai procedure),*** in which a segment of intestine is anastomosed to the resected porta hepatis to attempt bile drainage
- Postoperative antibiotic therapy
- Nutritional support with infant formulas that contain medium-chain triglycerides and essential fatty acids
- Supplementation with fat-soluble vitamins, a multivitamin, and minerals, including iron, zinc, and selenium
- Aggressive nutritional support with continuous tube feedings or TPN is indicated for moderate to severe growth failure (failure to thrive).
- Ursodeoxycholic acid to treat pruritus and hypercholesterolemia

Nursing Care Management
- Intraoperative care of family: Provide information about child's condition and what to expect after surgery.
- Pain management (postoperative)
- Family psychosocial support
- Nutritional support: special formulas, vitamin and mineral supplements, tube feedings, or parenteral nutrition

- Pruritus management
- Skin care

Patient and Family Teaching
- Care of child with chronic condition
- Administration of medications
- Nutritional support may entail family managing home TPN or tube feedings, administration of vitamins and supplements.

BOTULISM, INFANT
Description
Infant botulism is an acute flaccid paralysis caused by the pre-formed toxin produced by the anaerobic bacillus *Clostridium botulinum.*

Pathophysiology
Infant botulism occurs primarily in infants less than 6 months of age when spores or vegetative cells of *C. botulinum* are ingested with the subsequent release of the toxin from organisms colonizing the gastrointestinal tract. The symmetric descending paralysis associated with botulism occurs as a result of blockade of the neurotransmitter at the autonomic neuromuscular and voluntary motor junctions. *C. botulinum,* types A and B, are the most common causative strains of infant botulism. Common sources of botulism spores are soil and honey. Nonhuman milk substances are also believed to be the source of infant botulism spores.

Clinical Signs and Symptoms
- Variable: mild constipation to progressive sequential loss of neurologic function and respiratory failure
- Deep tendon reflexes diminished or absent
- Cranial nerve deficits common, as evidenced by loss of head control, absent facial expression, difficulty in feeding, weak cry, ocular palsies, and reduced gag reflex
- Lethargy
- Hypotonia
- Poor feeding
- May be mistakenly diagnosed as sepsis, metabolic condition or SMA Type 1

Diagnostic Evaluation

Diagnosis is made on the basis of the clinical history, physical examination, and laboratory detection of the organism in the patient's stool, and less commonly in the blood. EMG may be helpful in establishing the diagnosis; however, results may be normal early in the course of the illness.

Treatment

■ Administration of botulism immune globulin intravenously (BIG-IV; trade name BabyBIG)
■ Airway management (intubation and mechanical ventilation)
■ Nutritional support

Nursing Care Management

■ Observe for and report signs of neuromuscular weakness or impairment.
■ Provide supportive care including airway management and nutritional support.
■ Skin care for immobilized infant
■ Supportive emotional care of parents

Patient and Family Teaching

■ Avoidance of possible sources of botulism spores (e.g., honey), in infants less than 12 months old
■ Recognition of signs of feeding difficulty or decreased activity levels

BRONCHIOLITIS

Description

Bronchiolitis is an acute viral infection with maximum effect at the bronchiolar level. The infection occurs primarily in winter and spring, and it is the most frequent cause of hospitalization in children less than 1 year old. Although most cases of bronchiolitis are caused by RSV, adenoviruses, parainfluenza viruses are also implicated; recently, human metapneumovirus has also been associated with bronchiolitis in children.

Pathophysiology

The causative virus affects the epithelial cells of the respiratory tract. The ciliated cells swell, protrude into the lumen, and lose their cilia. RSV produces a fusion of the infected cell membrane with cell membranes of adjacent epithelial cells, thus forming a giant cell with multiple nuclei. At the cellular level, this fusion results in multinucleated masses of protoplasm, or *syncytia*.

The bronchiolar mucosa swells, and lumina are subsequently filled with mucus and exudate. The walls of the bronchi and bronchioles are infiltrated with inflammatory cells, and peribronchiolar interstitial pneumonitis is usually present. Because luminal epithelial cells are shed into the bronchioles when they die, the lumina are frequently obstructed, particularly on expiration. The varying degrees of obstruction produced in small air passages lead to hyperinflation, obstructive emphysema resulting from partial obstruction, and patchy areas of atelectasis. Dilation of bronchial passages on inspiration allows sufficient space for intake of air, but narrowing of the passages on expiration prevents air from leaving the lungs. Thus air is trapped distal to the obstruction and causes progressive overinflation (emphysema).

Clinical Signs and Symptoms
- Rhinorrhea
- Low-grade fever
- Cough
- Sneezing
- Poor feeding
- Slight lethargy or irritability
- Wheezing
- Possible ear or eye drainage

As diseases progresses
- Air hunger
- Tachypnea and retractions
- Cyanosis

Severe disease
- Tachypnea, greater than 70 breaths/min
- Listlessness
- Apnea
- Decreased air exchange
- Respiratory failure

Diagnostic Evaluation

Rapid immunofluorescent antibody–direct fluorescent antibody staining (DFA), or enzyme-linked immunosorbent assay (ELISA) techniques for RSV antigen detection, which are performed on nasal secretions

Treatment

- Ensure adequate fluid intake since infant has difficulty handling nasal secretions and nursing or taking a bottle.
- Airway maintenance-instillation of nasal saline drops into nares and suctioning.
- Humidified air; humidified oxygen as necessary
- Fever management: acetaminophen
- Treatment of concomitant illness such as otitis media with antibiotics
- Bronchodilator medications may be used.
- Racemic epinephrine (nebulized) may be used in some cases.

Prevention

- Administration of palivizumab (Synagis), a monoclonal antibody–intramuscular injection given once a month (November to March) to high-risk patients (preterm infants born before 32 weeks gestation, who required mechanical ventilation or oxygen; infants with bronchopulmonary dysplasia; children with severe immunodeficiencies [e.g., severe combined immunodeficiency or acquired immunodeficiency syndrome]; and children younger than 2 years of age with hemodynamically significant congenital heart disease)
- Handwashing and standard precautions in acute care facility
- Use of Ribavirin is controversial due to cost, questionable effectiveness, and side effects.

Nursing Care Management

- Contact and standard precautions in hospitalized infant to prevent spread
- Handwashing to prevent spread
- Parent teaching for home management (see next page)
- Maintaining patent airway
- Suction nares with normal saline drops
- Ensure adequate fluid intake: enteral, or parenteral if necessary.
- Parent support

- Administer bronchodilator medications.
- Encourage continuation of breastfeeding.

Patient and Family Teaching
- Teach prevention of spread to other household members: hand-washing.
- Therapies such as nasal suctioning, fever management, fluid intake with frequent small amounts
- Assist with and encourage breastfeeding mother.
- Provide reassurance.
- Signs and symptoms of increasing illness severity (when to seek immediate medical care)

BRONCHITIS
Description
Inflammation of the large airways: trachea and bronchi often in association with an upper respiratory infection

Pathophysiology
Viral agents and *Mycoplasma pneumoniae* are often the primary cause of the disease. The causative agents are inhaled into the upper airway and cause a local inflammatory response in the upper airway, producing the signs and symptoms.

Clinical Signs and Symptoms
- Dry, hacking cough
- Runny nose
- Dry, scratchy throat
- Fever

Diagnostic Evaluation
- Based on clinical presentation and physical examination

Treatment
- Primarily supportive: analgesics, antipyretics, humidity, cough suppressant may be used depending on age of child.

Nursing Care Management
- Medication administration: antipyretics, antitussives, analgesics
- Encourage increase in oral fluid intake.

- ▪ Parent teaching
- ▪ Prevent spread: close contact; avoid sneezing, coughing on infants or immunosuppressed persons.

Patient and Family Teaching
- ▪ Medication administration
- ▪ Comfort measures
- ▪ Prevent spread.

β-THALASSEMIA (COOLEY ANEMIA)
Description
β-Thalassemia is the most common of the thalassemias and occurs in four forms: two heterozygous forms: *thalassemia minor,* an asymptomatic silent carrier, and *thalassemia trait,* which produces a mild microcytic anemia; *thalassemia intermedia,* which is manifested as splenomegaly and moderate to severe anemia; and a homozygous form, *thalassemia major* (also known as *Cooley anemia*), which results in a severe anemia that would lead to cardiac failure and death in early childhood without transfusion support.

Pathophysiology
Normal postnatal Hgb is composed of 2 α- and 2 β-polypeptide chains. In β-thalassemia there is a partial or complete deficiency in the synthesis of the β-chain of the Hgb molecule. Consequently, there is a compensatory increase in the synthesis of α-chains, and γ-chain production remains activated, resulting in defective Hgb formation. This unbalanced polypeptide unit is very unstable; when it disintegrates, it damages RBCs, causing severe anemia. To compensate for the hemolytic process, an overabundance of erythrocytes is formed unless the bone marrow is suppressed by transfusion therapy. Excess iron from hemolysis of supplemental RBCs in transfusions and from the rapid destruction of defective cells is stored in various organs (*hemosiderosis*).

Clinical Signs and Symptoms
Anemia (Before Diagnosis)
- ▪ Pallor
- ▪ Unexplained fever
- ▪ Poor feeding
- ▪ Enlarged spleen or liver

Progressive Anemia
- Signs of chronic hypoxia
- Headache
- Precordial and bone pain
- Decreased exercise tolerance
- Listlessness
- Anorexia

Other Features
- Small stature
- Delayed sexual maturation
- Bronzed, freckled complexion (if not receiving chelation therapy)

Bone Changes (Older Children if Untreated)
- Enlarged head
- Prominent frontal and parietal bossing
- Prominent malar eminences
- Flat or depressed bridge of the nose
- Enlarged maxilla
- Protrusion of the lip and upper central incisors and eventual malocclusion
- Generalized osteoporosis

Diagnostic Evaluation
- Hematologic studies reveal the characteristic changes in RBCs (i.e., microcytosis, hypochromia, anisocytosis, poikilocytosis, target cells, and basophilic stippling of various stages).
- Low Hgb and Hct levels are seen in severe anemia, although they are typically lower than the reduction in RBC count because of the proliferation of immature erythrocytes.
- Hgb electrophoresis confirms the diagnosis, and radiographs of involved bones reveal characteristic findings.

Treatment
- The objective of supportive therapy is to maintain sufficient Hgb levels to prevent bone marrow expansion and the resulting bony deformities, and to provide sufficient RBCs to support normal growth and normal physical activity.
- Transfusions are used to maintain a child's Hgb level above 9.5 g/dL, a goal that may require transfusions as often as every

3 to 5 weeks. Advantages include (1) improved physical and psychologic well-being because of the ability to participate in normal activities, (2) decreased cardiomegaly and hepatosplenomegaly, (3) fewer bone changes, (4) normal or near-normal growth and development until puberty, and (5) fewer infections.

▪ One of the potential complications of frequent blood transfusions is iron overload. Because the body has no effective means of eliminating the excess iron, the mineral is deposited in body tissues. To minimize the development of hemosiderosis, the new oral iron chelators deferasirox or deferiprone have shown to be equivalent to *deferoxamine (Desferal),* a parenteral iron-chelating agent, and are much more tolerable by patients and families.

▪ In some children with severe splenomegaly who demonstrate increased transfusion requirements, a splenectomy may be necessary to decrease the disabling effects of abdominal pressure and to increase the lifespan of supplemental RBCs.

Nursing Care Management
▪ Promote compliance with transfusion and chelation therapy.
▪ Assist the child in coping with the anxiety-provoking treatments and the effects of the illness.
▪ Foster the child's and family's adjustment to a chronic illness.
▪ Observe for complications of multiple blood transfusions.

Patient and Family Teaching
▪ As with any chronic illness, the needs of the family must be met for optimal adjustment to the stresses imposed by the disorder.
▪ Genetic counseling for the parents and fertile offspring is mandatory, and both prenatal diagnosis using amniocentesis at 20 weeks of gestation or fetal blood sampling at 10 weeks and screening for thalassemia trait are available.

BULIMIA
Description
Bulimia is an eating disorder characterized by repeated episodes of binge eating followed by inappropriate compensatory behaviors, such as self-induced vomiting; misuse of laxatives, diuretics, or other medications; fasting; or excessive exercise. The binge behavior consists of secretive, frenzied consumption of large amounts of

high-calorie (or "forbidden") foods during a brief time (usually less than 2 hours). The binge is counteracted by a variety of weight control methods (purging), including self-induced vomiting, diuretic and laxative abuse, and rigorous exercise. These binge-purge cycles are followed by self-deprecating thoughts, a depressed mood, and an awareness that the eating pattern is abnormal.

Pathophysiology
The etiology and pathophysiology of the disorder is unclear. It appears to be caused by a combination of genetic, neurochemical, psychodevelopmental, and sociocultural factors. Patients with eating disorders commonly have psychiatric problems, including affective disorder, anxiety disorder, obsessive-compulsive disorder, and personality disorder. In addition, many experts associate the development of an eating disorder with family characteristics such as an adolescent perception of high parental expectations for achievement and appearance, difficulty managing conflict and poor communication styles, enmeshment and occasionally estrangement between family members, devaluation of the mother or the maternal role, and marital tension. Bulimia is observed more commonly in older adolescent girls and young women; males with bulimia are less common. BN patients may be of average or slightly above average weight.

Clinical Signs and Symptoms
- Low self-esteem
- Abnormal eating patterns
- Sudden weight gain and weight loss pattern within a matter of days or weeks
- Inordinate preoccupation with weight and food intake
- Excessive exercising

The following may be present and suggest the need for hospitalization (i.e., not all patients with bulimia will manifest the following):
- Syncope
- Serum potassium concentration <3.2 mmol/L
- Serum chloride concentration <88 mmol/L
- Esophageal tears
- Cardiac arrhythmias, including prolonged QT interval
- Hypothermia
- Suicide risk
- Intractable vomiting

- Hematemesis
- Failure to respond to outpatient treatment

Diagnostic Evaluation
The diagnosis is based on the American Psychiatric Association diagnostic criteria listed in Box 17-7 of the textbook. The diagnosis is confirmed by at least two binge-eating episodes per week for the preceding 3 months.

Treatment
- Medications: selective serotonin reuptake inhibitors (SSRIs); tricyclic antidepressants; Topiramate, an antiepileptic agent, and the selective serotonin antagonist, ondansetron
- Psychotherapy
- Dietary interventions—weight restoration

Nursing Care Management
- Monitor nutrition patterns and promote weight gain.
- Observance for fluid and electrolyte problems; cardiac manifestations
- Assist in implementing the behavioral contract.
- Positive reinforcement of healthy lifestyle including eating habits
- Emotional support
- Family support
- Monitor for suicide risk.
- Nutrition support
- Fluid and electrolyte replacement if severe imbalance exists

Patient and Family Teaching
- Positive self-esteem
- Setting boundaries and limitations
- Family teaching aimed at disengagement and redirection of malfunctioning processes in the family

CELIAC DISEASE
Description
Celiac disease, also known as *gluten-induced enteropathy, gluten-sensitive enteropathy, and celiac sprue,* is an immune-mediated enteropathy of the proximal small intestine triggered by inappropriate immune response to ingested gluten and gluten-related proteins found in wheat, rye, and barley.

Pathophysiology

Genetic predisposition is an essential factor in the development of celiac disease. Membrane receptors involved in preferential antigen presentation to CD4+ T cells play a crucial role in the immune response characteristic of celiac disease. Genes located on the HLA region of chromosome 6, namely HLA-DQ2 or DQ8, are found in almost 100% of those affected with celiac disease. Once the inflammatory reaction is activated by gluten, CD4+ T cells produce cytokines, which are likely to contribute to the intestinal damage. The damage consists of infiltration of the lamina propria, crypt hyperplasia, and villous atrophy and flattening. With sufficient villous atrophy, malabsorption occurs.

Clinical Signs and Symptoms

- Classic symptoms of celiac disease are GI manifestations usually noted several months after the introduction of gluten-containing grains into the diet, typically between the ages of 6 months and 2 years.
- Typically, children present with impaired growth, chronic diarrhea, abdominal distention, muscle wasting with hypotonia, poor appetite, and lack of energy.

Diagnostic Evaluation

Diagnosis of celiac disease is based on a biopsy of the small intestine demonstrating the characteristic changes of mucosal inflammation, crypt hyperplasia, and villous atrophy.

Treatment

- Treatment of chronic celiac disease is primarily dietary. Although the diet is called "gluten free," it is actually *low* in gluten, because it is impossible to remove every source of this protein.
- Because gluten is found primarily in the grains of wheat and rye, but also in smaller quantities in barley and oats, these four foods are eliminated. Corn and rice become substitute grain foods.

Nursing Care Management

- Provide strategies for the child to adhere to dietary m
- Dietary management includes a diet high in c teins, with simple carbohydrates, such as fruits but low in fats.

- Initially the bowel may be inflamed as a result of the pathologic process, so high-fiber foods, such as nuts, raisins, raw vegetables, and raw fruits with skin, are avoided until inflammation has subsided.
- A lactose-free diet is recommended, which necessitates eliminating most milk products.

Patient and Family Teaching
- Considerable time is involved in explaining to the child and the parents the disease process, the specific role of gluten in aggravating the condition, and those foods that must be restricted.
- The nurse must advise parents to read carefully all ingredients on labels to avoid hidden sources of gluten.
- Many gluten-containing products are easily eliminated from the infant's or young child's diet, but monitoring the diet of a school-age child or adolescent is more difficult.

CEREBRAL PALSY
Description
Cerebral palsy (CP) is defined as a group of permanent motor syndromes that occur as a result of disorders of early brain development. The condition involves motor disorders; disturbances of sensation, perception, communication, cognition, and behavior; secondary musculoskeletal problems; and epilepsy. The primary disturbance includes abnormal muscle tone and coordination. The majority of children with CP, however, do not have significant cognitive dysfunction.

Pathophysiology
The exact mechanism that causes the neurologic brain lesions of CP is often not identified. Some children with CP have congenital malformations of the brain; others may have evidence of vascular occlusion, atrophy, loss of neurons, and degeneration. Hypoxic infarction or hemorrhage adjacent to the lateral ventricles is often identified as a cause of CP. Ataxic CP may occur in relation to cerebral hypoplasia and, in some cases, severe hypoglycemia. Additional antenatal factors that contribute to CP include maternal chorioamnionitis, inflammation of placental membranes, umbilical cord inflammation, maternal sepsis, elevated maternal temperature prior to delivery, and urinary tract infection; however, not all infants born to mothers with these

clinical signs will develop CP. Preterm birth, low birthweight (less than 1000 grams), and the occurrence of intracerebral hemorrhage and periventricular leukomalacia are associated with an increased incidence of CP.

Clinical Signs and Symptoms
Spastic Type
- Increased muscle tone (hypertonicity)
- Increased deep tendon reflexes and *clonus*
- Flexor, adductor, and internal rotator muscles more involved than extensor, abductor, and external rotator muscles
- Difficulty with fine and gross motor skills
- Contracture of the heelcord
- Hip adductor contractures leading to progressive hip subluxation and dislocation
- Knee contractures
- Scoliosis
- Typical gait is crouched, intoeing, scissoring.
- Elbow, wrist, and fingers in flexed position with thumb adducted
- Motor weakness of antagonist muscle groups

Dyskinetic Type
- Purposeless, involuntary, uncontrollable movements of face and extremities
- Increased movements with stress and voluntary movements, absent during sleep

Ataxic Type
- Disturbed coordination
- Lack of equilibrium
- Unsteady gait
- Hyporeflexia
- Loss of ability to gauge distance, speed, power of movement
- Muscles hypotonic
- Speech slurred, jerky, explosive
- Nystagmus common

Other Manifestations
- Visual deficits (most common in spastic type)
- Hearing impairment (most common in dyskinetic type)

■ Oral motor involvement resulting in drooling and feeding problems
■ Developmental delay (40% to 60%; most common in atonic and rigid types and spastic quadriplegia)
■ Sensory impairment
■ Seizures (approximately 40% of those with spastic hemiplegia affected)

Diagnostic Evaluation

■ A neurologic examination and history are the primary modalities for diagnosis.
■ Neuroimaging of the child with suspected brain abnormality with magnetic resonance imaging (MRI)
■ Metabolic and genetic testing is recommended if no structural abnormality is identified by neuroimaging.
■ Persistence of primitive reflexes: A persistent Moro reflex or the crossed extensor reflex

Treatment

■ Early recognition and promotion of optimal development to enable affected children to attain normalization and their potential within the limits of their existing health problems
■ Five broad aims of therapy
  ■ Establish locomotion, communication, and self-help.
  ■ Gain optimal appearance and integration of motor functions.
  ■ Correct associated defects as effectively as possible.
  ■ Provide educational opportunities adapted to the individual child's needs and capabilities.
  ■ Promote socialization experiences with other affected and unaffected children.
■ Mobilization devices; AFOs (ankle foot othroses); wheelchairs, special walkers
■ Orthopedic surgery to correct contracture or spastic deformities
■ Medications to decrease spasticity: Dantrolene, Baclofen, dilantin; Botulinum toxin A (Botox)
■ AED medications: carbamazepime and valproic acid
■ Dental hygiene
■ Technical aides such as voice synthesizers

- Early intervention education
- Speech therapy and physical therapy
- Nutrition: may require special feeding techniques for oral motor skill; enteral feeding in severe cases.

Nursing Care Management
- Identification of infants at risk for development of CP
- Assist with diagnostic procedures.
- Prevent complications occurring as a result of motor impairments: contractures, skin breakdown, malnutrition.
- Seizures: prevent injury.
- Encourage parent participation in care of child.
- Encourage child to perform self-care and ADLs to capability.
- Parent support: explore expectations of child's capabilities; encourage education to fit child's capabilities.
- Medication administration

Patient and Family Teaching
- Medication administration
- Physical therapy and prevention of contractures
- Mobilization techniques
- Feeding techniques
- Injury prevention; falls prevention
- Seizure: safety; medication administration; oral care

CIRRHOSIS
Description
Cirrhosis occurs at the end stage of many chronic liver diseases, including biliary atresia and chronic hepatitis.

Pathophysiology
Cirrhosis can also result from infectious, autoimmune, or toxic factors and from chronic diseases such as hemophilia and cystic fibrosis. A cirrhotic liver is irreversibly damaged.

Clinical Signs and Symptoms
- Jaundice, poor growth, anorexia, muscle weakness, and lethargy are present.
- Ascites, edema, GI bleeding, anemia, and abdominal pain may be present with impaired intrahepatic blood flow.

- Pulmonary function may be impaired because of pressure against the diaphragm from hepatosplenomegaly and ascites.
- Dyspnea and cyanosis may occur, especially on exertion. Intrapulmonary arteriovenous shunts may develop and cause hypoxemia.
- Spider angiomas and prominent blood vessels are often present on the upper torso.

Diagnostic Evaluation
- Evaluation focuses on the underlying cause by clinical, biochemical, and liver histologic findings.
- Abdominal ultrasound and MRI may be performed.
- A liver biopsy can establish the histologic findings of cirrhosis and help identify the underlying cause.

Treatment
- Therapy is directed toward (1) frequent assessment of liver status with physical examination and liver function tests, (2) nutritional support, and (3) management of specific complications.
- The only successful treatment for end-stage liver disease and liver failure may be *liver transplantation,* which has improved the prognosis substantially for many children with cirrhosis.

Nursing Care Management
- Nutritional assessments are important to promote growth and development.
- Manage side effects such as pruritis, ascites, peritonitis, and GI bleeding.
  - Treat pruritis with medications; keep nails trimmed to prevent infection.
  - Manage acites: The amount of salt in the diet may be restricted to 2 grams per day and fluid to 1.2 liters per day. In most patients with cirrhosis, however, salt and fluid restriction is not enough, and diuretics have to be added.
  - Monitor lab studies closely for hematologic abnormalities and coagulation disorders.
  - Observe for signs of peritonitis: fever is a concern.

Patient and Family Teaching

- Teach family and child to avoid hepatotoxic drugs and toxins (i.e., avoid nonsteroidal antiinflammatory drugs [NSAIDs], such as ibuprofen).
- Instruct family on importance of high-protein, high-calorie diets.
- Teach family the importance of notifying health care provider when the child is febrile.
- Reinforce measures to manage side effects and monitor effectiveness of the interventions.

CLEFT LIP/CLEFT PALATE

Description

Clefts of the lip (CL) and palate (CP) are facial malformations that occur during embryonic development and are the most common congenital deformity of the head and neck. They may appear separately or, more often, together. Cleft lip and palate (CL/P) is more common than CP alone.

Pathophysiology

Cleft deformities represent a defect in cell migration that results in a failure of the maxillary and premaxillary processes to come together between the 3rd and 12th week of embryonic development. Although often appearing together, CL and CP are distinct malformations embryologically, occurring at different times during the developmental process. Merging of the upper lip at the midline is completed between the 7th and 11th weeks of gestation. Fusion of the secondary palate (hard and soft palate) takes place later, between the 7th and 12th weeks of gestation. In the process of migrating to a horizontal position, they are separated by the tongue for a short time. If there is delay in this movement, or if the tongue fails to descend soon enough, the remainder of development proceeds but the palate never fuses. CL and CP may be caused by exposure to teratogens such as alcohol, anticonvulsants, steroids, and retinoids, but there is little evidence to link isolated clefts to any single teratogenic agent with the exception of phenytoin. Use of phenytoin during pregnancy is associated with a tenfold increase in the incidence of CL. The incidence of CL among mothers who smoke during pregnancy is twice as great as the incidence in mothers who do not smoke during pregnancy.

Clinical Signs and Symptoms
- Isolated cleft of the upper lip
- Unilateral or bilateral cleft lip and unilateral or bilateral cleft hard palate

Diagnostic Evaluation
- Physical examination: palpation of the hard palate may reveal a cleft.
- Fetal ultrasound may reveal CL/CP in association with other anomalies.

Treatment
- Cleft lip: surgical closure—cheiloplasty; timing of surgery varies.
- Cleft lip/cleft palate: surgical closure (palatoplasty); performed before the child develops faulty speech habits; additional orthodontic surgery may be required.

Nursing Care Management
- Early identification of CP by physical exam
- Parent support and reassurance
- Demonstrate acceptance of infant.
- Preoperative care: feedings to promote weight gain—special feeding devices such as Breck feeder, Pigeon feeder, Haberman feeder; breastfeeding support
- Encourage maternal-infant contact pre- and postoperatively.
- Postoperative care
- Cleft lip: Protect operative site—avoid prone position; clean incision line; may use elbow restraints; manual aspiration of oral and nasal secretions; pain management.
- Cleft palate: Protect palatal repair; may be prone; avoid hard objects in mouth; may be cup fed; manual aspiration of secretions with soft-tipped catheter; pain management.

Patient and Family Teaching
- Holding and feeding positions: most important, secondary to maternal-infant contact
- Use of bulb syringe or other mucus and milk aspirator
- Use of soft restraints as required to protect surgical sites
- Feeding after surgical repair and long-term

■ Follow-up visits for evaluation
■ Referrals for further assistance as required

COARCTATION OF THE AORTA
Description
Localized narrowing near the insertion of the ductus arteriosus, which results in increased blood pressure proximal to the defect (head and upper extremities) and decreased blood pressure distal to the obstruction (body and lower extremities).

Pathophysiology
The effect of a narrowing within the aorta is increased pressure proximal to the defect (upper extremities) and decreased pressure distal to it (lower extremities).

Clinical Signs and Symptoms
There may be high blood pressure and bounding pulses in the arms, weak or absent femoral pulses, and cool lower extremities with lower blood pressure. There are signs of congestive heart failure (CHF) in infants (see Box 3-1). In infants with critical coarctation, the hemodynamic condition may deteriorate rapidly with severe acidosis and hypotension. In this situation, mechanical ventilation and inotropic support are often necessary before surgery. Older children may experience dizziness, headaches, fainting, and epistaxis resulting from hypertension. Patients are at risk for hypertension, ruptured aorta, aortic aneurysm, stroke, and bacterial endocarditis.

Diagnostic Evaluation
See Table 3-1.

Treatment
Surgical Treatment
Surgical repair is the treatment of choice for infants younger than 6 months of age and for patients with long-segment stenosis or complex anatomy, and may be performed for all patients with coarctation. Repair is by resection of the coarcted portion with an end-to-end anastomosis of the aorta or enlargement of the constricted section using a graft of prosthetic material or a portion of the left subclavian artery. Because this defect is outside the heart

and pericardium, cardiopulmonary bypass is not required, and a thoracotomy incision is used. Postoperative hypertension is treated with intravenous sodium nitroprusside, esmolol, or milrinone followed by oral medications, such as angiotensin-converting enzyme inhibitors or beta blockers. Residual permanent hypertension after repair of coarctation of the aorta (COA) seems to be related to age and time of repair. To prevent both hypertension at rest and exercise-provoked systemic hypertension after repair, elective surgery for COA is advised within the first 2 years of life. Percutaneous balloon angioplasty techniques have proved to be very effective in relieving residual postoperative coarctation gradients.

Nonsurgical Treatment

Balloon angioplasty is being performed as a primary intervention for COA in older infants and children. In adolescents, stents may be placed in the aorta to maintain patency. Recent studies have demonstrated that balloon angioplasty is effective in children and that aneurysm formation is rare. The high restenosis rate in young infants limits its application in this group (see Table 3-2).

Nursing Care Management
Assist in Measures to Assess and Improve Cardiac Function
Monitor Cardiac Function

- Vital signs monitoring
- Respiratory assessment
- Cardiac assessment
  - Cardiac output (color, pulses, perfusion, capillary refill, renal function, and neurologic function)
  - Heart sounds
  - Four-extremity blood pressures (If the subclavian artery is used in the repair, it is not possible to measure an accurate blood pressure in the left arm.)
  - Keep accurate record of intake and output.
- Weigh child or infant on same scale at same time of day.
- Monitor for signs and symptoms of postcoarctectomy syndrome.
  - Abdominal pain and/or distension
  - Ascites
  - Fever
  - Increased white blood cell count
  - Vomiting

- Monitor abdominal girth.
- Monitor for blood in gastric contents or stool.
- Monitor neurologic function.
  Administer Medications
- Review child's history related to cardiac management.
- Administer medications on schedule.
- Assess effectiveness of medications and any side effects noted.
- Be aware of drug-drug and drug-food interactions.
- Follow guidelines for medication administration.
  Manage Common Side Effects of Cardiac Defects
- Prevent fatigue during feeding; offer small frequent feedings to infant's or child's tolerance.
- Organize nursing care to allow child/infant uninterrupted rest.
- Promote activities that do not cause fatigue.
  Provide Support for the Child and Family
- Communicate with the child and family in an appropriate style.
- Provide the child and family with honest answers.
- Provide emotional support.
- Offer age-appropriate interventions.
- Provide information on available resources for support for the child and family.

Patient and Family Teaching
Prepare the Child and Family for Diagnostic and Operative Procedures
- Provide explanation of diagnostic tests and why each test is performed because many of them are invasive procedures.
- Prepare the child prior to the invasive procedure. Remember discussion is dependent upon the child's age and development.
- Use simple words or pictures to describe procedures and answer all questions the child and family may have.
- Postoperative wound care teaching as needed
- Post-cardiac catheterization wound care teaching as needed
- Assess and record results of teaching and family's participation in care.
  Educate the Child and Family
- Assess child's and family's level of knowledge regarding the COA.
- Assess child's and family's understanding of what they have heard about COA.

■ Assess child's and family's understanding of the surgery and/or cardiac catheterization.
■ Teach the child and/or family at least four characteristics of congestive heart failure that may occur because of the COA such as:
  ■ Fatigue after exertion
  ■ Fast heart rate
  ■ Fast breathing, shortness of breath, dyspnea
  ■ Retractions
  ■ Nasal flaring
  ■ Cool extremities
  ■ Diaphoresis
  ■ Decreased urinary output
  ■ Puffiness (edema)
  ■ Fussiness
  ■ Decreased appetite
■ Educate child and family about care such as medication preparation and administration.
■ Assess child's and family's access to appropriate pharmacy for any special preparation medications.
■ Educate child and family about when to notify their physician of any clinical changes.
■ Provide appropriate educational resources and review materials with them.
■ Clarify information presented by the health care team including appointment for follow-up visit.
■ Discuss SBE (subacute bacterial endocarditis) prophylaxis with pediatric cardiologist.

COLIC (PAROXYSMAL ABDOMINAL PAIN)
Description
Colic, or paroxysmal abdominal pain, is defined as duration of crying greater than 3 hours a day, occurring more than 3 days per week, and parental dissatisfaction with the child's behavior. The condition is generally described as paroxysmal abdominal pain or cramping that is manifested by loud crying and drawing the legs up to the abdomen. Colic has no particular affinity in regard to the gender, race, or socioeconomic status of the infant and family. Colic is more common in young infants under the age of 3 months than in older infants. There is no evidence of a residual effect of colic on older children, except perhaps a strained

parent-child relationship in some cases; in other words, infants who are colicky grow up to be normal children and adults.

Pathophysiology

There is no specific known cause for the condition. Among the theories that have been investigated as potential causes are too rapid feeding, overeating, swallowing excessive air, improper feeding technique (especially in positioning and burping), and emotional stress or tension between parent and child. Although all of these may occur, there is no evidence that one factor is consistently present. In some infants colic may be a sign of cow's-milk protein allergy or cow's-milk intolerance, and eliminating cow's milk products from the infant's diet and the diet of lactating mothers can reduce the symptoms; in some infants soy milk may cause the same discomfort as cow's milk. The consensus of most experts who study colic is that it is multifactorial in nature and that no single treatment for every colicky infant will be effective in alleviating the symptoms.

Clinical Signs and Symptoms
- Crying for up to as many as 3 or more hours a day
- Drawing the legs up to the abdomen.
- May occur at the evening mealtime or at any time of the day or night
- Infant appears to be in pain.

Diagnostic Evaluation
Diagnosis is based on the history and characteristic crying pattern. Other factors that are ruled out include:
- Constipation
- Hypertrophic pyloric stenosis (HTPS)
- Cow milk protein intolerance or allergy
- Intestinal obstruction
- Intussusception

Treatment
- Investigation of organic causes: cow milk intolerance or allergy; HTPS; or other
- Formula change: extensively hydrolyzed or amino acid based formula

- Medications are sometimes recommended: sedatives, antispasmodics, antihistamines, and antiflatulents, but trials show that not all medications work all the time for control of symptoms.
- Behavioral interventions to help parents cope with crying

Nursing Care Management
- Obtain detailed history regarding infant's diet, occurrence of symptoms, relationship of feeding to appearance of symptoms, activities in the household at time of crying, mother's diet if breastfeeding, family history of infant behavior, stooling pattern, method of feeding (breast or bottle).
- Discuss infant's diagnosis with parent and provide support.
- Recommend strategies for coping with crying.
- Parental reassurance that child is well despite crying

Patient and Family Teaching
- Special diet if prescribed
- Coping mechanisms
- Behavioral interventions to help parents cope with crying
- Interventions with child such as modifying environment, timing of feedings, carrying methods, riding in car

CONJUNCTIVITIS
Description
Conjunctivitis is an inflammation of the conjunctiva of the eye.

Pathophysiology
Bacterial infection is the common cause of conjunctivitis in newborn period usually from *Chlamydia trachomatis* or *Neisseria ghonorrheae;* herpes simplex may also cause the condition. A chemical conjunctivitis may occur within 24 hours of instillation of neonatal ophthalmic prophylaxis—the clinical features include mild lid edema and a sterile, nonpurulent eye discharge. In older children, the condition may be caused by bacterial or viral infection, nasolacrimal (tear) duct obstruction, allergies, or foreign body in the eye.

Clinical Signs and Symptoms
Bacterial Conjunctivitis ("Pink Eye")
- Purulent drainage
- Crusting of eyelids, especially on awakening

- Inflamed conjunctiva
- Swollen lids

Viral Conjunctivitis
- Usually occurs with upper respiratory tract infection
- Serous (watery) drainage
- Inflamed conjunctiva
- Swollen lids

Allergic Conjunctivitis
- Itching
- Watery to thick, stringy discharge
- Inflamed conjunctiva
- Swollen lids

Conjunctivitis Caused by Foreign Body
- Tearing
- Pain
- Inflamed conjunctiva
- Unilateral in most cases

Diagnostic Evaluation
- Diagnosis is made primarily from the clinical manifestations; cultures of purulent drainage may be obtained to identify the specific cause.

Treatment
- Bacterial—topical antibacterial ointment; oral erythromycin for *Chlamydia* conjunctivitis in newborn; prevention with neonatal ophthalmic prophylaxis (1% silver nitrate solution, or 1% tetracycline ophthalmic ointment, or 0.5% erythromycin ointment)
- Allergic—oral antihistamines
- Viral—usually self-limiting; keep eye clean; in some cases a topical antiviral agent may be administered.
- Foreign body—eye irrigation with saline

Nursing Care Management
- Identification of condition
- Medication administration; newborn eye prophylaxis
- Removal of crusts

Patient and Family Teaching
- Removal of crusts
- Medication administration
- Prevention of reinfection or transmission to others: handwashing; wash towels or cloths used to clean eyes in hot soapy water; avoid washcloth use by others in household; try to avoid child placing hands and fingers in eyes.

CONSTIPATION
Description
Constipation is an alteration in the frequency, consistency, or ease of passing stool. Parents often define constipation as passing less than 3 stools per week. It may also be defined as painful bowel movements, which are often blood streaked, or include the retention of stool, with or without soiling, even with a stool frequency of more than 3 stools per week.

Pathophysiology
Constipation may arise secondary to a variety of organic disorders or in association with a wide range of systemic disorders. Structural disorders of the intestine, such as strictures, ectopic anus, and Hirschsprung disease may cause the condition. Systemic disorders include hypothyroidism, hypercalcemia resulting from hyperparathyroidism or vitamin D excess, and chronic lead poisoning. Constipation may be associated with drugs such as antacids, diuretics, antiepileptics, antihistamines, opioids, and iron supplementation. Spinal cord lesions may be associated with loss of rectal tone and sensation; affected children are prone to chronic fecal retention and overflow incontinence. The majority of children have *idiopathic* or *functional constipation,* because no underlying cause can be identified. Chronic constipation may occur as a result of environmental or psychosocial factors, or a combination of both. Transient illness, withholding and avoidance secondary to painful or negative experiences with stooling, and dietary intake with decreased fluid and fiber all play a role in the etiology of constipation.

Clinical Signs and Symptoms
- Decreased frequency of stooling
- Straining to pass stool
- Stool passed is hard instead of soft and may be passed in small segments or pellets.

■ Loose liquid stool material may be passed if there is stool impaction in the colon.

Diagnostic Evaluation
■ Based on history of bowel movement pattern
■ Physical palpation of hard stool in colon

Treatment
■ Promotion of regular bowel movements
■ Increased fiber in diet
■ Eliminating constipating foods
■ Establishment of a bowel routine that allows for regular passage of stool
■ Medications: stool softeners (docusate or lactulose)
■ Polyethylene glycol (PEG) 3350 without electrolytes (Miralax)—a laxative

Nursing Care Management
■ Assessment of bowel habits, diet, drugs being taken, environmental conditions associated with stooling
■ Stool consistency, color, frequency, and other characteristics

Patient and Family Teaching
■ Dietary modifications, including increasing fiber, decreasing constipating foods, increasing fluid intake, increasing fruit and vegetable consumption
■ Parental reassurance
■ Establishment of regular bowel management program, especially in children with chronic or debilitating conditions (e.g., medications for some conditions may cause constipation); neuromuscular weakness
■ Administration of medications such as lactulose or Miralax
■ Caution regarding enemas to evacuate stool, especially in infants and toddlers, who may become easily water-intoxicated; caution regarding enemas containing high amounts of phosphates

CROUP
Description
Croup is a general term applied to a symptom complex characterized by hoarseness, a resonant cough described as "barking"

or "brassy" (croupy), varying degrees of inspiratory stridor, and varying degrees of respiratory distress resulting from swelling or obstruction in the region of the larynx; the trachea and bronchi may also be affected. Croup syndromes are described according to the primary anatomic area affected (e.g., epiglottitis [or supraglottitis], laryngitis, laryngotracheobronchitis [LTB], and tracheitis).

Table 3-3 provides a comparison of croup syndromes.

Pathophysiology

The cause of croup in children who have received childhood immunizations are viral, yet some croup may be bacterial. In general, there is inflammation of the affected area (see Table 3-3) with varying degrees of airway compromise. As the illness progresses, respiratory symptoms become more acute to the point of acute respiratory distress and failure; in some croup syndromes, the effects of the bacteria or virus may produce only mild symptoms such as a brassy cough and fever.

Clinical Signs and Symptoms

See Table 3-3.

Diagnostic Evaluation

Diagnosis is based on child's age and clinical presentation. A radiograph of the neck soft tissues may be obtained for acute epiglottitis and LTB.

Treatment

- Airway maintenance for acute epiglottitis
- Racemic epinephrine for some acute croup syndromes to decrease edema
- Oral dexamethasone (corticosteroid) is the drug of choice to treat croup.
- Oxygen and nebulization may be used.
- Cough suppressant may be used.
- Fluid intake: either oral or parenteral if acute croup
- Parent support
- Decrease child's anxiety.
- Antipyretic as necessary
- Antibiotics for bacterial croup (tracheitis)

TABLE 3-3

Comparison of Croup Syndromes

	ACUTE EPIGLOTTITIS	ACUTE LARYNGOTRA-CHEOBRONCHITIS (LTB)	ACUTE SPASMODIC LARYNGITIS	ACUTE TRACHEITIS
Age-group affected	2-8 years	Infant or child under 5 years	1-3 years	1 month-6 years
Etiologic agent	Bacterial	Viral	Viral with allergic component	Bacterial, usually *Staphylococcus aureus*
Onset	Rapidly progressive	Slowly progressive	Sudden; at night	Moderately progressive
Major symptoms	Dysphagia Stridor aggravated when supine Drooling High fever Toxic appearance Rapid pulse and respirations	URI Stridor Brassy cough Hoarseness Dyspnea Restlessness Irritability Low-grade fever Nontoxic appearance	URI Croupy cough Stridor Hoarseness Dyspnea Restlessness Symptoms awaken child Symptoms disappear during day Tends to recur	URI Croupy cough Purulent secretions High fever No response to LTB therapy
Treatment	Airway protection Racemic epinephrine Corticosteroids Fluids Reassurance	Racemic epinephrine Corticosteroids Fluids Reassurance	Cool mist	Antibiotics Fluids

Nursing Care Management
- Maintain patent airway.
- Assessment of respiratory status
- Oxygen or cool mist as required
- Medication administration, including nebulized treatments
- Decrease parent and child anxiety.
- Other supportive nursing measures as indicated: fever management; IV therapy; diagnostic evaluation

Patient and Family Teaching
- Reassurance
- Home management of viral croup syndromes without airway compromise: cool night air, cool mist humidifier
- Medication administration
- Prevent spread to other susceptible children.

CRYPTORCHIDISM
Description
Cryptorchidism is failure of one or both testes to descend normally through the inguinal canal into the scrotum. Absence of testes within the scrotum can be a result of (1) undescended (cryptorchid) testes, (2) retractile testes, or (3) anorchism (absence of testes).

Pathophysiology
Several processes may slow or arrest testicular descent, including endocrinologic abnormalities affecting the hypothalamic-pituitary-testicular axis, denervation of the genitofemoral nerve, traction of the gubernaculum, abnormal development of the epididymis, or premature birth. Cryptorchid testes are often accompanied by congenital hernias and abnormal testes, and they are at risk for subsequent torsion.

An ectopic testis emerges outside the inguinal ring into the perineum or femoral area, or lies in a transverse scrotal or prepenile location. Ectopia is postulated to occur because of obstruction of the scrotal inlet, scarring (fibrosis) of the gubernaculum, or other mechanical anomalies.

Anorchism is the complete absence of a testis. Anorchism is suspected whenever one or both testes cannot be palpated in the patient with apparent cryptorchidism. In some cases, bilateral an-orchism is associated with genotypic and phenotypic abnormalities, but it is commonly associated with a normal karyotype (46,XY) and normal genital development.

Retractile testes can be found at any level within the path of testicular descent, but they are most commonly identified in the groin. Fortunately, they are not truly cryptorchid; instead, they are introverted to an inguinal or abdominal position because of an overactive cremasteric reflex. The cremasteric reflex, observed as withdrawal of the testis above the scrotum and into the inguinal canal in response to various stimuli, including exposure to cool temperatures, is active during infancy and peaks around age 4 to 5 years. Unlike the cryptorchid testis, the retractile testis can be gently moved into the scrotum without residual tension and does not require treatment.

Clinical Signs and Symptoms
▪ Nonpalpable testis on physical examination

Diagnostic Evaluation
▪ Ultrasonography, CT, MRI, and abdominal laparoscopy

Treatment
▪ Retractile testes that can be manipulated into the scrotum require no treatment
▪ Hormone therapy with luteinizing hormone–releasing hormone (nasal spray) and human chorionic gonadotropin (injection) may be attempted.
▪ Orchiopexy, a surgical procedure in which the testes are brought down into the scrotum and secured in that position without tension or torsion; usually performed between 6 and 24 months of age

Nursing Care Management
▪ Early identification of condition
▪ Assist with diagnostic tests.
▪ Postoperative care—vital signs monitoring; pain management
▪ Parental support and reassurance

Patient and Family Teaching
- Child should avoid vigorous activity postoperatively.
- Area is cleansed carefully to prevent infection.
- Follow-up counseling regarding fertility

CUSHING SYNDROME
Description
Cushing syndrome is a characteristic group of manifestations caused by excessive circulating free cortisol.

Pathophysiology
Because the actions of cortisol are widespread, the etiology is equally profound and diverse and is described in Box 3-2.

Clinical Signs and Symptoms
- Weight gain, generalized or truncal with facial rounding
- Fatigue, muscle weakness
- Hirsutism, purple skin striae
- Growth restriction
- Glucose intolerance
- Hyperglycemia and hypokalemia
- Susceptibility to infection
- Hypertension

Diagnostic Evaluation
- Fasting blood glucose levels for hyperglycemia
- Serum electrolyte levels for hypokalemia and alkalosis
- 24-hour urinary levels of elevated 17-hydroxycorticoids and 17-ketosteroids
- Radiographic studies of bone for evidence of osteoporosis and of the skull for enlargement of the sella turcica
- Another procedure used to establish a more definitive diagnosis is the dexamethasone (cortisone) suppression test. Administration of an exogenous supply of cortisone normally suppresses ACTH production. However, in individuals with Cushing syndrome, cortisol levels remain elevated.

Treatment
- Treatment depends on the cause. In most cases, surgical intervention involves bilateral adrenalectomy and postoperative

BOX 3-2

Etiology of Cushing Syndrome

Pituitary: Cushing syndrome with adrenal hyperplasia, usually attributed to an excess of adrenocorticotropin hormone (ACTH)

Adrenal: Cushing syndrome with hypersecretion of glucocorticoids, generally a result of adrenocortical neoplasms

Ectopic: Cushing syndrome with autonomous secretion of ACTH, most often caused by extrapituitary neoplasms

Iatrogenic: Cushing syndrome, frequently a result of administration of large amounts of exogenous corticosteroids

Food dependent: Inappropriate sensitivity of adrenal glands to normal post-prandial increases in secretion of gastric inhibitory polypeptide

replacement of the cortical hormones (the therapy for this is the same as that outlined for chronic adrenal insufficiency).

■ If a pituitary tumor is found, surgical extirpation or irradiation may be chosen. In either of these instances, treatment of panhypopituitarism with replacement of GH, thyroid extract, ADH, gonadotropins, and steroids may be necessary for an indefinite period.

Nursing Care Management

■ Nursing care also depends on the cause.

■ Cushingoid features caused by steroid therapy may be lessened with administration of the drug early in the morning and on an alternate-day basis. Giving the drug early in the day maintains the normal diurnal pattern of cortisol secretion. If given during the evening, it is more likely to produce symptoms because endogenous cortisol levels are already low and the additional supply exerts more pronounced effects. An alternate-day schedule allows the anterior pituitary an opportunity to maintain more normal hypothalamic-pituitary-adrenal control mechanisms.

■ If an organic cause is found, nursing care is related to the treatment regimen. Although a bilateral adrenalectomy permanently solves one condition, it reciprocally produces another syndrome. Before surgery, parents need to be adequately informed of the operative benefits and disadvantages.

■ Postoperative complications of adrenalectomy are related to the sudden withdrawal of cortisol. Observe for shocklike symptoms (e.g., hypotension, hyperpyrexia).

Patient and Family Teaching
■ Teach parents to observe for sudden withdrawal of cortisol symptoms.
■ Teach parents signs and symptoms of infection.

CYSTIC FIBROSIS
Description
Cystic fibrosis (CF) is a condition characterized by exocrine (or mucus-producing) gland dysfunction that produces multisystem involvement. CF is inherited as an autosomal recessive trait; the affected child inherits the defective gene from both parents, with an overall 1 in 4 risk of contracting CF. The mutated gene responsible for CF is located on the long arm of chromosome 7. This gene codes a protein of 1480 amino acids called the *cystic fibrosis transmembrane regulator* (CFTR).

Pathophysiology
CF is characterized by increased viscosity of mucous gland secretions, a striking elevation of sweat electrolytes, an increase in several organic and enzymatic constituents of saliva, and abnormalities in autonomic nervous system function. The defect appears to be primarily a result of abnormal chloride movement; the CFTR appears to function as a chloride conductance channel. The primary factor is mechanical obstruction caused by the increased viscosity of mucous gland secretions. Instead of forming a thin, freely flowing secretion, the mucous glands produce a thick, mucoprotein that accumulates and dilates them. Small passages in organs such as the pancreas and bronchioles become obstructed as secretions precipitate or coagulate to form concretions in glands and ducts.

Clinical Signs and Symptoms
■ Meconium ileus in the newborn
■ Bulky stools that are frothy from undigested fat *(steatorrhea)* and foul smelling from putrefied protein *(azotorrhea)* as a result of pancreatic necrosis

- Pancreatic enzyme deficiency because of duct blockage
- Rectal prolapse from large bulky stools
- Stagnation of mucus in the airways with subsequent bacterial growth
- Bronchiectasis, atelectasis, and hyperinflation from mucus in airways
- Cough
- Reproductive infertility in men
- Problems with labor in childbearing female
- GI malabsorption of fats
- Growth failure (failure to thrive)
- Cystic fibrosis-related diabetes mellitus
- High salt concentration in sweat; skin has salty taste
- Anorexia
- Depression
- Hemoptysis
- Repetitive bacterial and viral pulmonary infections
- Fatigue
- Sleep disruption
- Nasal polyps

Diagnostic Evaluation
- DNA analysis with presence of F508 mutation or other mutations (newborn screening)
- In newborn, elevated immunoreactive trypsinogen analysis
- Sweat chloride test (>60 mEq/L)
- Pulmonary radiograph shows characteristic patchy atelectasis and obstructive emphysema.
- Absence of pancreatic enzymes

Treatment
- Prevent or minimize pulmonary complications: removal of secretions; prevention and treatment of pulmonary infections (antibiotics); improve pulmonary aeration with bronchodilators, CPT, mucus-removal devices; oxygen administration as required.
- Ensure adequate nutrition for growth: pancreatic enzyme administration; well-balanced high-protein, high-caloric diet; administer vitamins A, D, E, and K.
- Endocrine management: Monitor blood sugar; administration of exogenous insulin; carbohydrate counting; exercise.

- Promote a reasonable quality of life for the child and the family: Encourage school participation and other age-appropriate activities.
- Lung and heart transplantation is an option for some children and adults with CF.
- Prevent other associated complications.

Nursing Care Management
- Assist with diagnostic testing.
- Thorough physical assessment and evaluation of affected systems: pulmonary, GI, pancreatic, skin
- Treatments: oxygen, aerosolized medications, CPT, mucus clearing devices
- Medication administration: vitamins, insulin, supplements, pancreatic enzymes, antibiotics, antifungal, anti-inflammatory
- Provide emotional support for child with chronic illness, which is also terminal in many cases (median predicted survival age for the CF patient in 2005 was 36.5 years).
- Encourage well-balanced nutrition.
- May benefit from nighttime enteral feedings to prevent excessive weight loss
- Prevent infections, especially pulmonary.

Patient and Family Teaching
- Disease management of affected systems; treatments; medication administration; diet and exercise; management of illness exacerbations; emotional support of child
- Compliance with therapeutic regimen including involvement in age-appropriate activities such as school and sports, according to medical condition

DERMATITIS, DIAPER
Description
Diaper dermatitis is very common in infants and one of several acute inflammatory skin disorders caused either directly or indirectly by the wearing of diapers.

Pathophysiology
Diaper dermatitis is caused by prolonged and repetitive contact with an irritant (e.g., urine, feces, soaps, detergents, ointments,

friction). Although the irritant in the majority of cases is urine and feces, the specific components that contribute to irritation include a combination of factors. The irritant quality of urine is related to an increase in pH from the breakdown of urea in the presence of fecal urease. The increased pH promotes the activity of fecal enzymes, principally proteases and lipases, which act as irritants. Fecal enzymes also increase the permeability of skin to bile salts, another potential irritant in feces.

Prolonged contact of the skin with diaper wetness produces higher friction, greater abrasion damage, increased transepi-dermal permeability, and increased microbial counts. Perianal involvement is usually the result of chemical irritation from feces, especially diarrheal stools. Risk factors for development of *Candida* infection are an altered immune status and antibiotic therapy.

Clinical Signs and Symptoms
- The eruption of diaper dermatitis is manifested primarily on convex surfaces or in folds.
- The lesions represent a variety of types and configurations.
- *Candida albicans* infection produces perianal inflammation and a maculopapular rash with satellite lesions that may cross the inguinal fold.
- Erythematous eruptions involving the skin in most intimate contact with the diaper (e.g., the convex surfaces of buttocks, inner thighs, mons pubis, scrotum); however, lesions not involving the folds are likely to be caused by chemical irritants, especially from urine and feces.

Diagnostic Evaluation
- Differential diagnosis includes contact dermatitis, bacterial, viral or monilial infection, atopic dermatitis, psoriasis, seborrhea, scabies, or congenital syphilis.

Treatment
- Keep area dry and clean.
- Use absorbent diapers with frequent diaper changes.
- Treatment is specific for the cause of the dermatitis.
- Emollients such as zinc oxide preparations provide protection from urine and feces.
- Hydrocortisone 1% ointment can be used for severe dermatitis.

- For *Candida albicans,* topical anticandidal therapy; adding hydrocortisone 1% to the antifungal agent may promote healing.
- Avoid potent topical corticosteroids.

Nursing Care Management
- Nursing interventions are aimed at altering the three factors that produce dermatitis: wetness, pH, and fecal irritants.

Patient and Family Teaching
- Teaching parents to change the diaper as soon as it becomes wet eliminates a large part of the problem, and removing the diaper to expose healthy skin to air facilitates drying. The use of a hair dryer or heat lamp is *not recommended* because these devices can cause burns.
- A common misconception about using cornstarch on skin is that it promotes the growth of *Candida albicans.* Neither cornstarch nor talc promotes the growth of fungi under conditions normally found in the diaper area. Cornstarch is more effective in reducing friction and tends to cake less than talc when the skin is wet.

DIABETES INSIPIDUS
Description
The principal disorder of posterior pituitary hypofunction is diabetes insipidus (DI), also known as neurogenic DI, resulting from undersecretion of ADH, or vasopressin (Pitressin), and producing a state of uncontrolled diuresis.

Pathophysiology
Primary causes are familial or idiopathic; of the total cases, approximately 45% to 50% are idiopathic. Secondary causes include trauma (accidental or surgical), tumors, granulomatous disease, infections (meningitis or encephalitis), and vascular anomalies (aneurysm). Certain drugs, such as alcohol or phenytoin (diphenylhydantoin), can cause a transient polyuria.

Clinical Signs and Symptoms
- The cardinal signs of DI are polyuria and polydipsia.
- In the older child, signs such as excessive urination accompanied by a compensatory insatiable thirst may be so intense

that the child does little more than go to the toilet and drink fluids.

Diagnostic Evaluation
- The simplest test used to diagnose this condition is restriction of oral fluids and observation of consequent changes in urine volume and concentration. In DI, fluid restriction has little or no effect on urine formation but causes weight loss from dehydration. Accurate results from this procedure require strict monitoring of fluid intake and urinary output, measurement of urine concentration (specific gravity or osmolality), and frequent weight checks. A weight loss between 3% and 5% indicates significant dehydration and requires termination of the fluid restriction.
- If this test is positive, the child should be given a test dose of injected aqueous vasopressin, which should alleviate the polyuria and polydipsia.

Treatment
- Hormone replacement, either with an intramuscular or subcutaneous injection of vasopressin tannate in peanut oil or with a nasal spray of aqueous lysine vasopressin
- Desmopressin acetate (DDAVP) has fewer side effects, and is administered intranasally by way of a flexible tube to achieve adequate control. The child's response pattern is variable, with duration ranging from 6 to 24 hours. It is usually administered twice daily—at bedtime to allow the child to sleep through the night and in the morning to allow fewer interruptions in the school day.
- The injectable form of vasopressin has the advantage of lasting for 48 to 72 hours, which affords the child a full night's sleep. However, it has the disadvantage of requiring frequent injections and proper preparation of the drug.

Nursing Care Management
- The initial objective is identification of the disorder. Because an early sign may be sudden enuresis in a child who is toilet trained, excessive thirst with bed-wetting is an indication for further investigation.

■ Parent education is needed on how to administer intranasal DDAVP, or intramuscular or subcutaneous injection vasopressin.
■ Vasopressin must be thoroughly resuspended in the oil by being held under warm running water for 10 to 15 minutes and shaken vigorously before being drawn into the syringe. If this is not done, the oil may be injected minus the ADH. Small brown particles, which indicate drug dispersion, must be seen in the suspension.

Patient and Family Teaching
■ Parents need a thorough explanation regarding the condition with specific clarification that DI is a different condition from DM.
■ If children are to receive the injectable vasopressin (Pitressin), ideally two caregivers should be taught the correct procedure for preparation and administration of the drug.
■ For emergency purposes, children should wear medical alert identification.
■ Older children should carry the nasal spray with them for temporary relief of symptoms.
■ School personnel need to be aware of the problem so they can grant children unrestricted use of the lavatory.

DIABETES MELLITUS
Description
Diabetes mellitus (DM) is a chronic disorder of metabolism characterized by a partial or complete deficiency of the hormone insulin. Type 1 DM is the predominant form of diabetes in the pediatric age-group, and type 2 DM is more uncommon. However, changes in food consumption and exercise patterns have increased the rate of type 2 DM in children and adolescents in the United States.

Pathophysiology
Insulin is needed to support the metabolism of carbohydrates, fats, and proteins, primarily by facilitating the entry of these substances into the cell. Insulin is needed for the entry of glucose into the muscle and fat cells, prevention of mobilization of fats from fat cells, and storage of glucose as glycogen in the cells of liver and muscle. With a deficiency of insulin, glucose is unable to enter the cell, and its concentration in the bloodstream increases. The increased concentration of glucose (hyperglycemia) produces an osmotic gradient that causes the movement of body fluid from the intracellular space

to the interstitial space, then to the extracellular space and into the glomerular filtrate in order to "dilute" the hyperosmolar filtrate. When the glucose concentration in the glomerular filtrate exceeds the renal threshold (6180 mg/dl), glucose spills into the urine (glycosuria) along with an osmotic diversion of water (polyuria), a cardinal sign of diabetes. The urinary fluid losses cause the excessive thirst (polydipsia) observed in diabetes. Protein is also wasted during insulin deficiency. Because glucose is unable to enter the cells, protein is broken down and converted to glucose by the liver (glucogenesis); this glucose then contributes to the hyperglycemia. Without the use of carbohydrates for energy, fat and protein stores are depleted as the body attempts to meet its energy needs. The hunger mechanism is triggered, but increased food intake (polyphagia) enhances the problem by further elevating blood glucose.

Clinical Signs and Symptoms
The 3 cardinal symptoms of DM are the 3 "Ps" —polyphagia, polydipsia, and polyuria. Others include:
- Abdominal discomfort
- Fatigue
- Irritability
- Enuresis
- Weight loss
- Hyperglycemia
- Shortened attention span
- Lowered frustration tolerance
- Dry skin
- Blurred vision
- Poor wound healing
- Flushed skin
- Headache
- Frequent infections

Diagnostic Evaluation
- An 8-hour fasting blood glucose level of 126 mg/dl or more
- A random blood glucose value of 200 mg/dl or more accompanied by classic signs of diabetes
- Or, an oral glucose tolerance test (OGTT) finding of 200 mg/dl or more in the 2-hour sample
- Serum insulin levels may be normal or moderately elevated.

BOX 3-3

Types of Insulin

There are four types of insulin, based on the following criteria:
- How soon the insulin starts working (onset)
- When the insulin works the hardest (peak time)
- How long the insulin lasts in the body (duration)

However, each person responds to insulin in his or her own way. That is why onset, peak time, and duration are given as ranges.

- **Rapid-acting insulin** reaches the blood within 15 minutes after injection. The insulin peaks 30 to 90 minutes later and may last as long as 5 hours (e.g., NovoLog®).
- **Short-acting (regular) insulin** usually reaches the blood within 30 minutes after injection. The insulin peaks 2 to 4 hours later and stays in the blood for about 4 to 8 hours (e.g., Novolin® R).
- **Intermediate-acting insulins** reach the blood 2 to 6 hours after injection. The insulins peak 4 to 14 hours later and stay in the blood for about 14 to 20 hours. (e.g., Novolin® N).
- **Long-acting insulin** takes 6 to 14 hours to start working. It has no peak or a very small peak 10 to 16 hours after injection. The insulin stays in the blood between 20 and 24 hours (e.g., Lantus®).

Some insulins come mixed together. (e.g. Novolin® 70/30). For example, you can buy regular insulin and NPH insulins already mixed in one bottle, which makes it easier to inject two kinds of insulin at the same time. However, you cannot adjust the amount of one insulin without also changing how much you get of the other insulin.

- Glycosylated hemoglobin (hemoglobin A1c), which reflects the average blood glucose levels over the previous 2 to 3 months; method for assessing control, detecting incorrect testing, monitoring effectiveness of changes in treatment, defining patients' goals, and detecting nonadherence; Hgb A1c, however, is not considered to be a diagnostic tool.

Treatment
- Insulin therapy (to maintain near normal glucose levels <126 mg/dL, and HbA1c of 7% or less) with subcutaneous injections or via portable insulin pump (see Box 3-3)
- Self blood glucose monitoring (SBGM): Insulin administration is based on the blood glucose level—target range is 80 to 120 mg/dl.

- Nutrition: Three balanced meals to provide sufficient calories to balance daily expenditure for energy and to satisfy the requirement for growth and development
- Timing of food consumption regulated to correspond to the time and action of the insulin prescribed
- Snacks between meals
- Fat reduced to 30% or less of the total caloric requirement
- Increase in dietary fiber
- Exercise—lowers blood glucose levels; must be tailored to child's abilities and needs; child may need an additional snack with strenuous exercise; SBGM to evaluate carbohydrate needs
- Hypoglycemia and hyperglycemia prevention (see signs and symptoms in Table 3-4). The best way to prevent is to monitor blood glucose levels and maintain a log of activity, food intake, insulin needs, and symptoms.
- Illness often increases insulin needs, therefore it is important to continue SBGM during illness to evaluate insulin requirements.

TABLE 3-4

Comparison of Manifestations of Hypoglycemia and Hyperglycemia

VARIABLE	HYPOGLYCEMIA	HYPERGLYCEMIA
Onset	Rapid (minutes)	Gradual (days)
Mood	Labile, irritable, nervous, weepy	Lethargic
Mental status	Difficulty concentrating, speaking, focusing, coordinating Nightmares	Dulled sensorium Confusion
Inward feeling	Shaky feeling, hunger Headache Dizziness	Thirst Weakness Nausea and vomiting Abdominal pain
Skin	Pallor Sweating	Flushed Signs of dehydration
Mucous membranes	Normal	Dry, crusty

Continued

▍**TABLE 3-4—cont'd**

Comparison of Manifestations of Hypoglycemia and Hyperglycemia

VARIABLE	HYPOGLYCEMIA	HYPERGLYCEMIA
Respirations	Shallow, normal	Deep, rapid (Kussmaul)
Pulse	Tachycardia, palpitations	Less rapid, weak
Breath odor	Normal	Fruity, acetone
Neurologic	Tremors	Diminished reflexes Paresthesia
Ominous signs	Late: hyperreflexia, dilated pupils, seizure Shock, coma	Acidosis, coma
Blood:		
Glucose	Low: <60 mg/dl	High: ≥250 mg/dl
Ketones	Negative	High, large
Osmolarity	Normal	High
pH	Normal	Low (≤7.25)
Hematocrit	Normal	High
Bicarbonate	Normal	<20 mEq/L
Urine:		
Output	Normal	Polyuria (early) to oliguria (late)
Glucose	Negative	Enuresis, nocturia
Ketones	Negative/trace	High
Visual	Diplopia	Blurred vision

▪ Prevent long-term complications: nephropathy, retinopathy, and neuropathy.

Nursing Care Management
▪ Assist with diagnostic testing.
▪ Child and parent teaching
▪ Acute care during diabetic ketoacidosis (see Diabetic Ketoacidosis)
▪ Child and family support

- Care during hospitalization: hydration, SBGM, insulin administration, antibiotics, prevention of complications

Patient and Family Teaching
- SBGM
- Insulin administration
- Nutrition: meal planning, snacks, carbohydrate counting to regulate insulin administration
- Prevention and recognition of hypoglycemia, hyperglycemia, and appropriate interventions
- Living and coping with chronic disease
- Illness management
- Exercise: importance; regulating CHO intake and insulin to fit type of exercise
- Self-care and prevention of skin breakdown and infection, especially in extremities (feet)
- Regular ophthalmologic evaluations for retinopathy
- Involvement in regular activities such as school, sports, camps

DIABETIC KETOACIDOSIS
Description
Diabetic ketoacidosis (DKA) is a state of relative insulin insufficiency and may include the presence of hyperglycemia (blood glucose level ≥330 mg/dl), ketonemia (strongly positive), acidosis (pH <7.30 and bicarbonate <15 mmol/L), glycosuria, and ketonuria. DKA constitutes an emergency medical situation.

Pathophysiology
When insulin is absent or there is an altered insulin sensitivity, glucose is unavailable for cellular metabolism, and the body chooses alternate sources of energy, principally fat. Fats break down into fatty acids, and glycerol in the fat cells is converted by the liver to ketone bodies (β-hydroxybutyric acid, acetoacetic acid, acetone). Any excess is eliminated in the urine (ketonuria) or the lungs (acetone breath). The ketone bodies in the blood (ketonemia) are strong acids that lower serum pH, producing ketoacidosis.

Ketones are organic acids that readily produce excessive quantities of free hydrogen ions, causing a fall in plasma pH. Then, chemical buffers in the plasma, principally bicarbonate, combine with the hydrogen ions to form carbonic acid, which readily dissociates into water and carbon dioxide. The respiratory system attempts to eliminate the excess carbon dioxide by increased depth and rate—Kussmaul respirations, or the hyperventilation characteristic of metabolic acidosis. The ketones are buffered by sodium and potassium in the plasma. The kidney attempts to compensate for the increased pH by increasing tubular secretion of hydrogen and ammonium ions in exchange for fixed base, thus depleting the base buffer concentration.

With cellular death, potassium is released from the cell (intracellular fluid) into the bloodstream (extracellular fluid) and excreted by the kidney, where the loss is accelerated by osmotic diuresis. The total body potassium is then decreased, even though the serum potassium level may be elevated as a result of the decreased fluid volume in which it circulates. Alteration in serum and tissue potassium can lead to cardiac arrest.

Clinical Signs and Symptoms
- Kussmaul respirations
- Increased urinary output initially, then decreased as cells become dehydrated
- Abdominal pain, nausea and vomiting
- Mental confusion, altered LOC
- Serum blood glucose >330 mg/dl
- Ketotic breath (sweet or fruity smelling)
- Ketonuria and glycosuria
- Dry mouth, mucous membranes

Diagnostic Evaluation
- Based in part on clinical presentation and history
- Serum blood glucose level
- Arterial blood gases
- Urine specific gravity, presence of ketones and glucose
- Serum electrolytes, CBC, BUN, calcium
- ECG

Treatment
- Prompt recognition
- Intravenous access
- Hydration bolus with 0.9% NS bolus (correct dehydration)
- Evaluation and correction of electrolyte imbalance
- Monitor for hypokalemia once fluid balance has been restored.
- Monitor renal function.

- Place on cardiac monitor, and evaluate cardiac status with potassium replacement.
- Continuous insulin administration (IV) once serum blood glucose is known and after initial rehydration bolus.
- Correct acidosis (use $NaHCO_3$ judiciously).
- Monitor for cerebral edema.

Nursing Care Management
- Diagnostic tests
- Vital signs
- Obtain intravenous access.
- Administer fluids, electrolyte replacements, and medications (insulin); titrate as necessary.
- Monitor serum blood glucose levels: urine ketones and urine glucose.
- Monitor serum electrolyte levels.
- Place on cardiac monitor.
- Monitor urinary output.
- Monitor level of consciousness and other neurologic signs.
- Provide family support, information about child's status, and reassurance.

Patient and Family Teaching
- Recognition of DKA signs and symptoms
- When to access immediate medical attention if signs and symptoms are present.
- Prevention of DKA; diabetic therapeutic regimen maintenance
- Keep parents informed of child's progress.
- Once acute care period has passed, involve parents in care of child.

DOWN SYNDROME
Description
Down syndrome (DS) is the most common chromosomal abnormality of a generalized syndrome.

Pathophysiology
The cause of Down syndrome is not known, but evidence from cytogenetic and epidemiologic studies supports the concept of multiple causality. Approximately 95% of all cases of Down syndrome are attributable to an extra chromosome 21 (group G).

Clinical Signs and Symptoms

Clinical manifestations of Down syndrome are described in Box 3-4.

▌**BOX 3-4**

Clinical Signs of Down Syndrome

HEAD / EYES
*Separated sagittal suture
Brachycephaly
Rounded and small skull
Flat occiput
Enlarged anterior fontanel
*Oblique palpebral fissures (upward, outward slant)
Inner epicanthal folds
Speckling of iris (Brushfield spots)

NOSE / EARS
*Small nose
*Depressed nasal bridge (saddle nose)
Small ears and narrow canals
Short pinna (vertical ear length)
Overlapping upper helices
Conductive hearing loss

MOUTH / NECK
*High, arched, narrow palate
Protruding tongue
Hypoplastic mandible
Delayed teeth eruption and microdontia
Alignment teeth abnormalities common
Periodontal disease
*Neck skin excess and laxity
Short and broad neck

CHEST / HEART
Shortened rib cage
Twelfth rib anomalies
Pectus excavatum/carinatum
Congenital heart defects common (e.g. atrial septal defect, ventricular septal defect)

ABDOMEN / GENITALIA
Protruding, lax, and flabby abdominal muscles
Diastasis recti abdominis
Umbilical hernia
Small penis
Cryptorchidism
Bulbous vulva

HANDS / FEET
Broad, short hands and stubby fingers
Incurved little finger (clinodactyly)
Transverse palmar crease
*Wide space between big and second toes
*Plantar crease between big and second toes
Broad, short feet and stubby toes

MUSCULOSKELETON / SKIN
Short stature
*Hyperflexibility and muscle weakness
Hypotonia
Atlantoaxial instability
Dry, cracked, and frequent fissuring
Cutis marmorata (mottling)

OTHER
Reduced birth weight
Learning difficulty (average intelligence quotient is 50)
Hypothyroidism common
Impaired immune function
Increased risk of leukemia
Early-onset dementia (in one third)

---

*Most common findings

Diagnostic Evaluation

Down syndrome can usually be diagnosed by the clinical manifestations alone, but a chromosomal analysis should be done to confirm the genetic abnormality.

Treatment

Although no cure exists for Down syndrome, a number of therapies are advocated.

- Surgery to correct serious congenital anomalies (e.g. heart defects, strabismus)
- Children with Down Syndrome also benefit from an evaluative echocardiogram soon after birth.
- Evaluation of sight and hearing is essential, and treatment of otitis media is required to prevent auditory loss, which can influence cognitive function.
- Periodic testing of thyroid function is recommended, especially if growth is severely delayed.
- Children participating in sports that may involve stress on the head and neck, such as gymnastics, diving, butterfly stroke in swimming, high jump, and soccer, should be evaluated radiologically for *atlantoaxial instability*.

Nursing Care Management

- Support family at time of diagnosis.
  - Allow the parents to express their feelings.
- Assist family in preventing physical problems. Many of the physical characteristics of Down syndrome present nursing problems.
  - Hypotonicity of muscles and hyperextensibility of joints complicate positioning.
  - Decreased muscle tone compromises respiratory expansion.
  - Underdeveloped nasal bone can cause inadequate drainage of mucus.
  - Decreased muscle tone affects gastric motility, predisposing the child to constipation. Use dietary measures such as increased fiber and fluid promote evacuation.

Patient and Family Teaching

- Teach parents how to physically care for the infant.
  - Encourage swaddling the infant tightly in a blanket before picking up the child to provide security and warmth.

■ Prevent respiratory problems by clearing the nose with a bulb-type syringe, rinsing the mouth with water after feedings, increasing fluid intake, and using a cool-mist vaporizer to keep the mucous membranes moist and the secretions liquefied.
■ Other helpful measures include changing the child's position frequently; infants should sleep supine.

■ When eating solids, the child may gag on the food because of mucus in the oropharynx.
■ Advise parents to clear the nose before each feeding, give small, frequent feedings, and allow opportunities for rest during mealtime.

■ The protruding tongue also interferes with feeding, especially of solid foods. Parents need to know that the tongue thrust is not an indication of refusal to feed, but a physiologic response.
■ Advise parents to use a small but long, straight-handled spoon to push the food toward the back and side of the mouth.

DYSMENORRHEA

Description

Primary dysmenorrhea is painful menses not related to any pelvic disease. *Secondary dysmenorrhea* is defined as painful menses with a pathologic condition such as endometriosis, salpingitis, or congenital anomalies.

Pathophysiology

Primary dysmenorrhea usually begins at the time of menarche or within 6 to 12 months. The exact etiology is unknown but the pain is clearly related to ovulatory cycles. The overproduction of uterine prostaglandins has been implicated, and women with dysmenorrhea have higher levels of prostaglandins. Overproduction of vasopressin (a hormone that stimulates the contraction of muscular tissue) may also contribute to dysmenorrhea.

Clinical Signs and Symptoms

■ Pain begins with menstrual flow or hours before the onset of bleeding each month, usually continuing for 48 to 72 hours.
■ Associated symptoms include nausea, vomiting, diarrhea, and leg and back pain.

Diagnostic Evaluation

A careful history should include the onset of symptoms; the duration, type of pain, and relationship to menstrual flow; age at menarche; family history of dysmenorrhea; and sexual history.

Treatment

- First-line treatment for adolescents with dysmenorrhea is the administration of NSAIDs that block the formation of prostaglandins for 2 to 3 days of the menstrual cycle.
- Cyclic estrogen therapy and oral contraceptives are also effective.
- Additional therapies which may be beneficial include: dietary changes, supplements, and herbal medications; vitamins B_1 and E.

Nursing Care Management

- Begin the medication at the first sign of cramping or bleeding.
- Girls with regular menstrual cycles benefit from beginning the medication 1 to 2 days before the onset of their menses.
- Medications should be taken with food.

Patient and Family Teaching

- All adolescent girls need reassurance that menstruation is a normal function.
- Adequate personal hygiene, participation in regular activities, and methods to decrease stress should be discussed with the adolescent.
- Medication administration

ENCEPHALITIS

Description

Encephalitis is an inflammatory process of the CNS that is caused by a variety of organisms, including bacteria, spirochetes, fungi, protozoa, helminths, and viruses.

Pathophysiology

Encephalitis can occur as a result of (1) direct invasion of the CNS by a virus or (2) postinfectious involvement of the CNS after a viral disease. The majority of cases of known etiology are associated with the childhood diseases of measles, mumps, varicella, and rubella and, less often, with the enteroviruses, herpes viruses, and

West Nile virus. Viral encephalitis can cause devastating neurologic injury.

Clinical Signs and Symptoms
▪ Manifestations can range from a mild benign form that resembles aseptic meningitis, lasts a few days, and is followed by rapid and complete recovery, to a fulminating encephalitis with severe CNS involvement.
▪ The onset may be sudden or may be gradual with malaise, fever, headache, dizziness, apathy, nuchal rigidity, nausea and vomiting, ataxia, tremors, hyperactivity, and speech difficulties.
▪ In severe cases, the patient has high fever, stupor, seizures, disorientation, spasticity, and coma that may proceed to death. Ocular palsies and paralysis also may occur.

Diagnostic Evaluation
▪ Early in the course of encephalitis, CT scan results may be normal. Later, hemorrhagic areas in the frontotemporal region may be seen.
▪ Herpes, mumps, measles, and enteroviruses may be found in the CSF.
▪ Serologic blood testing may be required. The first blood sample should be drawn as soon as possible after onset, with the second sample drawn 2 or 3 weeks later.

Treatment
▪ Treatment is primarily supportive and includes conscientious nursing care, control of cerebral manifestations, and adequate nutrition and hydration, with observations and management as for other cerebral disorders.
▪ Cerebral hyperemia occurs in severe viral encephalitis, and ICP monitoring as well as aggressive treatment to reduce pressure may be needed.

Nursing Care Management
▪ Observe for deterioration in consciousness.
▪ Isolation of the child is not necessary; however, good handwashing technique must be followed.
▪ A main focus of nursing management is the control of rapidly rising ICP.
▪ Neurologic monitoring

- Administration of medications
- Support of the child and parents are the major aspects of care.

Patient and Family Teaching
Parents need to be aware that very young children (younger than 2 years of age) may have neurologic disability, including learning difficulties and seizure disorders.

ENCOPRESIS
Description
Encopresis is the repeated voluntary or involuntary passage of feces of normal or near-normal consistency into places not appropriate for that purpose according to the individual's own sociocultural setting. *Primary encopresis* is identified by age 4 when the child has not achieved fecal continence. *Secondary encopresis* is fecal incontinence occurring in a child older than 4 years of age after a period of established fecal continence. The disorder is more common in boys than in girls.

Pathophysiology
Can be caused by untreated long-standing constipation. Unsuccessful toilet training as a toddler with significant struggles and subsequent voluntary withholding can be a factor. There is often a history of painful bowel movements (from mucosal tear or infection). Emotional causes such as limited access to toilets, shyness over its use, stress at school or in family, are common factors.

Clinical Signs and Symptoms
- Child resists having bowel movements, causing impacted stool to collect in the colon and rectum.
- When a child's colon is full of impacted stool, liquid stool can leak around the impacted stool then out of the anus, staining the child's underwear.

Diagnostic Evaluation
- Diagnostic tests are not routinely ordered.
- Urinalysis may be done if a urinary tract infection is suspected. Radiographic imaging studies may be ordered if there is suspicion of structural or organic causes of constipation.

Treatment
■ The treatment goals are to:
  ■ Establish regular bowel habits in the child.
  ■ Reduce stool retention.
  ■ Restore normal physiological control over bowel function.
  ■ Diffuse conflicts and reduce concerns within the family brought on by the child's symptoms.
■ The intestinal tract has to be cleansed with medications. For the first week or two, the child may need enemas, strong laxatives, or suppositories to empty the intestinal tract so it can shrink to a more normal size.
■ Next, it is important to schedule regular times to use the toilet along with daily laxatives like mineral oil or milk of magnesia.
■ Proper diet is important, too, with sufficient fluids and high-fiber foods. These steps will keep the stool soft and prevent constipation.

Nursing Care Management
■ Combine an aggressive pharmacotherapy regimen along with intense behavioral program.
■ Monitor diet, encourage fiber and water intake, use prune juice daily.
■ Decrease milk intake.
■ Establish regular bowel habits, reduce stool retention, restore normal physiological control over bowel function.
■ Help reduce conflicts and reduce concern within the family.

Patient and Family Teaching
■ Education regarding the physiology of normal defecation, toilet training as a developmental process, and the treatment outlined for the particular family is essential to a successful outcome.
■ Teach parents to use rewards to encourage development of normal bowel habits.

ENDOCARDITIS, BACTERIAL (INFECTIVE)
Description
Bacterial endocarditis (BE), or infective endocarditis (IE), also referred to as *subacute bacterial endocarditis (SBE),* is an infection of the valves and inner lining of the heart. Although it can

occur without underlying heart disease, it is most often a sequela of bacteremia in the child with acquired or congenital anomalies of the heart or great vessels. It especially affects children with valvular abnormalities, prosthetic valves, shunts, recent cardiac surgery with invasive lines, and rheumatic heart disease with valve involvement.

Pathophysiology
The most common causative agent is *Streptococcus viridans;* other causative agents are *Staphylococcus aureus,* gram-negative bacteria, and fungi such as *Candida albicans.* The microorganisms grow on the endocardium, forming vegetations (verrucae), deposits of fibrin, and platelet thrombi. The lesion may invade adjacent tissues, such as aortic and mitral valves, and may break off and embolize elsewhere, especially in the spleen, kidney, and central nervous system.

Clinical Signs and Symptoms
- Subacute endocarditis: the child may be ill for a month or longer with low-grade fever and fatigue.
- Acute endocarditis
    - Fever
    - Heart failure, regurgitant murmur, chest pain, arrhythmias
    - Skin symptoms: petechiae, Osler nodes (small painful red-blue nodules on the tufts of the fingers), Janeway lesions (painless purple macules on the soles of the feet), splenomegaly
    - Musculoskeletal symptoms: back pain, arthralgias, synovitis
    - Splenomegaly

Diagnostic Evaluation
- Blood cultures (definitive diagnosis rests on growth and identification of the causative agent in the blood)
- ECG (prolonged P-R interval)
- CXR (evidence of cardiomegaly)
- Echocardiogram (vegetations on the valve and abnormal valve function)
- CBC (leukocytosis)
- Erythrocyte sedimentation rate (increased)
- Urinalysis (microscopic hematuria)

Treatment

- Treatment should be instituted immediately and consists of administration of high doses of appropriate antibiotics intravenously for 2 to 8 weeks.
- Blood cultures are taken periodically to evaluate response to antibiotic therapy.
- Prophylaxis with dental procedures recommended for*:
  - Previous episode of infective endocarditis
  - Prosthetic cardiac valve
  - Congenital heart disease (CHD) including only:
    - Unrepaired cyanotic CHD, including palliative shunts and conduits
    - Completely repaired congenital heart defect with prosthetic material or device, whether placed by surgery or by catheter intervention, during the first 6 months after the procedure
    - Repaired CHD with residual defects at the site or adjacent to the site of a prosthetic patch or prosthetic device (which inhibit endotheliazation)
    - Cardiac transplantation recipients who develop cardiac valvulopathy
- Drugs of choice for prophylaxis include amoxicillin, ampicillin, clindamycin, cephalexin, cefadroxil, azithromycin, and clarithromycin.

Nursing Care Management

- Treatment of endocarditis requires long-term parenteral drug therapy. In many cases, IV antibiotics may be administered at home with nursing supervision for part of the treatment course.
- Nursing management includes:
  - Preparation of the child for IV infusion, usually with an intermittent-infusion device, and several venipunctures for blood cultures
  - Observation for side effects of antibiotics, especially inflammation at venipuncture sites
  - Observation for complications, including embolism and CHF

*Adapted from Wilson, W., Taubert, K., Gewitz, M. et al. Prevention of Infective Endocarditis. Guidelines from the American Heart Association. *Circulation*, May 8, 2007, pp. 1-19.

- Education regarding the importance of follow-up visits for cardiac evaluation, echocardiographic monitoring, and blood cultures

Patient and Family Teaching
- The family's regular dentist should be advised of the child's cardiac diagnosis as an added precaution to ensure preventive treatment. SBE prophylaxis is now reserved for very high-risk patients.
- Parents should also have a high index of suspicion regarding potential infections. Stress that any unexplained fever, weight loss, or change in behavior (lethargy, malaise, anorexia) must be brought to the practitioner's attention.

ENURESIS
Description
Enuresis is the intentional or involuntary passage of urine into bed (usually at night) or into clothes during the day in children.

Pathophysiology
In some cases, the bladder has not grown as quickly as the rest of the body and needs time to catch up. Enuresis has a strong family tendency. If one parent wet the bed as a child, there is a 40% chance that their child will have nighttime accidents. If both parents wet the bed, the odds can rise to 70%. Many children sleep so soundly that they just do not realize when their bladder is full. Each night the body secretes an anti-diuretic hormone (ADH) that slows down the production of urine by the kidneys. Some children who wet the bed are in a stage where they produce too little of this hormone.

Clinical Signs and Symptoms
- Inappropriate voiding of urine must occur at least twice a week for at least 3 months, and the chronologic or developmental age of the child must be at least 5 years.
- Predominant symptom is urgency that is immediate and accompanied by acute discomfort, restlessness, and urinary frequency.
- Enuresis is more common in boys; nocturnal bed-wetting usually ceases between 6 and 8 years of age.

Diagnostic Evaluation
■ Organic causes that may be related to enuresis should be ruled out before psychogenic factors are considered.
■ These include structural disorders of the urinary tract; urinary tract infection; neurologic deficits; disorders that increase the normal output of urine, such as diabetes; and disorders that impair the concentrating ability of the kidneys, such as chronic renal failure or sickle cell disease.

Treatment
■ Medications, bladder training, restriction or elimination of fluids after the evening meal, interruption of sleep to void, and various devices designed to establish a conditioned reflex response to awaken the child at the initiation of voiding
■ Three types of drugs are used to treat enuresis: tricyclic antidepressants, antidiuretics, and antispasmodics. The drug used most frequently to inhibit urination is the tricyclic antidepressant, imipramine (Tofranil). Another anticholinergic drug, oxybutynin, reduces uninhibited bladder contractions and may be helpful for children with daytime urinary frequency. Desmopressin (DDAVP) nasal spray, an analog of vasopressin, reduces nighttime urine output to a volume less than functional bladder capacity.

Nursing Care Management
■ Provide consistent support and encouragement to help sustain both the child and the parents through the inconsistent and unpredictable treatment process.
■ Evaluate parent and child's ability to administer medications.

Patient and Family Teaching
■ Help parents and child understand the problem of enuresis, the treatment plan, and the difficulties they may encounter in the process.
■ Provide strategies for bladder training: set up a schedule for restriction or elimination of fluids after the evening meal, discuss importance of interruption of sleep to void, and review various devices designed to establish a conditioned reflex response to awaken the child at the initiation of voiding.

- Parents need to understand that punishment is contraindicated because of its negative emotional impact and limited success in reducing the behavior.
- Children need to believe that they are helping themselves, and they need to sustain feelings of confidence and hope.

EPIGLOTTITIS, ACUTE
Description
Acute epiglottitis, or *acute supraglottitis,* is a serious obstructive inflammatory process that occurs predominantly in children 2 to 8 years of age, but can occur from infancy to adulthood. It is a part of the croup syndromes. The obstruction is supraglottic as opposed to the subglottic obstruction of laryngitis.

Pathophysiology
Haemophilus influenzae has historically been the most common cause of acute epiglottitis, however with the advent of HiB vaccine, most cases in children are caused by a viral agent. The disease progresses rapidly, and without prompt recognition and intervention, supraglottic obstruction may occur, resulting in severe respiratory distress.

Clinical Signs and Symptoms
- Onset is abrupt; may rapidly progress to severe respiratory distress.
- The child usually goes to bed asymptomatic to awaken later, complaining of sore throat and pain on swallowing.
- The child has a fever; insists on sitting upright and leaning forward, with the chin thrust out, mouth open, and tongue protruding *(tripod position)*.
- Drooling of saliva is common because of the difficulty or pain on swallowing and excessive secretions.
- Three clinical observations that are predictive of epiglottitis are absence of spontaneous cough, presence of drooling, and agitation.
- Irritable and extremely restless and has an anxious, apprehensive, and frightened expression
- Thick, muffled voice, with a froglike croaking sound on inspiration, but the child is not hoarse.
- Suprasternal and substernal retractions may be evident.

■ Throat is red and inflamed, and a distinctive large, cherry red, edematous epiglottis is visible on careful throat inspection. (See comment below regarding throat inspection!)

Diagnostic Evaluation
■ Clinical symptoms are suggestive.
■ Lateral neck radiograph including soft tissue to evaluate for supraglottic obstruction; anterior radiograph to rule out other acute respiratory condition
■ Throat inspection *should be attempted only when immediate endotracheal intubation can be performed if needed.*

Treatment
■ Establish adequate airway; if there is suspicion of emergent respiratory compromise, endotracheal intubation may be required.
■ In otherwise healthy child with no respiratory compromise: administration of humidified cool mist
■ Racemic epinephrine may be administered initially to decrease edema.
■ Oral corticosteroid administration; may be administered IM or IV if child unable to take oral dose
■ Observation for respiratory distress

Nursing Care Management
■ Respiratory assessment
■ Allow child to remain in position of comfort for breathing.
■ Reassure child and parents of interventions to decrease discomfort and allay anxiety.
■ Avoid throat inspection if above signs are present.
■ Administer treatments such as humidified mist, racemic epinephrine, oral and parenteral medications.
■ Assist with intubation and airway maintenance as required (may also include IV hydration and medications to decrease anxiety, edema).

Patient and Family Teaching
■ Recognition of condition clinical signs and symptoms
■ Comforting and calming measures to decrease child's anxiety

- Therapy: administration of oral medications; administration of humidified mist or aerosolized medications
- Importance of routine childhood immunizations (HiB)

EPILEPSY/SEIZURE DISORDER

Description

Epilepsy is a condition characterized by two or more unprovoked seizures and can be caused by a variety of pathologic processes in the brain. Seizures are a symptom of an underlying disease process. A single seizure event should not be classified as epilepsy.

Seizures are caused by excessive and disorderly neuronal discharges in the brain. The manifestation of seizures depends on the region of the brain in which they originate and may include unconsciousness or altered consciousness; involuntary movements; and changes in perception, behaviors, sensations, and posture.

Pathophysiology

Regardless of the etiologic factor or type of seizure, the basic mechanism is the same. Abnormal electrical discharges (1) may arise from central areas in the brain that affect consciousness; (2) may be restricted to one area of the cerebral cortex, producing manifestations characteristic of that particular anatomic focus; or (3) may begin in a localized area of the cortex and spread to other portions of the brain, which, if sufficiently extensive, produce generalized seizure activity.

Seizure activity is believed to be caused by spontaneous electrical discharges initiated by a group of hyperexcitable cells referred to as the *epileptogenic focus*. As evidenced on EEG tracings, these cells display increased electric excitability but may remain quiescent over time while discharging intermittently. Normally these discharges are restrained from spreading beyond the focal area by normal inhibitory mechanisms.

In response to physiologic stimuli, such as cellular dehydration, severe hypoglycemia, electrolyte imbalance, sleep deprivation, emotional stress, and endocrine changes, these hyperexcitable cells activate normal cells in surrounding areas and in distant, synaptically related cells. A generalized seizure develops when the neuronal excitation from the epileptogenic focus spreads to the brainstem, particularly the midbrain and reticular formation. These centers within the brainstem, known as the *centrencephalic system*, are responsible for the spread of the epileptic potentials. The discharges can originate spontaneously in the centrencephalic system or be triggered by a focal area in the cortex. On the basis of these characteristic neuronal discharges (as recorded by the EEG), seizures are designated as partial, generalized, and unclassified epileptic seizures. In a large proportion of children focal seizures spread to other areas, ultimately becoming generalized with loss of consciousness.

Clinical Signs and Symptoms
Classification and Clinical Manifestations of Seizures
Partial Seizures
Simple Partial Seizures with Motor Signs
- Characterized by:
  - Localized motor symptoms
  - Somatosensory, psychic, and autonomic symptoms
  - Combination of these
  - Abnormal discharges remaining unilateral
- Manifestations
  - Aversive seizure (most common motor seizure in children)
  - Eye or eyes and head turn away from the side of the focus
  - Awareness of movement or loss of consciousness
  - Rolandic (Sylvan) seizure
  - Tonic-clonic movements involving the face
  - Salivation
  - Arrested speech
  - Most common during sleep
  - Jacksonian march (rare in children)
    - Orderly, sequential progression of clonic movements beginning in a foot, hand, or face and moving, or "marching," to adjacent body parts

Simple Partial Seizures with Sensory Signs
- Characterized by various sensations, including:
  - Numbness, tingling, prickling, paresthesia, or pain originating in one area (e.g., face or extremities) and spreading to other parts of the body
  - Visual sensations or formed images
  - Motor phenomena such as posturing or hypertonia
  - Uncommon in children younger than 8 years of age

Complex Partial Seizures (Psychomotor Seizures)
- Observed more often in children from 3 years through adolescence
- Characterized by:
  - Period of altered behavior
  - Amnesia for event (no recollection of behavior)
  - Inability to respond to environment
  - Impaired consciousness during event
  - Drowsiness or sleep usually following seizure
  - Confusion and amnesia possibly prolonged
  - Complex sensory phenomena (aura)
  - Most frequent sensation: strange feeling in the pit of the stomach that rises toward the throat
  - Often accompanied by:
    Odd or unpleasant odors or tastes
    Complex auditory or visual hallucinations
    Ill-defined feelings of elation or strangeness (e.g., déjà vu, a feeling of familiarity in a strange environment)
    Strong feelings of fear and anxiety; distorted sense of time and self
    In small children, emission of a cry or attempt to run for help
- Patterns of motor behavior
  - Stereotypic
  - Similar with each subsequent seizure
  - May suddenly cease activity, appear dazed, stare into space, become confused and apathetic, and become limp or stiff or display some form of posturing
  - May be confused
  - May perform purposeless, complicated activities in a repetitive manner (automatisms), such as walking, running, kicking, laughing, or speaking incoherently, most often followed by postictal confusion or sleep; may exhibit oropharyngeal activities, such as smacking, chewing, drooling, swallowing, and nausea or abdominal pain followed by stiffness, a fall, and postictal sleep; rarely manifests actions such as rage or temper tantrums; aggressive acts uncommon during seizure

Generalized Seizures
Tonic-Clonic Seizures (Formerly Known as Grand Mal)
- Most common and most dramatic of all seizure manifestations
- Occur without warning

- Tonic phase: lasts approximately 10 to 20 seconds
- Manifestations
  - Eyes roll upward.
  - Immediate loss of consciousness
  - If standing, falls to floor or ground
  - Stiffens in generalized, symmetric tonic contraction of entire body musculature
  - Arms usually flexed
  - Legs, head, and neck extended
  - May utter a peculiar piercing cry
  - Apneic, may become cyanotic
  - Increased salivation and loss of swallowing reflex

Clonic phase: lasts about 30 seconds but can vary from only a few seconds to a half hour or longer
- Manifestations
  - Violent jerking movements as the trunk and extremities undergo rhythmic contraction and relaxation
  - May foam at the mouth
  - May be incontinent of urine and feces
  - As event ends, movements less intense, occurring at longer intervals, then ceasing entirely
  - Status epilepticus: series of seizures at intervals too brief to allow the child to regain consciousness between the time one event ends and the next begins
  - Requires emergency intervention
  - Can lead to exhaustion, respiratory failure, and death
- Postictal state
  - Appears to relax
  - May remain semiconscious and difficult to arouse
  - May awaken in a few minutes
  - Remains confused for several hours
  - Poor coordination
  - Mild impairment of fine-motor movements
  - May have visual and speech difficulties
  - May vomit or complain of severe headache
  - When left alone, usually sleeps for several hours
  - On awakening is fully conscious
  - Usually feels tired and complains of sore muscles and headache
  - No recollection of entire event

Absence Seizures (Formerly Called Petit Mal or Lapses)
■ Characterized by:
  ■ Onset usually between 4 and 12 years of age
  ■ More common in girls than boys
  ■ Usually cease at puberty
  ■ Brief loss of consciousness
  ■ Minimum or no alteration in muscle tone
  ■ May go unrecognized because of little change in child's behavior
  ■ Abrupt onset; suddenly develops 20 or more attacks daily
  ■ Event often mistaken for inattentiveness or daydreaming
  ■ Events possibly precipitated by hyperventilation, hypoglycemia, stresses (emotional and physiologic), fatigue, or sleeplessness
■ Manifestations
  ■ Brief loss of consciousness
  ■ Appear without warning or aura
  ■ Usually last about 5 to 10 seconds
  ■ Slight loss of muscle tone may cause child to drop objects
  ■ Ability to maintain postural control; seldom falls
  ■ Minor movements such as lip smacking, twitching of eyelids or face, or slight hand movements
  ■ Not accompanied by incontinence
  ■ Amnesia for episode
  ■ May need to reorient self to previous activity

Atonic and Akinetic Seizures (Also Known as Drop Attacks)
■ Characterized by:
  ■ Onset usually between 2 and 5 years of age
  ■ Sudden, momentary loss of muscle tone and postural control
  ■ Events recurring frequently during the day, particularly in the morning hours and shortly after awakening
■ Manifestations
  ■ Loss of tone causing child to fall to the floor violently
  ■ Unable to break fall by putting out hand
  ■ May incur a serious injury to the face, head, or shoulder
  ■ Loss of consciousness only momentary

Myoclonic Seizures
■ A variety of seizure episodes
■ May be isolated as benign essential myoclonus

- May occur in association with other seizure forms
- Characterized by:
  - Sudden, brief contractures of a muscle or group of muscles
  - Occur singly or repetitively
  - No postictal state
  - May or may not be symmetric
  - May or may not include loss of consciousness

Infantile Spasms

- Also called *infantile myoclonus, massive spasms, hypsarrhythmia, salaam episodes,* or *infantile myoclonic spasms*
- Most commonly occur during the first 6 to 8 months of life
- Twice as common in boys as in girls
- Numerous seizures during the day without postictal drowsiness or sleep
- Poor outlook for normal intelligence
- Manifestations
  - Possible series of sudden, brief, symmetric, muscular contractions
  - Head flexed, arms extended, and legs drawn up
  - Eyes sometimes rolling upward or inward
  - May be preceded or followed by a cry or giggling
  - May or may not include loss of consciousness
  - Sometimes flushing, pallor, or cyanosis
- Infants who are able to sit but not stand
  - Sudden dropping forward of the head and neck with trunk flexed forward and knees drawn up—the *salaam* or *jackknife* seizure
  - Less often: alternate clinical forms
  - Extensor spasms rather than flexion of arms, legs, and trunk, and head nodding
  - Lightning events involving a single, momentary, shocklike contraction of the entire body

Diagnostic Evaluation

- Comprehensive neurologic exam and history
- Lumbar puncture
- Blood lead level
- Complete blood count
- Serum blood glucose
- Serum amino acids

- Magnetic Resonance Imaging (MRI)
- Electroencephalogram (EEG): with the child asleep, awake, awake with provocative stimulation (flashing lights, noise), and hyperventilating (as needed)
- CT scan
- Electrolytes
- Urine organic acids
- Toxicology blood screen
- Chromosomal analysis

Treatment

The goal of treatment of seizure disorders is to control the seizures or to reduce their frequency and severity, discover and correct the cause when possible, and help the child live as normal a life as possible. Management of epilepsy has four treatment options: drug therapy, the ketogenic diet, vagus nerve stimulation, and epilepsy surgery.

Nursing Care Management

- Identify seizure activity.
- Protect from harm during seizure and observe characteristics of same; prevent aspiration; vital signs monitoring.
- Provide comfort and reassurance to child experiencing seizure and to parents.
- AED administration
- Child in *status epilepticus*: a continuous seizure that lasts more than 30 minutes or a series of seizures from which the child does not regain a premorbid level of consciousness. Administer appropriate AED—rectal diazepam, intranasal midazolam pre-hospital or home; in hospital—IV diazepam or lorazepam (if IV not immediately available administer AEDs listed above); IV fosphenytoin, IV or rectal valproic acid; phenobarbital; additional care in status includes maintenance of ABCs (airway, breathing, circulation) of life support; vital signs monitoring

Patient and Family Teaching

- Management of seizures in home setting
- Administration of AEDs; adverse effects of AEDs
- Management of status epilepticus
- Personal safety: wear helmet; swim only with close supervision; avoid heights.

- Prevent triggering factors: emotional stress, sleep deprivation, fatigue, fever, and illness.
- Encourage involvement in school and ADLs.

ESOPHAGEAL ATRESIA/ TRACHEOESOPHAGEAL FISTULA
Description
Congenital atresia of the esophagus and tracheoesophageal fistula (TEF) are rare malformations that result from failed separation of the esophagus and trachea by the fourth week of gestation. These defects occur as separate entities or in combination. EA/TEF is often present with the VATER or VACTERL syndromes, which are acronyms that describe the associated anomalies. These syndromes involve a combination of vertebral, anorectal, cardiovascular, tracheoesophageal, renal, and limb abnormalities.

Pathophysiology
The cause of EA/TEF is unknown. In the most frequently encountered form of esophageal atresia and TEF, the proximal esophageal segment terminates in a blind pouch, and the distal segment is connected to the trachea or primary bronchus by a short fistula at or near the bifurcation. The second most common variety consists of a blind pouch at each end, widely separated and with no communication to the trachea. Less frequently, an otherwise normal trachea and esophagus are connected by a common fistula. Extremely rare anomalies involve a fistula from the trachea to the upper esophageal segment or to both the upper and lower segments.

Clinical Signs and Symptoms
- Maternal polyhydramnios is often a clue to suspect EA or TEF.
- Varies according to the type of defect; when there is an esophageal atresia (EA) or a connecting fistula between the esophagus and trachea, the most common clinical manifestation in the newborn is gasping and frothy mucus from the mouth and nose, which may be accompanied by spitting up, cyanosis, apnea, and coughing.
- With EA and distal TEF, the stomach becomes distended with air; thoracic and abdominal compression (especially during crying) causes the gastric contents to be regurgitated through the fistula and into the trachea, producing a chemical pneumonitis.

▪ The child with the distal "H" type EA may not present until later in life with signs of chronic respiratory problems, recurrent pneumonia, and signs of gastroesophageal reflux; cyanosis or choking during feeding may be the only symptom of this type.

Diagnostic Evaluation
▪ Passage of a soft flexible feeding tube (nasal or oral route) through the esophagus may be met with resistance as the tube coils in the closed segment of the proximal esophagus.
▪ Radiographic studies to determine exact type of defect
▪ Bronchoscopic examination

Treatment
▪ Maintenance of patent airway
▪ Gastric decompression with double-lumen catheter
▪ Prevention of pneumonia
▪ Surgical correction of defect
▪ Staged repair for complex defect or infant instability; placement of gastrostomy is first surgical procedure.
▪ Treatment of long-term complications and associated midline defects such as cleft lip/palate and gastrointestinal or cardiac anomaly

Nursing Care Management
▪ Early detection and airway maintenance: withhold feedings if clinical signs cited above evident
▪ Newborn care: temperature maintenance; vitamin K administration
▪ Assist with diagnostic procedures.
▪ Preparation for surgery
▪ Encourage maternal-infant contact (and paternal), even though infant may be NPO.
▪ Vital signs monitoring; intravenous access; fluid monitoring; effective gastric decompression; positioning to prevent aspiration
▪ Postoperative care: pain management; vital signs monitoring; fluid and electrolytes; gastrostomy care; initiation of feedings and observation for complications (fistulae); incision care; chest tube care (if applicable)
▪ Keep parents informed of infant's progress during surgery; discuss recovery and expectations.

Patient and Family Teaching
- Newborn care
- Involvement in care activities as infant's condition allows
- Special care needs such as suctioning airway to clear secretions (as applicable)
- Postoperative care: pain management; feeding; gastrostomy feeding (as applicable)
- Long-term follow up care needs

EWING SARCOMA (PRIMITIVE NEUROECTODERMAL TUMOR [PNET] OF THE BONE)

Description
Ewing sarcoma, classified as a PNET, is the second most common malignant bone tumor (after osteosarcoma) in childhood.

Pathophysiology
Ewing sarcoma arises in the marrow spaces of the bone rather than from osseous tissue. The tumor originates in the shaft of long and trunk bones, most often affecting the femur, tibia, fibula, humerus, ulna, vertebra, scapula, ribs, pelvic bones, and skull. It occurs almost exclusively in individuals under age 30, with the majority being between 4 and 25 years of age.

Clinical Signs and Symptoms
- Most malignant bone tumors produce localized pain in the affected site, which may be severe or dull and may be attributed to trauma or the vague complaint of "growing pains."
- Pain is often relieved by a flexed position, which relaxes the muscles overlying the stretched periosteum. Frequently it draws attention when the child limps, curtails physical activity, or is unable to hold heavy objects.

Diagnostic Evaluation
- CT to determine the extent of the lesion; MRI to assess soft tissue, tumor boundaries, nerve and vessel involvement
- Radioisotope bone scans to evaluate metastasis; and either needle or surgical bone biopsy to determine the histologic pattern
- Radiologic findings are characteristic for each type of tumor. At present, there is no reliable biochemical test for bone cancers.

- Lung tomography is usually a standard procedure, because pulmonary metastasis is the most common complication of primary bone tumors.
- Bone marrow aspiration and biopsy is helpful in diagnosing Ewing sarcoma in the rare event that the child has bone marrow metastasis.

Treatment

Surgical amputation is not routinely recommended but may be considered when the results of radiotherapy render the extremity useless or deformed (e.g., from restricted growth in young children) or the tumor appears resectable. The treatment of choice is intensive irradiation of the involved bone combined with chemotherapy.

Nursing Care Management
Prepare the Child and Family for Diagnostic and Operative Procedures

The psychologic adjustment to PNET of the bone is typically less traumatic than it is to osteogenic sarcoma because of the preservation of the affected limb. Many families accept the diagnosis with a sense of relief in knowing that this type of bone cancer does not necessitate amputation, and initially they may not be aware of the damaging effects on the irradiated site.

- Once a diagnosis of PNET of the bone is suspected, a battery of diagnostic tests is ordered. The family needs an explanation of why each test is performed because many of them, such as bone marrow aspiration and biopsy, are invasive procedures.
- Appropriate preparation for the child prior to the invasive procedure is dependent upon the child's age and development. Use simple words to describe procedures, and answer all questions the child and family may have.

Administer Therapy
- Review child's history related to previous tolerance to therapy.
- Determine appropriate premedication prior to therapy.
- Be aware of drug-specific interactions.
- Assess the child's laboratory findings prior to therapy administration.

- Ensure that the chemotherapy doses are correct by checking orders according to the institution's policies and procedures.
- Follow the guidelines for chemotherapy administration.
- If the treatment is given intravenously, observe the IV site for signs of irritation or infiltration.
- Follow the institution's policy for safe handling of chemotherapy wastes, including the patient's bodily fluids.
- Observe the child for signs of reaction during and following treatment.

Manage Common Side Effects of Cancer Treatment
- Assess for toxicities specific to the cancer treatment.
- Monitor for signs of infection and obtain cultures and initiate antibiotics if indicated.
- Monitor nutrition and weight changes and alternative methods of nutrition if appropriate.
- Monitor fluid and electrolytes.
- Evaluate child's response to treatment.
- Manage central line care.

Monitor for Complications Related to PNET of the Bone and Treatment
- Assess for symptoms related to PNET of the bone and treatment.
- Review laboratory findings.
- Obtain a complete history evaluating the incidence and duration of symptoms.
- Perform a complete physical examination; assess for fever, night sweats, weight loss, pallor, signs of infection, and lymphadenopathy.

Patient and Family Teaching
Educate the Child and Family
- Assess child's and family's level of knowledge regarding the PNET of the bone and treatment.
- Assess child's and family's understanding of what they have heard about PNET of the bone and treatment.
- Explain that chemotherapeutic reactions vary with the specific drug regimen. Explain that the most common side effects from chemotherapy include nausea and vomiting, body image changes, neuropathy, and mucosal ulceration.

■ If the child is to receive radiation therapy, review the common side effects associated with radiation therapy and precautions that should be followed during treatment: high-dose radiotherapy often causes a skin reaction of dry or moist desquamation followed by hyperpigmentation. The child should wear loose-fitting clothes over the irradiated area to minimize additional skin irritation. Because of increased sensitivity, the area is protected from sunlight and sudden changes in temperature, such as from heating pads or ice packs. The child is encouraged to use the extremity as tolerated. Occasionally an active exercise program may be planned by the physical therapist to preserve maximum function.

■ Educate the family regarding neutropenia, anemia, and thrombocytopenia, the signs and symptoms of infection and fever precautions.

■ Provide appropriate educational resources, and review materials with them.

■ Clarify information presented by the health care team.

Provide Support for the Child and Family

■ Communicate with the child and family in an appropriate style.

■ Provide the child and family with honest answers.

■ Provide emotional support.

■ Offer age-appropriate interventions.

■ Provide information on available resources for support for the child and family.

FAILURE TO THRIVE (GROWTH FAILURE)
Description

Failure to thrive (FTT), or growth failure, is a sign of inadequate growth resulting from inability to obtain or use calories required for growth. FTT has no universal definition, although one of the more common parameters is a weight (and sometimes height) that falls below the 5th percentile for the child's age. Another definition of FTT includes a weight for age (height) z-value of less than -2.0 (a z-value is a standard deviation value that represents anthropometric data normalizing for sex and age with greater precision than growth percentile curves). A third way to define FTT is a weight curve that crosses more than 2 percentile lines on the National

Center for Health Statistics (NCHS) growth charts after previous achievement of a stable growth pattern.

Pathophysiology

A chronic decrease in the consumption or absorption of an adequate amount of calories in infants during the period of rapid body growth becomes apparent when the child fails to show signs of physical growth in height and weight parameters. In particular, subcutaneous fat deposits become noticeably absent as catabolism occurs. In some instances, a combination of psychosocial and physical factors may contribute to growth failure; the child may not consume adequate amounts of calories, and there may be a disturbance in the maternal-child relationship, which further contributes to growth failure. Organic causes of growth failure include malabsorption of nutrients in the GI tract as a result of extensive surgical resection of the intestine.

Clinical Signs and Symptoms

- Underweight
- Dull affect
- Lack of subcutaneous fat on arms and legs
- Decreased activity level

Diagnostic Evaluation

- History and physical examination
- Anthropometric measurements
- Dietary intake history
- Parental height and weight
- Evaluate for organic causes such as malabsorption, metabolic disease.

Treatment

- Initiate healthy feeding program with increased caloric intake.
- Behavioral modification for child and family if causes are psychosocial
- Environmental modification: if assessment reveals unhealthy pattern that is not conducive to appropriate feeding
- Identify the cause(s) of the problem and treat.
- Change environment if child's life is at risk.
- Caretaker or parent teaching (see the next page)

Nursing Care Management
- Evaluate (through history) child's feeding and living environment.
- Provide positive feeding environment.
- Observe parent food preparation and feeding of child.
- Provide positive reinforcement for parent behaviors that are positive.
- Behavioral modification as noted above
- Evaluate infant's response to parental feeding behaviors.

Patient and Family Teaching
- Depending on the cause of the growth failure, teaching may be aimed at preparation of formula or food, or teaching parents infant feeding cues and behaviors.
- Environmental and feeding changes as assessment reveals
- Teach parent or caretaker infant care techniques.

FEBRILE SEIZURES
Description
A febrile seizure is defined by the International League Against Epilepsy as a seizure in association with a febrile illness in the absence of a central nervous system infection or acute electrolyte imbalance in children older than 1 month of age without prior afebrile seizures.

Pathophysiology
The cause of febrile seizures is still uncertain. Both animal and human studies demonstrate an age-specific susceptibility to seizures induced by fever and that it is the peak temperature that is important, not the rapidity of the temperature elevation. The temperature usually exceeds 38.8° C (101.8° F), and the seizure occurs during the temperature rise rather than after a prolonged elevation. Sometimes it constitutes the dramatic beginning of an illness, often an upper respiratory or gastrointestinal infection.

Clinical Signs and Symptoms
- Tonic clonic, generalized
- Possible series of sudden, brief, symmetric, muscular contractions

BOX 3-5

Emergency Treatment for Seizures   *(Tonic-Clonic Seizure)*

DURING THE SEIZURE
- Remain calm.
- Time seizure episode.
- If child is standing or seated, ease child down to the floor.
- Place pillow or folded blanket under child's head.
- Loosen restrictive clothing.
- Remove eyeglasses.
- Clear area of any hazards or hard objects.
- Allow seizure to end without interference.
- If vomiting occurs, turn child to one side.

DO NOT
- Attempt to restrain child or use force
- Put anything in child's mouth
- Give any food or liquids

AFTER THE SEIZURE
- Time postictal period.
- Check for breathing. Check position of head and tongue.
- Reposition if head is hyperextended. If breathing is not present, give rescue breathing and call emergency medical services (EMS).
- Keep child on side.
- Remain with child.
- Do not give food or liquids until child is fully alert and swallowing reflex has returned.
- Call EMS when necessary.
- Look for medical identification, and determine what factors occurred before onset of seizure that may have been triggering factors.
- Check head and body for possible injuries.
- Check inside of mouth to see if tongue or lips have been bitten.

- Eyes sometimes rolling upward or inward
- May or may not include loss of consciousness
- Sometimes flushing, pallor, or cyanosis
- Postictal confusion and drowsiness; young child may cry and be fearful.
- Lasts a few seconds to usually no more than 10 minutes

Diagnostic Evaluation

Based on history and physical examination; may be based in part on description of seizure activity

Treatment

- Control the seizure with IV or rectal diazepam
- Lower temperature with acetaminophen

Nursing Care Management

- Identify seizure activity.
- Prevent harm during seizure (see Box 3-5).
- Administer AEDs if witnessed.
- Parent support and education: tepid sponge baths are discouraged.

Patient and Family Teaching

- Reassurance of benign nature of febrile seizures
- Protect the child during seizure, and observe exactly what happens during the seizure.
- Acetaminophen to lower temperature
- Medical evaluation after seizure occurs

FLUID AND ELECTROLYTE DISORDERS
Description

Alterations in fluid volume affect the electrolyte component, and changes in electrolyte concentration influence fluid movement. Because intracellular water and electrolytes move to and from the ECF compartment, any imbalance in the ICF is reflected by an imbalance in the ECF. The two most common fluid alterations in children are dehydration and water intoxication. Dehydration is a body fluid disturbance that occurs whenever the total output of fluid exceeds the total intake, regardless of the cause. Dehydration may result from a number of diseases that cause insensible losses through the skin and respiratory tract, through increased renal excretion, and through the GI tract. Dehydration can result from lack of oral intake (especially in elevated environmental temperatures), but more often it is a result of abnormal losses, such as those that occur in vomiting or diarrhea (gastroenteritis). Because sodium is the primary osmotic force that controls fluid movement between the major fluid compartments, dehydration is often described according to plasma sodium concentrations (i.e., isonatremic, hyponatremic, or hypernatremic) (see Table 3-5).

Water intoxication, or water overload, may occur in children who ingest excessive amounts of electrolyte-free water and subsequently develop a concurrent decrease in serum sodium accompanied by central nervous system (CNS) symptoms. There is a large urinary output and, because water moves into the brain more rapidly than sodium moves out, the child may also exhibit irritability, somnolence, headache, vomiting, diarrhea, or generalized seizures. The affected child usually appears well hydrated but may be edematous or even dehydrated. Fluid intoxication may also occur during acute IV water overloading, too rapid dialysis, tap water enemas, feeding of incorrectly mixed formula,

TABLE 3-5

Clinical Manifestations of Dehydration

	ISOTONIC (LOSS OF WATER AND SALT)	HYPOTONIC (LOSS OF SALT IN EXCESS OF WATER)	HYPERTONIC (LOSS OF WATER IN EXCESS OF SALT)
Skin Color	Gray	Gray	Gray
Temperature	Cold	Cold	Cold or hot
Turgor	Poor	Very poor	Fair
Feel	Dry	Clammy	Thickened, doughy
Mucous membranes	Dry	Slightly moist	Parched
Tearing and salivation	Absent	Absent	Absent
Eyeball	Sunken	Sunken	Sunken
Fontanel	Sunken	Sunken	Sunken
Body temperature	Subnormal or elevated	Subnormal or elevated	Subnormal or elevated
Pulse	Rapid	Very rapid	Moderately rapid
Respirations	Rapid	Rapid	Rapid
Behavior	Irritable to lethargic	Lethargic or comatose; convulsions	Marked lethargy with extreme hyperirritability on stimulation

excess water ingestion, or with too rapid reduction of glucose levels in diabetic ketoacidosis. Patients with CNS infections occasionally retain excessive amounts of water. Administration of inappropriate hypotonic solutions (e.g., 0.45% sodium chloride) may cause a rapid reduction in sodium and result in symptoms of water overload.

The major fluid and electrolyte disturbances, their usual causes, and clinical manifestations are outlined in Table 3-6. Problems of fluid and electrolyte disturbance always involve both water and electrolytes; therefore replacement includes administration of both, calculated on the basis of ongoing processes and laboratory serum electrolyte values.

TABLE 3-6
Disturbances of Fluid and Electrolyte Balance

CLINICAL MANIFESTATIONS	NURSING CARE MANAGEMENT
WATER EXCESS	
Edema	Limit fluid intake.
▪ Generalized	Administer diuretics.
▪ Pulmonary (moist rales or crackles)	Monitor vital signs.
▪ Intracutaneous (noted especially in loose areolar tissue)	Determine and treat cause of water excess.
Elevated venous pressure	Analyze laboratory electrolyte measurements frequently.
Hepatomegaly	
Slow, bounding pulse	
Weight gain	
Lethargy	
Increased spinal fluid pressure	
Central nervous system manifestations (seizures, coma)	
Laboratory findings	
▪ Low urine specific gravity	
▪ Decreased serum electrolytes	
▪ Decreased hematocrit	
▪ Variable urine volume	
SODIUM DEPLETION (HYPONATREMIA)	
Associated with water loss:	Determine and treat cause.
Same as with water loss—dehydration, weakness, dizziness, nausea, abdominal cramps, apprehension	Administer IV fluids with appropriate saline concentration.

Continued

TABLE 3-6—cont'd	

Disturbances of Fluid and Electrolyte Balance

CLINICAL MANIFESTATIONS	NURSING CARE MANAGEMENT
Mild—apathy, weakness, nausea, weak pulse Moderate—decreased blood pressure, lethargy Laboratory findings: ■ Sodium concentration <130 mEq/L (may be normal if volume loss) ■ Urine specific gravity depends on water deficit or excess	
SODIUM EXCESS (HYPERNATREMIA)	
Intense thirst Dry, sticky mucous membranes Flushed skin Temperature possibly increased Hoarseness Oliguria Nausea and vomiting Possible progression to disorientation, convulsions, muscle twitching, nuchal rigidity, lethargy at rest, hyperirritability when aroused Laboratory findings: ■ Serum sodium concentration ≥150 mEq/L ■ High plasma volume ■ Alkalosis	Determine and treat cause. Administer prescribed fluids. Measure intake and output. Monitor laboratory data. Monitor neurologic status.
POTASSIUM DEPLETION (HYPOKALEMIA)	
Muscle weakness, cramping, stiffness, paralysis, hyporeflexia Hypotension Cardiac arrhythmias, gallop rhythm Tachycardia or bradycardia Ileus Apathy, drowsiness Irritability Fatigue Laboratory findings: ■ Decreased serum potassium concentration ≤3.5 mEq/L	Determine and treat cause. Monitor vital signs, including ECG. Administer supplemental potassium. ■ Assess for adequate renal output before administration. ■ For IV replacement, administer potassium slowly. Always monitor ECG for IV bolus potassium replacement.

TABLE 3-6—cont'd
Disturbances of Fluid and Electrolyte Balance

CLINICAL MANIFESTATIONS	NURSING CARE MANAGEMENT
■ Abnormal ECG—notched or flattened T waves, decreased ST segment, premature ventricular contractions	■ For oral intake, offer high-potassium fluids and foods. ■ Evaluate acid-base status.

POTASSIUM EXCESS (HYPERKALEMIA)

Muscle weakness, flaccid paralysis	Determine and treat cause.
Twitching	Monitor vital signs, including
Hyperreflexia	ECG.
Bradycardia	Administer exchange resin, if
Ventricular fibrillation and cardiac arrest	prescribed.
Oliguria	Administer IV fluids as
Apnea: respiratory arrest	prescribed.
Laboratory findings	Administer IV insulin (if
■ High serum potassium concentration ≥5.5 mEq/L	ordered) to facilitate movement of potassium into cells.
■ Variable urine volume	Monitor potassium levels.
■ Flat P wave on ECG, peaked T waves, widened QRS complex, increased PR interval	Evaluate acid-base status.

Diagnostic Evaluation
- Based on clinical manifestations and history
- Physical examination
- Serum electrolytes
- Body weight

Treatment
- Dehydration: Ascertain degree of fluid loss; replace fluids (oral or IV replacement); monitor electrolytes; treat cause of fluid loss (e.g., vomiting, insensible water losses via respiratory system or skin).
- Water excess: Determine cause; restrict intake of electrolyte-free water; correct electrolyte imbalance.
- Electrolyte imbalance: Treat cause; replace deficient electrolytes or restrict fluid intake; prevent complications.

Nursing Care Management
General Care
- Provide replacement of fluid losses commensurate with volume depletion.
- Provide maintenance fluids and electrolytes (oral replacement or IV).

Daily Maintenance Fluid Requirements

BODY WEIGHT	AMOUNT OF FLUID PER DAY
1-10 kg	100 ml/kg
11-20 kg	1000 ml plus 50 ml/kg for each kg >10 kg
>20 kg	1500 ml plus 20 ml/kg for each kg >20 kg

- Measure intake and output.
- Monitor vital signs.
- Monitor urine specific gravity.
- Monitor IV site status.
- Monitor for complications of fluid and electrolyte imbalance.
- Parent and patient teaching for hydration

Patient and Family Teaching
- Ensure parent knows how to mix infant powder formula appropriately.
- Discourage administration of electrolyte-free water; monitor infants and small children swimming and taking baths for taking in large amounts of water.
- Fluid replacement: Oral administration of small amounts (5 to 10 ml—depends on weight) of fluid such as Pedialyte with vomiting; encourage breastfeeding, even with vomiting.
- Signs of moderate to severe dehydration requiring medical intervention: no urine output in 12 hours; listless; seizures; unable to take any oral fluids

GASTROESOPHAGEAL REFLUX
Description
Gastroesophageal reflux (GER) is defined as the transfer of gastric contents into the esophagus. This phenomenon is physiologic, occurring throughout the day, most frequently after meals

and at night. This "physiological" GER usually resolves spontaneously by 1 year of age. GER becomes a disease when complications such as failure to thrive (growth failure), bleeding, or dysphagia develop. Gastroesophageal reflux disease (GERD) represents symptoms or tissue damage that result from GER and it is associated with respiratory symptoms, including apnea, bronchospasm, laryngospasm, and pneumonia. Heartburn is also a frequent symptom in children.

Pathophysiology
The pathogenesis of GER is multifactorial; the primary causative mechanism involves inappropriate transient relaxation of the lower esophageal sphincter. Factors that increase abdominal pressure such as coughing and sneezing, scoliosis, and overeating may contribute to GERD. Esophageal symptoms occur as a result of inflammation caused by the acid in the gastric refluxate.

Clinical Signs and Symptoms
Infants
- Spitting up, regurgitation, vomiting (may be forceful)
- Excessive crying, irritability, arching of the back, stiffening
- Weight loss, growth failure (failure to thrive)
- Respiratory problems (cough, wheeze, stridor, gagging, choking with feedings)
- Hematemesis
- Apnea or apparent life-threatening event (ALTE)

Children
- Heartburn
- Abdominal pain
- Noncardiac chest pain
- Chronic cough
- Dysphagia
- Nocturnal asthma
- Recurrent pneumonia

Diagnostic Evaluation
- Based in part on history and physical examination
- Upper GI series to evaluate the presence of anatomic abnormalities

- 24-hour intraesophageal pH monitoring study is the gold standard in the diagnosis of GER.
- Other exams may include: endoscopy with biopsy; scintigraphy.

Treatment
- Depends in part on the severity
- No therapy is needed for the infant who is thriving and has no respiratory complications.
- Thickened feedings and upright positioning in infants
- Avoidance of foods that exacerbate symptoms in older children
- Pharmacologic therapy: H2-receptor antagonists (cimetidine [Tagamet], ranitidine [Zantac], or famotidine [Pepcid]) and proton pump inhibitors (esomeprazole [Nexium], lansoprazole [Prevacid], omeprazole [Prilosec], pantoprazole [Protonix], and rabeprazole [Aciphex]) reduce gastric hydrochloric acid secretion and may stimulate some increase in LES tone. Use of available prokinetic drugs (e.g., urecholine [Bethanechol] and metoclopramide [Reglan]) remains controversial.
- Surgical management for severe complications: Nissen fundoplication

Nursing Care Management
- Identification of infant or child with symptoms
- Assist with diagnostic tests.
- Reassure parents and provide emotional support (see Patient and Family Teaching).
- Educate parents regarding management.
- Provide nursing care: pre-and postoperative, for child undergoing surgery; pain management; intravenous fluids; vital signs monitoring; care of child in acute care setting with severe disease and complications such as:
  - Esophagitis
  - Esophageal stricture
  - Laryngitis
  - Recurrent pneumonia
  - Anemia
  - Growth failure (failure to thrive)

Patient and Family Teaching

- Management in regards to feedings and preparation of same; positioning after feedings; medication administration
- Skin care if child spits up frequently
- Coping strategies (parents may feel helpless when particular nonsurgical strategies fail and child continues to spit up and not gain weight).

GIARDIASIS
Description

Giardiasis is an intestinal parasitic infection caused by the protozoan *Giardia lamblia*. Childcare centers and institutions providing care for persons with developmental disabilities are common sties for urban giardiasis, and the children may pass cysts for months. Chief modes of transmission are person to person; contaminated water, especially in mountain lakes and streams; and swimming or wading pools frequented by diapered infants; food; and animals, especially puppies.

Pathophysiology

Giardia is a flagellate protozoan that causes infection in the small intestine and biliary tract. In children, person-to-person transmission is the most likely cause. Many persons may remain asymptomatic.

Clinical Signs and Symptoms
Infants and Young Children

- Diarrhea
- Vomiting
- Anorexia
- Growth failure/failure to thrive

Children Older than Five Years of Age

- Abdominal cramps
- Intermittent loose stools
- Constipation
- Stools may be malodorous, watery, pale, and greasy.
- Rarely, chronic form occurs.
  - Intermittent loose, foul-smelling stools
  - Possibility of abdominal bloating, flatulence, sulfur-tasting belches, epigastric pain, vomiting, headache, and weight loss

Diagnostic Evaluation
- Microscopic examination of stool specimens or duodenal fluid, or by identification of *G. lamblia* antigens in these specimens by techniques such as enzyme immunoassay (EIA)
- The string test: The child swallows a gelatin capsule with a nylon string attached; after several hours, the string is withdrawn and the contents are sent for laboratory analysis.

Treatment
Pharmacotherapy
- Metronidazole (Flagyl)
- Tinidazole (Tindamax)
- Nitazoxanide (Alinia)
- Quinacrine (Atabrine): has many undesirable side effects
- Furazolidone (Furoxone)
- Albendazole

Nursing Care Management
- Prevention by education of parents, childcare workers, and those caring for persons with disabilities
- Handwashing
- Standard precautions

Patient and Family Teaching
- Sanitation practices to prevent giardiasis:
    - Handwashing
    - Changing diapers using gloves and away from food items
    - Children should avoid swimming in stagnant water.
    - Children who are infected or who have diarrhea should be discouraged from swimming in community or private pools until they are infection-free.
    - Avoid drinking water that may be contaminated with *Giardia;* boil or filter water if in doubt, or drink bottled water.

GLOMERULONEPHRITIS, ACUTE POSTSTREPTOCOCCAL
Description
Acute poststreptococcal glomerulonephritis (APSGN) is an immune-complex disease that occurs after an antecedent streptococcal infection with certain strains of the group A β-hemolytic streptococcus.

Pathophysiology

The pathophysiology of APSGN is still uncertain. Immune complexes are deposited in the glomerular basement membrane. The glomeruli become edematous and infiltrated with polymorphonuclear leukocytes, which occlude the capillary lumen. The resulting decrease in plasma filtration results in an excessive accumulation of water and retention of sodium that expands plasma and interstitial fluid volumes, leading to circulatory congestion and edema. The cause of the hypertension associated with AGN cannot be completely explained by fluid retention. Excess renin may also be produced.

Clinical Signs and Symptoms

- Common features include oliguria, edema, hypertension and circulatory congestion, hematuria, and proteinuria.
- Typically, affected children are in good health until they experience the streptococcal infection. In some instances, there is a history of only a mild cold or no previous infection at all. The onset of glomerulonephritis appears after an average latent period of about 10 days.

Diagnostic Evaluation

- Urinalysis during the acute phase characteristically shows hematuria and proteinuria. Proteinuria generally parallels the hematuria and may be 3+ or 4+ in the presence of gross hematuria.
- Gross discoloration of the urine (tea colored) reflects red blood cell and hemoglobin content. Microscopic examination of the sediment shows many red blood cells, leukocytes, epithelial cells, and granular and red blood cell casts. Bacteria are not seen.
- Azotemia that results from impaired glomerular filtration is reflected in elevated blood urea nitrogen and creatinine levels in at least 50% of cases.
- Occasionally proteinuria is excessive and the patient may have nephrotic syndrome (i.e., hypoproteinemia and hyperlipidemia).
- Cultures of the pharynx are rarely positive for streptococci, because the renal disease occurs weeks after the infection.
- All patients with APSGN have reduced serum complement (C3) activity in the early stages of the disease. Rising C3 levels are

used as a guide to indicate improvement of the disease and should be normal in almost all patients 8 weeks after the disease onset.

▪ Chest x-ray may show cardiac enlargement, pulmonary congestion, or pleural effusion during the edematous phase of acute disease.

▪ Renal biopsy for diagnostic purposes is seldom required but may be useful in the diagnosis of atypical cases.

Treatment

▪ Management consists of general supportive measures and early recognition and treatment of complications.

▪ Children who have normal blood pressure and a satisfactory urine output can often be treated at home.

▪ Children with substantial edema, hypertension, gross hematuria, or significant oliguria are hospitalized because of the unpredictability of complications.

▪ Dietary restrictions depend on the stage and severity of the disease, especially the extent of edema. Moderate sodium restriction and even fluid restriction may be instituted for children with hypertension and edema. Foods with substantial amounts of potassium are generally restricted during the period of oliguria.

▪ Acute hypertension must be anticipated and identified early. Blood pressure measurements are taken every 4 to 6 hours. A variety of antihypertensive medications, as well as diuretics, are used to control hypertension.

▪ Antibiotic therapy is indicated only for those children with evidence of persistent streptococcal infections.

Nursing Care Management

▪ Careful assessment of the disease status, with regular monitoring of vital signs (including frequent measurement of blood pressure), fluid balance, and behavior

▪ Evaluate and record the volume and character of urine, and weigh the child daily.

▪ Observe for signs of dehydration in children with restricted fluid intake, especially those who are not severely edematous or those who have lost weight.

▪ For most children a regular diet is allowed, but it should contain no added salt. Foods high in sodium and salted treats are

eliminated, and parents and friends are advised not to bring snacks such as potato chips or pretzels.
- Fluid restriction, if prescribed, is more difficult, and the amount permitted should be evenly divided throughout the waking hours.

Patient and Family Teaching
- Collaborate with parents and the dietitian and special consideration for food preferences and facilitate meal planning.
- Provide parent education and support in preparation for discharge and home care; include education in home management and the need for follow-up care and health supervision.

HEMOPHILIA
Description
The two most common forms of the disorder are factor VIII deficiency (hemophilia A, or classic hemophilia) and factor IX deficiency (hemophilia B, or Christmas disease). von Willebrand disease (vWD) is another hereditary bleeding disorder characterized by a deficiency, abnormality, or absence of the protein called von Willebrand factor (vWF) and a deficiency of factor VIII. Unlike hemophilia, vWD affects both males and females. The following discussion is primarily concerned with factor VIII deficiency, which accounts for 80% to 85% of all hemophilia cases and has an X-linked recessive inheritance pattern.

Pathophysiology
The basic defect of hemophilia A is a deficiency of *factor VIII (antihemophilic factor [AHF])*. AHF is produced by the liver and is necessary for the formation of thromboplastin in phase I of blood coagulation. The less AHF found in the blood, the more severe the disease. Individuals with hemophilia have two of the three factors required for coagulation: vascular influence and platelets. Therefore, they may bleed for longer periods, but not at a faster rate.

Clinical Signs and Symptoms
- Bleeding into subcutaneous and intramuscular tissue is common.
- Hemarthrosis, which is bleeding into a joint space, is the most frequent type of internal bleeding. Signs of hemarthrosis are swelling, warmth, redness, pain, and loss of movement.
- Bony changes and crippling deformities occur after repeated bleeding episodes over several years.

- Bleeding in the neck, mouth, or thorax is serious, because the airway can become obstructed.
- Intracranial hemorrhage can have fatal consequences and is one of the major causes of death.

Diagnostic Evaluation

- The diagnosis is usually made from a history of bleeding episodes, evidence of X-linked inheritance (only one third of the cases are new mutations), and laboratory findings.
- The tests specific for hemophilia plasma depend on specific factors for a reaction to occur, such as the partial thromboplastin time (PTT).
- Specific determination of factor deficiencies requires assay procedures normally performed in specialized laboratories.
- Carrier detection is possible in classic hemophilia using DNA testing and is an important consideration in families in which female offspring may have inherited the trait.

Treatment

- The primary therapy for hemophilia is replacement of the missing clotting factor. The products available are factor VIII concentrate from pooled plasma or a genetically engineered recombinant, to be reconstituted with sterile water immediately before use, and DDAVP (1-deamino-8-d-arginine vasopressin), a synthetic form of vasopressin that increases plasma factor VIII and vWF levels and is the treatment of choice in mild hemophilia and vWD if the child shows an appropriate response. DDAVP is not effective in the treatment of severe hemophilia A, severe vWD, or any form of hemophilia B.
- A regular program of exercise and physical therapy is an important aspect of management. Physical activity within reasonable limits strengthens muscles around joints and may decrease the number of spontaneous bleeding episodes.

Nursing Care Management

- The earlier a bleeding episode is recognized, the more effectively it can be treated.
- Factor replacement therapy should be instituted according to established medical protocol, and supportive measures may be implemented, such as RICE, which is (1) rest, (2) ice, (3) compression, and (4) elevation.

- During bleeding episodes, the joint is elevated and immobilized. Active range-of-motion exercises are usually instituted after the acute episode. This allows the child to control the degree of exercise and discomfort.
- Prevention of bleeding episodes is geared mostly toward appropriate exercises to strengthen muscles and joints and to allow age-appropriate activity.
- To prevent oral bleeding, some readjustment in terms of dental hygiene may be needed to minimize trauma to the gums, such as use of a water irrigating device, softening the toothbrush in warm water before brushing, or using a sponge-tipped disposable toothbrush.
- The subcutaneous route is substituted for IM injections whenever possible.
- Venipunctures for blood samples are usually preferred for these children. There is usually less bleeding after the venipuncture than after finger or heel punctures.

Patient and Family Teaching
- Early recognition of a bleeding episode and how to administer factor replacement therapy are important components of patient and family education.
- Children should wear medical identification, and older children should be encouraged to recognize situations in which disclosing their condition is important, such as during dental extraction or injections.
- Use of protective equipment, such as padding and helmets, is particularly important, and noncontact sports, especially swimming, walking, jogging, tennis, golf, fishing, and bowling are encouraged.
- Neither aspirin nor any aspirin-containing compound should be used. Acetaminophen (Tylenol) is a suitable aspirin substitute, especially for use during control of pain at home.

HEPATITIS
Description
Hepatitis is an acute or chronic inflammation of the liver that can result from several different causes (e.g. virus, chemical or drug reaction, or other diseases). Nonviral causes of hepatitis include autoimmune hepatitis, Wilson disease, alpha-1 antitrypsin deficiency, and steatohepatitis.

Pathophysiology

The following six viruses cause 90% of viral hepatitis:

- ▪ Hepatitis A virus (HAV)
- ▪ Hepatitis B virus (HBV)
- ▪ Hepatitis C virus (HCV)
- ▪ Hepatitis D virus (HDV)
- ▪ Hepatitis E virus (HEV)
- ▪ Hepatitis G virus (HGV)

HAV is the most common form of acute viral hepatitis in most parts of the world. The virus produces a contagious disease transmitted primarily in contaminated stool spread via the fecal-oral route from person to person. HBV infection is the second most common form and can occur as an acute or chronic infection and may range from being asymptomatic and limited to causing fatal fulminant (rapid and severe) hepatitis. HBV transmission is usually via the parenteral route, through the exchange of blood or any bodily secretion or fluid. HBV-infected mothers can transmit the HBV virus to the child at birth. Another common route of infection is by percutaneous and permucosal exposure to infectious body fluids; transmission may also occur through transfusion of contaminated blood or blood products, transplantation of organs or tissues, or through sharing used needles. HCV is primarily transmitted by intravenous exposure to HCV-infected blood. Transfusion-associated HCV infection is low, but a common cause of infection is injection drug use. Perinatal HCV transmission risk is reported to be lower than HBV transmission.

Clinical Signs and Symptoms

- ▪ Initial anicteric (absence of jaundice) phase usually lasts 5 to 7 days and is often mistaken for influenza.
- ▪ Symptoms include nausea, vomiting, extreme anorexia, malaise, easy fatigability, arthralgia, skin rashes, slight to moderate fever, and epigastric or upper right quadrant abdominal pain.
- ▪ Dark urine is a symptom of the icteric (jaundice) phase.
- ▪ Pruritus may accompany jaundice and can be bothersome, but many children with acute viral hepatitis do not develop jaundice.

Diagnostic Evaluation

- ▪ History (especially regarding possible exposure to a hepatitis virus), physical examination, and serologic markers (antibodies

or antigens) indicating the presence of active infection with hepatitis A, B, or C or previous infection
- Diagnosis of viral hepatitis is based on the presence of specific viral markers.
- Diagnosis of acute HAV infection is based on the presence of anti-HAV immunoglobulin (IgM) antibody in the serum.
- HBV diagnosis depends on the presence of hepatitis B surface antigen (HBsAG) or anti-HBV core (anti-HBc) IgM antibody.
- Chronic HBV infection is associated with the persistence of HBsAg and HBV DNA markers.
- The diagnosis of HCV is based on the detection of anti-HCV antibodies and confirmation by polymerase chain reaction for hepatitis C RNA.

Treatment
- Treatment options for viral hepatitis are limited.
- The goals of management include early detection, recognition of chronic liver disease, support and monitoring, and prevention of spread of the disease.
- Interferons are used to treat HBV and HCV.

Nursing Care Management
Prevention
- Proper handwashing and standard isolation precautions can prevent the spread of hepatitis.
- Prophylactic use of standard immune globulin (IG) is effective in preventing HAV infection in situations of pre-exposure (e.g., anticipated travel to areas where HAV is prevalent) or in situations of post-exposure during the early part of the incubation period.
- Hepatitis B immune globulin (HBIG) is effective in preventing HBV infection after exposure. IG or HBIG must be administered less than 2 weeks after exposure.
- Vaccines have been developed to prevent HAV and HBV infection. HBV vaccination is recommended for all newborns and for high-risk groups. HAV is also recommended for high-risk groups.

Disease Management
- Encourage a well-balanced diet.
- Establish a realistic schedule of rest and activity adjusted to the child's condition.

- If on medications, assure proper dose and administration.
- HAV is not infectious within a week after the onset of jaundice, and children may feel well enough to resume school.

Patient and Family Teaching
- Parents should be cautioned about administering any medication to the child, because normal doses of many drugs may become dangerous because of the liver's inability to detoxify and excrete them.
- Emphasize handwashing as the single most critical measure in reducing risk of transmission.
- Explain to parents and children the ways in which HAV (oral-fecal route) and HBV (parenteral route) are spread.

HERNIA, CONGENITAL DIAPHRAGMATIC
Description
Congenital diaphragmatic hernia (CDH) results when the diaphragm does not form completely, resulting in an opening between the thorax and the abdominal cavity.

Pathophysiology
If the diaphragm does not form completely, the intestines and other abdominal structures, such as the liver, can enter the thoracic cavity, compressing the lung. Lung growth may be arrested on the affected side and to a lesser degree on the contralateral side. Ventilation is further compromised by hypoplasia and compression of the lung, including the airways and blood vessels. Pulmonary hypoplasia and pulmonary hypertension are also components in the pathology of CDH.

Clinical Signs and Symptoms
- Acute respiratory distress in the newborn—dyspnea, apnea, scaphoid abdomen, respiratory failure, profound cyanosis, absence of breath sounds, decreased cardiac output, shock; in some cases, the respiratory distress may not be manifested until later in infancy once feedings are initiated.

Diagnostic Evaluation
- Antenatal diagnosis by ultrasonography
- Postnatal diagnosis: radiography shows fluid- and air-filled loops of intestine in the affected side of the chest, and

possibly a mediastinum that may be shifted to the unaffected side.

Treatment
- Fetal surgery in some major centers
- Postnatal: Provide oxygenation with immediate endotracheal intubation and supplemental oxygen; GI decompression; IV hydration; maintain acid base balance and prevention of pulmonary hypertension; maintenance of thermoregulatory status; surfactant replacement.
- Ventilation and stabilization strategies: Permissive hypercapnia; ECMO (extracorporeal membrane oxygenation) for stabilization; high-frequency ventilation
- Once stable, surgical correction of the defect, including placement of abdominal organs in abdominal cavity, is performed.

Nursing Care Management
- Early identification in postnatal period, intervention and provision of oxygenation and hemodynamic stabilization; care of central lines; IV fluids; vital signs monitoring; blood gas monitoring; skin care for prolonged immobilization and sedation; medication administration; postoperative care; ECMO care; developmental care, feedings and discharge planning
- Parent support and provision of information regarding infant's condition; allow parent-infant contact as infant condition allows to minimize effects of separation on mother-infant dyad; assist mother with breast milk pumping and storage for later use as appropriate.

Patient and Family Teaching
- Information about the course of the illness, recovery, expectations about prognosis
- Newborn care as appropriate for recovering infant: feeding, handling, holding, breastfeeding, managing complications such as GER

HIRSCHPRUNG DISEASE
Description
Hirschsprung disease (congenital aganglionic megacolon) is a mechanical obstruction caused by inadequate motility of part of the intestine. It is usually an isolated birth defect, but it

has been associated with other syndromes including Down syndrome.

Pathophysiology

HD is a developmental disorder of the enteric nervous system that is characterized by the absence of ganglion cells, originating from the neural crest, in both the Auerbach's myenteric and Meissner's submucosal plexuses of the distal intestine. The length of the aganglionic distal bowel is dependent on the timing of the arrest in craniocaudal migration of ganglion cells. The aganglionic bowel is chronically contracted, which results in absent peristalsis in the affected bowel and the development of a functional intestinal obstruction. Intestinal distention and ischemia may also occur as a result of distention of the bowel wall, which contributes to the development of enterocolitis (inflammation of the small bowel and colon). Enterocolitis is characterized by fever, abdominal distention, and diarrhea that may be severe and lead to life-threatening dehydration or sepsis.

Clinical Signs and Symptoms
Newborn Period
- Failure to pass meconium within 24 to 48 hours after birth
- Refusal to feed
- Bilious vomiting
- Abdominal distention

Infancy
- Growth failure (failure to thrive)
- Constipation
- Abdominal distention
- Episodes of diarrhea and vomiting
- Signs of enterocolitis
  - Explosive, watery diarrhea
  - Fever
  - Appears significantly ill

Childhood
- Constipation
- Ribbonlike, foul-smelling stools

- Abdominal distention
- Visible peristalsis
- Easily palpable fecal mass
- Undernourished anemic appearance

Diagnostic Evaluation
- Clinical signs and symptoms
- Radiographic contrast enema
- Anorectal manometric examination
- Rectal biopsy demonstrating the absence of ganglion cells in the myenteric and submucosal plexus

Treatment
- Surgical removal of the aganglionic portion of the bowel to relieve obstruction and restore normal bowel motility and function of the internal anal sphincter
- If two-stage surgery required, a temporary ostomy is created proximal to the aganglionic segment to relieve obstruction and allow the normally enervated and dilated bowel to return to its normal size; corrective surgery is performed later, and the ostomy is removed with anastomosis of distal and proximal bowel segments.

Nursing Care Management
- Dependent on age and condition at time of diagnosis
- Neonatal: surgical consents, IV access, NPO, keep parents informed of condition
- If malnourished, older child: symptomatic treatment with enemas; a low-fiber, high-calorie, and high-protein diet; and in severe situations, the use of total parenteral nutrition (TPN)
- Bowel preparation preoperatively with colonic irrigation; systemic antibiotics; fluid and electrolyte management
- If enterocolitis present: observe for symptoms of bowel perforation, such as fever, increasing abdominal distention, vomiting, increased tenderness, irritability, dyspnea, and cyanosis; vital signs monitoring.
- Postoperative care: vital signs monitoring; pain management; bowel function; observe for signs of complications.
- With ostomy: stoma care and skin care; application of appliance (colostomy bag)

■ Parent teaching: ostomy care (see Patient and Family Teaching); discharge teaching; nutrition
■ Parent support

Patient and Family Teaching
■ Colostomy care—reassurance of temporary nature of most colostomies
■ Skin and stoma care; appliance care
■ Intraoperative information for surgical procedures
■ Medication administration: pain; bowel preparation or cleansing

HODGKIN DISEASE
Description
Hodgkin disease originates in the lymphoid system and primarily involves the lymph nodes. It predictably metastasizes to nonnodal or extralymphatic sites, especially the spleen, liver, bone marrow, lungs, and mediastinum (mass of tissues and organs separating the lungs; includes the heart and its vessels, trachea, esophagus, thymus, and lymph nodes), although no tissue is exempt from involvement.

Pathophysiology
It is classified according to four histologic types: (1) lymphocytic predominance, (2) nodular sclerosis, (3) mixed cellularity, and (4) lymphocytic depletion. With present treatment protocols, the histologic stage of the disease has less prognostic significance.

Clinical Signs and Symptoms
■ Hodgkin disease is characterized by painless enlargement of lymph nodes. The most common finding is enlarged, firm, nontender, movable nodes in the supraclavicular or cervical area. In children, the "sentinel" node located near the left clavicle may be the first enlarged node. Enlargement of axillary and inguinal lymph nodes is less frequent.
■ Mediastinal lymphadenopathy may cause a persistent nonproductive cough.
■ Enlarged retroperitoneal nodes may produce unexplained abdominal pain.
■ Systemic symptoms include low-grade or intermittent fever (Pel-Ebstein disease), anorexia, nausea, weight loss, night sweats, and pruritis.

Diagnostic Evaluation

- A lymph node biopsy is essential to establish histologic diagnosis and staging. The presence of Sternberg-Reed cell is considered diagnostic of Hodgkin disease because it is absent in the other lymphomas; however, it may occur in infectious mononucleosis (see Box 3-6).
- Bone marrow aspiration and biopsy
- CT scans of the neck, chest, abdomen, and pelvis; gallium scan (identifies metastatic/ recurrent disease); chest radiograph
- Complete blood count, uric acid levels, liver function tests, erythrocyte sedimentation rate, serum copper, ferritin level, fibrinogen, immunoglobulins, T-cell function studies, and urinalysis

Treatment

- The primary modalities of therapy are irradiation and chemotherapy. Each may be used alone or in combination, based on the clinical staging. One of the major concerns with combined radiation and antineoplastic drug therapy is the serious late effects in children with an excellent prognosis.
- Radiation may involve involved field (IF), extended field (EF) radiation (involved areas plus adjacent nodes), or total nodal

BOX 3-6
Stages of Hodgkin Disease

Stage I: Lesions are limited to one lymph node area or only one additional extralymphatic site (IE), such as the liver, lungs, kidney, or intestines.

Stage II: Two or more lymph node regions on the same side of the diaphragm or one additional extralymphatic site or organ (IIE) on the same side of the diaphragm is involved.

Stage III: Lymph node regions on both sides of the diaphragm are involved, or one extralymphatic site (IIIE), spleen (IIIS), or both (IIISE).

Stage IV: Cancer has metastasized diffusely throughout the body to one or more extralymphatic sites with or without involvement of associated lymph nodes.

Each stage is further subdivided into A or B. A denotes absence of associated general symptoms. B indicates presence of symptoms such as night sweats, fever (38° C [100.4° F]), or weight loss of 10% or more during the preceding 6 months. In stages II and III, subtype B has a significantly poorer prognosis than subtype A.

irradiation (TNI) (the entire axial lymph node system), depending on the extent of involvement. In stage IV disease, chemotherapy is the primary form of treatment, although limited irradiation may be given to areas of bulky disease.

■ Follow-up care of children no longer receiving therapy is essential to identify relapse and second malignancies. In children with splenectomy by laparotomy, prophylactic antibiotics are administered for an indefinite period. Also, immunizations against pneumococci and meningococci are recommended before the splenectomy.

Nursing Care Management
Prepare the Child and Family for Diagnostic and Operative Procedures
■ Once the diagnosis of Hodgkin disease is suspected, a battery of diagnostic tests is ordered. The family needs an explanation of why each test is performed because many of them, such as bone marrow aspiration and lymph node biopsy, are invasive procedures.

■ Appropriate preparation of the child prior to the invasive procedure is dependent upon the child's age and development. Use simple words to describe procedures, and answer all questions the child and family may have.

Administer Therapy
■ Review child's history related to previous tolerance to therapy.
■ Determine appropriate premedication prior to therapy.
■ Be aware of drug-specific interactions.
■ Assess the child's laboratory findings prior to therapy administration.
■ Ensure that the chemotherapy doses are correct by checking orders according to the institution's policies and procedures.
■ Follow the guidelines for chemotherapy administration.
■ If the treatment is given intravenously, observe the IV site for signs of irritation or infiltration.
■ Follow the institution's policy for safe handling of chemotherapy wastes, including the patient's body fluids.
■ Observe the child for signs of reaction during and following treatment.

Manage Common Side Effects of Cancer Treatment
- Assess for toxicities specific to the cancer treatment.
- Monitor for signs of infection and obtain cultures; initiate antibiotics if indicated.
- Monitor nutrition and weight changes and alternative methods of nutrition if appropriate.
- Monitor fluid and electrolytes.
- Evaluate child's response to treatment.
- Manage central line care.

Monitor for Complications Related to Hodgkin Disease and Treatment
- Assess for symptoms related to Hodgkin disease and treatment.
- Review laboratory findings.
- Obtain a complete history evaluating the incidence and duration of symptoms.
- Perform a complete physical examination; assess for fever, night sweats, weight loss, pallor, signs of infection, lymphadenopathy.

Patient and Family Teaching
Educate the Child and Family
- Assess child's and family's level of knowledge regarding Hodgkin disease and treatment.
- Assess child's and family's understanding of what they have heard about Hodgkin disease and treatment.
- Explain that chemotherapeutic reactions vary with the specific drug regimen. Explain that the most common side effects from chemotherapy include nausea and vomiting, body image changes, neuropathy, and mucosal ulceration.
- Review the common side effects associated with radiation therapy and precautions that should be followed during treatment.
- Educate the family regarding neutropenia, anemia, and thrombocytopenia, the signs and symptoms of infection, and fever precautions.
- Provide appropriate educational resources, and review materials with them.
- Clarify information presented by the health care team.

Provide Support for the Child and Family
- Communicate with the child and family in an appropriate style.
- Provide the child and family with honest answers.
- Provide emotional support.
- Offer age-appropriate interventions.
- Provide information on available resources for support for the child and family.

HUMAN IMMUNODEFICIENCY VIRUS INFECTION
Description
Human immunodeficiency virus (HIV) is a retrovirus that is transmitted by lymphocytes and monocytes. It is found in the blood, semen, vaginal secretions, and breast milk. It has an incubation period of months to years.

Pathophysiology
The HIV virus primarily infects a specific subset of T lymphocytes, the CD_4^+ T cells. The virus takes over the machinery of the CD_4^+ lymphocyte, using it to replicate itself, rendering the CD_4^+ cell dysfunctional. The CD_4^+ lymphocyte count gradually decreases over time, leading to progressive immune deficiency. The count eventually reaches a critical level below which there is substantial risk of opportunistic illnesses followed by death.

Clinical Signs and Symptoms
Common Clinical Manifestations of HIV Infection in Children
- Lymphadenopathy
- Hepatosplenomegaly
- Oral candidiasis
- Chronic or recurrent diarrhea
- Growth failure/Failure to thrive
- Developmental delay
- Parotitis

Common Defining Conditions for Acquired Immunodeficiency Syndrome in Children
- *Pneumocystis carinii* pneumonia
- Lymphoid interstitial pneumonitis
- Recurrent bacterial infections
- Wasting syndrome

- Candidal esophagitis
- Human immunodeficiency virus encephalopathy
- Cytomegalovirus disease
- *Mycobacterium avium*-intracelulare complex (MAC) infection
- Pulmonary candidiasis
- Herpes simplex disease
- Cryptosporidiosis

Diagnostic Evaluation
- For children 18 months of age and older, the HIV enzyme-linked immunosorbent assay (ELISA) and Western blot immunoassay are performed to determine HIV infection.
- In infants born to HIV-infected mothers, these assays will be positive because of the presence of maternal antibodies derived transplacentally.
- Maternal antibodies may persist in the infant up to 18 months of age. Therefore, other diagnostic tests are employed, most commonly the HIV polymerase chain reaction (PCR) for detection of proviral DNA.

Treatment
- The goals of therapy for HIV infection include slowing the growth of the virus, preventing and treating opportunistic infections, and providing nutritional support and symptomatic treatment.
- Antiretroviral drugs work at various stages of the HIV life cycle to prevent reproduction of functional new virus particles.
- Infants born to HIV-infected women should receive pneumocystis prophylaxis during the first year of life; after 1 year of age, the need for prophylaxis is determined by the presence of severe immunosuppression or a history of *Pneumocystis carinii* pneumonia.
- Prophylaxis is often employed for other opportunistic infections, such as disseminated *Mycobacterium avium*-intracelulare complex (MAC), candidiasis, or herpes simplex.
- Immunization against common childhood illnesses is recommended.

Nursing Care Management
- Nutritional management is a challenge because of recurrent illness, diarrhea, and other physical problems. Intensive nutritional

interventions should be instituted when the child's growth begins to slow or weight begins to decrease.
■ Parents and the child must be taught how and when to administer the antiretroviral drugs.
■ Aggressive pain management is essential for these children to have an acceptable quality of life. Their pain may be due to infections (e.g., otitis media, dental abscess), encephalopathy (e.g., spasticity), adverse effects of medications (e.g., peripheral neuropathy), or an unknown source (e.g., deep musculoskeletal pain).

Patient and Family Teaching
■ Education concerning transmission and control of infectious diseases, including HIV infection, is essential for children with HIV infection and anyone involved in their care. Safety issues, including appropriate storage of special medications and equipment (e.g., needles and syringes), are emphasized.
■ Parents and legal guardians have the right to decide whether they inform these agencies of their child's HIV diagnosis.
■ School personnel receive current HIV information.

HYDROCEPHALUS
Description
Hydrocephalus is a condition caused by an imbalance in the production and absorption of CSF in the ventricular system. When production is greater than absorption, CSF accumulates within the ventricular system, usually under increased pressure, producing passive dilation of the ventricles.

Pathophysiology
The causes of hydrocephalus are varied, but the result is either (1) impaired absorption of CSF fluid within the subarachnoid space, obliteration of the subarachnoid cisterns, or malfunction of the arachnoid villi; or (2) obstruction to the flow of CSF through the ventricular system. Although rare, a tumor of the choroid plexus may cause increased CSF secretion. Any imbalance of secretion and absorption causes an increased accumulation of CSF in the ventricles, which become dilated (ventriculomegaly) and compress the brain substance against the surrounding rigid bony cranium. When this occurs before fusion of the cranial sutures, it causes enlargement of the skull, as well as dilation of the

ventricles. Developmental defects (e.g., Arnold-Chiari malformations [ACMs], aqueduct stenosis, aqueduct gliosis, and atresia of the foramina of Luschka and Magendie [Dandy-Walker syndrome]) account for most cases of hydrocephalus from birth to 2 years of age. Other causes include neoplasms, infections, intracranial hemorrhage (neonatal), and trauma. An obstruction to the normal flow can occur at any point in the CSF pathway to produce increased pressure and dilation of the pathways proximal to the site of obstruction. In older children, hydrocephalus is most often a result of space-occupying lesions, intracranial infections, hemorrhage, or preexisting developmental defects, such as aqueduct stenosis or the Arnold-Chiari malformation.

Clinical Signs and Symptoms
Infants
- Abnormal head growth
- Bulging fontanels
- Dilated scalp veins
- Separated sutures
- Macewen sign (cracked-pot sound on percussion)
- Thinning of skull bones
- Frontal cranial enlargement, or bossing
- Setting sun sign (sclera visible above the iris)
- Pupils sluggish, with unequal response to light
- Irritability
- Lethargy
- Weak, shrill cry
- Early infantile reflexes may persist.
- Change in level of consciousness
- Opisthotonos (often extreme)
- Lower extremity spasticity
- Vomiting
- Advanced cases:
  - Difficulty in sucking and feeding
  - Shrill, brief, high-pitched cry
  - Cardiopulmonary embarrassment

Older Children
- Headache on awakening; improvement following emesis or upright posture

- Papilledema
- Strabismus
- Extrapyramidal tract signs (e.g., ataxia)
- Irritability
- Lethargy
- Apathy
- Confusion
- Incoherence
- Vomiting

Diagnostic Evaluation
Infants
- Based on head circumference that crosses one or more grid lines on the head measurement chart within a period of 2 to 4 weeks and on associated neurologic signs that are present and progressive
- Echoencephalography

Older Children
- CT scan
- MRI

Treatment
- Surgical placement of a shunt that provides primary drainage of the CSF from the ventricles to an extracranial compartment, usually the peritoneum (ventriculoperitoneal [VP] shunt)
- Endoscopic third ventriculostomy in children with noncommunicating hydrocephalus. In this procedure, an endoscope is used to make a small opening in the floor of the third ventricle that allows the CSF to flow freely through the previously blocked ventricle.
- Removal of tumor if present

Nursing Care Management
- Identification of increasing head growth OFC (occipital frontal circumference) in children at high risk for hydrocephalus (e.g., preterm infant with intracranial bleed; child with meningitis)
- Monitoring for signs of increased intracranial pressure (ICP) in older child
- Neurologic signs monitoring

- Observe and monitor for signs of shunt complications (infection and mechanical failure [blockage, kinking, disconnection]), which are signs of increased ICP in older child; in an infant, signs are nonspecific and resemble sepsis—poor feeding, lethargy, irritability, bulging anterior fontanel.
- Prepare and assist with diagnostic procedures.
- Pain management postoperatively
- Observation for increased ICP postoperatively: may signal shunt failure
- Care of EVD (extraventricular drainage) device if infection present
- Provide family support and education (see Patient and Family Teaching).

Patient and Family Teaching
- Educate family about condition and treatment.
- Signs of shunt malfunction—infection and mechanical failure (blockage, kinking)
- Keep family updated on child's progress intraoperatively.
- Child's activity restrictions after shunt placement
- Importance of follow up visits with neurosurgeon
- Developmental interventions if developmental delays noted or if child is at high risk for same

HYPERBILIRUBINEMIA
Description
The term *hyperbilirubinemia* refers to an excessive level of accumulated bilirubin in the blood and is characterized by *jaundice*, a yellowish discoloration of the skin and sclerae. Hyperbilirubinemia is a common finding in the newborn and in most instances is relatively benign.

Pathophysiology
In the newborn, an imbalance between bilirubin production and bilirubin metabolism or clearance from the body results in an excess of circulating bilirubin, and thus jaundice is common. Bilirubin is one of the breakdown products of hemoglobin that results from red blood cell (RBC) destruction. When RBCs are destroyed, the breakdown products are released into the circulation, where the hemoglobin splits into two fractions: heme and

globin. The globin (protein) portion is used by the body, and the heme portion is converted to unconjugated bilirubin, an insoluble substance bound to albumin.

In the liver, the bilirubin is detached from the albumin molecule and, in the presence of the enzyme glucuronyl transferase, is conjugated with glucuronic acid to produce a highly soluble substance, conjugated bilirubin, which is then excreted into the bile. In the intestine, bacterial action reduces the conjugated bilirubin to urobilinogen, the pigment that gives stool its characteristic color. Most of the reduced bilirubin is excreted through the feces; a small amount is eliminated in the urine. The sterile and less motile newborn bowel is initially less effective in excreting urobilinogen; the enzyme β-glucuronidase is able to convert conjugated bilirubin into the unconjugated form, which is subsequently reabsorbed by the intestinal mucosa and transported to the liver. This process, known as *enterohepatic circulation,* or *shunting,* is accentuated in the newborn. Newborn conditions wherein excessive amounts of bilirubin are produced, such as hemolysis (congenital spherocytosis; G6PD; Rh incompatibility), or bruising (cephalhematoma), increases circulating levels and causes more jaundice. Illness factors such as intestinal obstruction or preterm birth, wherein bowel motility is compromised, increase circulating levels of bilirubin via enterohepatic shunting. Some syndromes are associated with increased bilirubin levels in the newborn period, namely Gilbert syndrome, Lucey-Driscoll syndrome, and Crigler Najjar type I and II. Breast feeding is also associated with increasing levels of bilirubin. Unconjugated bilirubin is highly toxic to neurons; therefore, an infant with severe jaundice is at risk of developing kernicterus or bilirubin encephalopathy, a syndrome of severe brain damage resulting from the deposition of unconjugated bilirubin in brain cells.

Clinical Signs and Symptoms
■ Jaundice: yellow tint of skin
■ Sclerae may also be yellow.
■ Dark-yellow urine

Diagnostic Evaluation
■ Serum bilirubin: total and direct
■ Transcutaneous bilirubin monitoring

- Direct Coombs test
- If hemolysis is present or suspected, other tests may be appropriate: CBC, G6PD, RBC morphology, albumin, reticulocyte count, PT, PTT.
- End-tidal carbon monoxide (ETCO) levels (measured in exhaled breath) may be of value in determining the presence of hemolysis and the rate of heme degradation and bilirubin production in some infants.

Treatment
- Close monitoring: Appearance of jaundice in any newborn in the first 24 hours of life requires further evaluation and monitoring.
- Bilirubin nomogram for hour-specific risk evaluation
- Phototherapy
- Severe cases may require exchange transfusion.
- In healthy newborn, early initiation of breast feeding, formula feeding, and promotion of stooling
- Medications: metalloporphyrins; Phenobarbital
- Prevention of complications

Nursing Care Management
- Early detection of jaundice
- Initiate early feedings in healthy newborn.
- Encourage and assist breastfeeding mother–infant pair.
- Diagnostic tests: serum bilirubin and transcutaneous bilirubin monitoring
- Parent education (see Patient and Family Teaching); support and reassurance
- Treatments: phototherapy—light intensity, eye protection (infant), observation for complications (dehydration, temperature instability); maternal and paternal—newborn contact during treatment; skin care (perianal and general); use of fiberoptic biliblanket phototherapy as appropriate

Patient and Family Teaching
- Avoid newborn exposure to direct sunlight.
- Feeding healthy newborn to promote stooling
- Features of jaundice requiring medical attention once discharged home

- Contact phone number for questions regarding routine newborn care and jaundice
- Reassurance and support
- Management during phototherapy if required
- Importance of follow-up appointments for jaundice evaluation (TSB or TcB)

HYPERTHYROIDISM
Description
The largest percentage of hyperthyroidism in childhood is caused by Graves disease, which is usually associated with an enlarged thyroid gland and exophthalmos.

Pathophysiology
The hyperthyroidism of Graves disease is apparently caused by an autoimmune response to TSH receptors, but no specific etiology has been identified. There is definitive evidence for familial association, with a high concordance incidence in twins.

Clinical Signs and Symptoms
Cardinal Signs
- Emotional lability
- Physical restlessness, characteristically at rest
- Decelerated school performance
- Voracious appetite with weight loss in 50% of cases
- Fatigue

Physical Signs
- Tachycardia
- Widened pulse pressure
- Dyspnea on exertion
- Exophthalmos (protruding eyeballs)
- Wide-eyed, staring expression with lid lag
- Tremor
- Goiter (hypertrophy and hyperplasia)
- Warm, moist skin
- Accelerated linear growth
- Heat intolerance (may be severe)

- Hair fine and unable to hold a curl
- Systolic murmur

Diagnostic Evaluation
- The presence of a thyroid mass in a child requires a thorough history, including inquiry into prior irradiation to the head and neck and exposure to a goitrogen.
- The diagnosis is established on the basis of increased levels of T_4 and T_3. TSH is suppressed to unmeasurable levels.

Treatment
- Therapy for hyperthyroidism is controversial, but all methods are directed toward retarding the rate of hormone secretion.
- The three acceptable modes available are the antithyroid drugs, subtotal thyroidectomy, or ablation with radioiodine.
- Surgery in most centers is reserved for children who do not respond to or comply with the use of antithyroid drugs or who are prone to recurrences.

Nursing Care Management
- Dietary requirements should be adjusted to meet the child's increased metabolic rate. Although the need for calories is increased, these should be provided in wholesome foods rather than "junk" foods.
- Heat intolerance is common. Preferring a cooler environment than others, the child is likely to open windows, complain about the heat, wear minimum clothing, and remove blankets while sleeping.
- A regular routine is beneficial in providing frequent rest periods.

Patient and Family Teaching
- Inform the patient and family that academic difficulties are common and result from a short attention span and inability to sit still.
- Unexplained fatigue and sleeplessness, and difficulty with fine-motor skills such as writing is common.
- Parents need help in understanding the uncontrollable nature of these outbursts and ways of minimizing them through decreased environmental stimulation, stress, and frustration.

HYPERTROPHIC PYLORIC STENOSIS
Description
Hypertrophic pyloric stenosis (HPS) is an obstructive disorder that occurs when the circumferential muscle of the pyloric sphincter becomes thickened, resulting in elongation and narrowing of the pyloric channel. This produces an outlet obstruction and compensatory dilation, hypertrophy, and hyperperistalsis of the stomach. This condition usually develops in the first 2 to 5 weeks of life.

Pathophysiology
The precise etiology of HPS is unknown. The circular muscle of the pylorus thickens as a result of hypertrophy (increased size) and hyperplasia (increased mass). This produces severe narrowing of the pyloric canal between the stomach and the duodenum, causing partial obstruction of the lumen. Over time, inflammation and edema further reduce the size of the opening, resulting in complete obstruction. The hypertrophied pylorus may be palpable as an olive-like mass in the upper abdomen.

Clinical Signs and Symptoms
- Projectile nonbilious vomiting
- Dehydration
- Metabolic alkalosis
- In severe cases, growth failure (failure to thrive)

Diagnostic Evaluation
- Diagnosis is often made after the history and physical examination.
- Ultrasonography
- Upper GI radiography if US is inconclusive

Treatment
- Surgical pyloromyotomy (via laparotomy or laparoscopy): consists of longitudinal incision through the circular muscle fibers of the pylorus down to, but not including, the submucosa
- Preoperative IV hydration to correct any fluid or electrolyte imbalance

Nursing Care Management
- Assist with diagnostic tests.
- Obtain IV access.
- Prepare infant for surgery—IV fluids, NPO, operative consents.
- Provide parent information of condition, and pre- and postoperative care.
- Pain management in postoperative period
- Vital sign monitoring postoperatively
- Involve parents in care of child.
- Discharge education

Patient and Family Teaching
- Pain management
- Feeding method
- Care of incision
- Observe for complications: persistent HPS, wound dehiscence, GER.

HYPOPITUITARISM
Description
Hypopituitarism is diminished or deficient secretion of pituitary hormones.

Pathophysiology
The most common organic cause of pituitary undersecretion is tumors in the pituitary or hypothalamic region, especially the craniopharyngiomas. Idiopathic hypopituitarism, or idiopathic pituitary growth failure, is usually related to GH deficiency, which inhibits somatic growth in all cells of the body. The extent of idiopathic GH deficiency may be complete or partial, but the cause is unknown. It is frequently associated with other pituitary hormone deficiencies, such as deficiencies of TSH and ACTH; thus it is theorized that the disorder is probably secondary to hypothalamic deficiency.

Hypopituitarism may be congenital (a condition present at birth) and caused by birth trauma, genetic (inherited) disorders, defective, underdeveloped, or absent pituitary gland.

Clinical Signs and Symptoms
Newborns
- Small genital organs
- Jaundice

- Hypoglycemia
- Irritability due to diabetes insipidus (a condition in which excessive amounts of urine are passed)

Older Infants and Children
- Short stature and slow growth; may be associated with delayed tooth development and delayed tooth eruption. Children may fall off their growth curve both in height and/or weight.
- Mental development delay
- Increased thirst and urination
- Fatigue
- Weight gain out of proportion to growth
- Absent or delayed puberty
- Visual and nervous system problems, such as decreased visual acuity, abnormalities in peripheral vision, or headache

Diagnostic Evaluation
- Diagnostic evaluation is aimed at isolating organic causes.
- A complete diagnostic evaluation should include a family history, a history of the child's growth patterns and previous health status, physical examination, psychosocial evaluation, radiographic surveys, and endocrine studies.
- Definitive diagnosis is based on absent or subnormal reserves of pituitary GH.

Treatment
Treatment of hypopituitarism depends on its cause. The goal of treatment is to restore the pituitary gland to normal function, producing normal levels of hormones. Treatment may include specific hormone replacement therapy, surgical tumor removal, and/or radiation therapy.

Nursing Care Management
- Growth cessation or restriction in a child whose growth has previously been normal should alert the observer to the possibility of hypothyroidism.
- Family education concerning medication preparation and storage, injection sites, injection technique, and syringe disposal
- Parent should be taught the importance of administering TH replacement; optimum dosing is often achieved when GH is

administered at bedtime. Physiologic release is more normally stimulated as a result of pituitary release of GH during the first 45 to 90 minutes after the onset of sleep.

Patient and Family Teaching
- Once a diagnosis is made confirming the cause of the problem, the parents and child need an opportunity to express their thoughts and feelings.
- Children undergoing hormone replacement require additional support. The nurse should provide education for patient self-management during the school-age years.
- Administration of GH is facilitated by family routines that include a specific time of day for the injection. Younger children may enjoy using a calendar and colorful stickers to designate received injections.

HYPOPLASTIC LEFT HEART SYNDROME (HLHS)
Description
A cyanotic heart defect that is characterized by the underdevelopment of the left-sided heart structures resulting in a range of defects including hypoplastic left ventricle with aortic and mitral valve atresia or aortic and mitral stenosis. A mixture of oxygenated and deoxygenated blood flows from the left atrium across the patent foramen ovale to the right atrium, to the right ventricle, and out the pulmonary artery. The descending aorta receives blood from the patent ductus arteriosus (PDA). Ductal patency is critical to survival until surgical palliation early in the newborn period.

Pathophysiology
An ASD or patent foramen ovale allows saturated blood from the left atrium to mix with desaturated blood from the right atrium and to flow through the right ventricle and out into the pulmonary artery. From the pulmonary artery, the blood flows both to the lungs and through the ductus arteriosus into the aorta and out to the body. The amount of blood flow to the pulmonary and systemic circulations depends on the relationship between the pulmonary and systemic vascular resistances. The coronary and cerebral vessels receive blood by retrograde flow through the hypoplastic ascending aorta.

Clinical Signs and Symptoms

There is mild cyanosis and signs of congestive failure until the patent ductus arteriosus closes, then progressive deterioration with cyanosis and decreased cardiac output, leading to cardiovascular collapse (see Box 3-1). The condition is usually fatal in the first months of life without intervention.

Diagnostic Evaluation

See Table 3-1.

Treatment

Neonates require stabilization with mechanical ventilation and inotropic support preoperatively. A prostaglandin E_1 infusion is needed to maintain ductal patency and ensure adequate systemic blood flow.

Surgical Treatment

Staged palliation. The first stage is a Norwood procedure, which involves an anastomosis of the main pulmonary artery to the aorta to create a new aorta, shunting to provide pulmonary blood flow (usually with a modified Blalock-Taussig shunt), and creation of a large atrial septal defect. Postoperative complications include imbalance of systemic and pulmonary blood flow, bleeding, low cardiac output, and persistent heart failure. A new modification of the first stage repair is the use of a right ventricle–to–pulmonary artery homograft conduit instead of a shunt to supply pulmonary blood flow (Sano procedure). The second stage is often a bidirectional Glenn shunt procedure or a hemi-Fontan operation. Both involve anastomosing the superior vena cava to the right pulmonary artery so superior vena cava flow bypasses the right atrium and flows directly to the lungs. The procedure is usually done at 3 to 6 months of age to relieve cyanosis and reduce the volume load on the right ventricle. The final repair is a modified Fontan procedure.

Transplantation

Heart transplantation in the newborn period is another option for these infants. Problems include the shortage of newborn organ donors, risk of rejection, long-term problems with chronic immunosuppression, and infection.

Nursing Care Management
Assist in Measures to Assess and Improve Cardiac Function
Monitor Cardiac Function
- Vital signs monitoring
  - After the Norwood operation, monitor 4-extremity blood pressures to identify a blood pressure gradient if one occurs.
- Respiratory assessment
  - Monitor oxygen saturation. Patients with HLHS will not have normal oxygen saturations after the first and second stage surgeries. SpO$_2$ should be 75-80% before and after the first surgery. This signifies a balance between the pulmonary and systemic circulations.
  - After the Norwood, monitor for an increase in saturations >80-85%. This may signify an increase in systemic vascular resistance that needs to be explored. Also monitor for excessive cyanosis with SpO$_2$ <75%.
  - After the bidirectional Glenn or hemi-Fontan, oxygen saturations will be in the 80s; following the Fontan, the saturations will be close to normal (depending on the presence of a fenestration).
- Following shunt placement
  - Monitor shunt patency by auscultating over the shunt and hearing the "shunt murmur."
  - Monitor for increased cyanosis.
  - Monitor platelets.
- Monitor cardiac output (color, pulses, perfusion, capillary refill, renal function, and neurologic function).
- Monitor for dysrhythmias.
- Monitor for excessive sweating.
- Monitor for any neurologic changes.
- Monitor for any fussiness or inconsolability.
- Keep accurate record of intake and output.
- Weigh child or infant on same scale at same time of day.
- Monitor for any difficulty feeding or swallowing after the Norwood operation.

Administer Medications
- Review child's history related to cardiac management.
- Administer medications on schedule.
- Assess effectiveness of medications and any side effects noted.

▪ Be aware of drug-drug interactions and drug-food interactions.
▪ Follow guidelines for medication administration.

Manage Common Side Effects of Cardiac Defects
▪ Prevent fatigue during feeding; offer small frequent feedings to infant's or child's tolerance.
▪ Organize nursing care to allow child/infant uninterrupted rest.
▪ Promote activities that do not cause fatigue.

Provide Support for the Child and Family
▪ Communicate with the child and family in an appropriate style.
▪ Provide the child and family with honest answers.
▪ Provide emotional support.
▪ Offer age-appropriate interventions.
▪ Provide information on available resources for support for the child and family.

Patient and Family Teaching
Prepare the Child and Family for Diagnostic and Operative Procedures
▪ Provide explanation of diagnostic tests and why each test is performed because many of them are invasive procedures.
▪ Prepare the child prior to the invasive procedure. Remember discussion is dependent upon the child's age and development.
▪ Use simple words to describe procedures, and answer all questions the child and family may have.

Educate the Child and Family
▪ Assess child's and family's level of knowledge regarding HLHS.
▪ Assess child's and family's understanding of what they have heard about HLHS.
▪ Assess child's and family's understanding of the surgery.
▪ Teach the child and/or family at least four characteristics of heart failure that may occur because of HLHS such as:
    ▪ Fatigue after exertion
    ▪ Fast heart rate
    ▪ Fast breathing, shortness of breath, dyspnea
    ▪ Retractions

- Nasal flaring
- Cool extremities
- Diaphoresis
- Decreased urine output
- Puffiness (edema)
- Fussiness
- Decreased appetite
- Educate child and family about medication administration.
- Provide appropriate educational resources, and review materials with them.
- Clarify information presented by the health care team.
- Postoperative wound care teaching as needed
- Post-cardiac catheterization wound care teaching as needed
- Assess and record results of teaching and family's participation in care.

HYPOSPADIAS AND EPISPADIAS
Description
Hypospadias is a condition in which the urethral opening is located below the glans penis or anywhere along the ventral surface (underside) of the penile shaft.

Epispadias is a condition in which the urethral opening is located on the dorsal surface (top side) of the penile shaft, including the glans. Epispadias may occur as a simple defect or as a component of complex congenital anomalies of GU development, including exstrophy of the bladder.

Pathophysiology
Both occur as a result of failure of the tissue forming the urethra to fold and close during embryologic formation.

Clinical Signs and Symptoms
- Urethral opening evidenced on the ventral or dorsal surface of the penis; in hypospadias, there may be an associated chordee or ventral curvature of the penis; in severe cases, the urethral opening may be located on the perineum between the halves of the scrotum (bifid scrotum).
- Epispadias: bladder exstrophy or eventration of the bladder externalized on the abdomen with a meatal opening on the micropenis or on the perineum

Diagnostic Evaluation

■ Based on physical examination and observation of urination from the meatal opening

Treatment

■ Hypsopadias: surgical correction; glans approximation procedure (GAP) or a meatal advancement and glanuloplasty (MAGPI) procedure; urethral reconstruction with or without stint; preferred time for surgical repair is 6 to 12 months of age, before the child has developed body image.

■ Epispadias—simple defect requires surgical reconstruction of the urethra; complex defect involves bladder closure and the pelvic diastasis is corrected with an osteotomy; later, repair of the epispadias and creation of a urethral sphincter mechanism.

Nursing Care Management

■ Hypsopadias: preoperative care—detection by observing location of neonate's meatal opening and urine stream; postoperative care of a urinary stent in some cases; pain management; care of urine collection drainage device in some cases; parental information and support before and after surgery

■ Epispadias—detection by observing urinary meatal opening location; preoperative care—prevention of damage to tissues of bladder (exstrophy) and prevention of infection; IV access and fluid management if exstrophy present; intraoperative care of parents and information regarding child's progress; postoperative care involves pain management, preserving pelvic immobility, maintaining ureteric catheter patency, and maintaining the operative site intact. Family support is particularly important with bladder exstrophy or persistent cloaca as child's external and internal genitalia is altered and there will be questions regarding urinary and bowel function (with cloaca in females), as well as sexual and reproductive function; the child's external genitalia may require numerous surgical repairs.

Patient and Family Teaching

■ Hypopadias—postoperative care of child with urinary stent (as applicable); care of urine drainage device as applicable; prevention of damage to operative site

- Epispadias—prevention of bladder infection; prevention of tissue trauma of unrepaired bladder; postoperative pain management; care of child with urinary diversion; recognition of signs and symptoms of urinary tract infection; provide realistic expectations regarding the appearance of the external genitalia after surgery; reality of child's handicap may overwhelm parents; therefore, counseling is offered as well as details regarding physical care.

HYPOTHYROIDISM, JUVENILE
Description
Hypothyroidism is one of the most common endocrine problems of childhood. It may be either congenital or acquired and represents a deficiency in secretion of TH.

Pathophysiology
Beyond infancy, primary hypothyroidism may be caused by a number of defects. For example, a congenital hypoplastic thyroid gland may provide sufficient amounts of TH during the first year or two but be inadequate when rapid body growth increases demands on the gland. A partial or complete thyroidectomy for cancer or thyrotoxicosis can leave insufficient thyroid tissue to furnish hormones for body requirements. Radiotherapy for Hodgkin disease or other malignancies may lead to hypothyroidism. Infectious processes may cause hypothyroidism. It can also occur when dietary iodine is deficient.

Clinical Signs and Symptoms
Clinical manifestations depend on the extent of dysfunction and the child's age at onset. Box 3-7 describes the clinical signs of juvenile hypothyroidism.

Diagnostic Evaluation
- The GNRH test and baseline measurement of gonadotropin and sex hormone serum concentrations at 3 months of age are promising options for assessment of hypothalamic-pituitary-gonadal function in infants with congenital hypothyroidism.

Treatment
- Therapy is TH replacement, the same as for hypothyroidism in the infant, although the prompt treatment needed in the infant is not required in the child.

BOX 3-7
Clinical Signs of Juvenile Hypothyroidism
DECELERATED GROWTH Less when acquired at later age
MYXEDEMATOUS SKIN CHANGES Dry skin Puffiness around eyes Sparse hair Constipation Sleepiness Mental decline

- In children with severe symptoms, the restoration of euthyroidism is achieved more gradually with administration of increasing amounts of L-thyroxine over a period of 4 to 8 weeks to avoid symptoms of hyperthyroidism, which can occur with treatment of chronic hypothyroidism.

Nursing Care Management
- Growth cessation or retardation in a child whose growth has previously been normal should alert the observer to the possibility of hypothyroidism.
- Parent should be taught the importance of administering TCH replacement.

Patient and Family Teaching
- After diagnosis and implementation of thyroxine therapy, the importance of compliance and periodic monitoring of response to therapy should be stressed to parents.

IDIOPATHIC THROMBOCYTOPENIC PURPURA
Description
Idiopathic thrombocytopenic purpurea (ITP) is an acquired hemorrhagic disorder characterized by (1) ***thrombocytopenia,*** excessive destruction of platelets, (2) ***purpura,*** a discoloration caused by petechiae beneath the skin, and (3) a ***normal bone marrow with normal or increased number of immature platelets (megakaryocytes) and eosinophils.***

Pathophysiology

Although the cause is unknown, it is believed to be an autoimmune response to disease-related antigens. It is the most frequently occurring thrombocytopenia of childhood. The disease occurs in one of two forms: an acute, self-limiting course or a chronic condition (greater than 6 months' duration). The acute form is most often seen after upper respiratory infections; after the childhood diseases measles, rubella, mumps, and chickenpox; or after infection with parvovirus B19.

The greatest frequency of occurrence is between 2 and 10 years of age.

Clinical Signs and Symptoms

- Easy bruising
- Petechiae
- Ecchymoses
- Most often over bony prominences
- Bleeding from mucous membranes
- Epistaxis
- Bleeding gums
- Internal hemorrhage evidenced by:
  - Hematuria
  - Hematemesis
  - Melena
  - Hemarthrosis
  - Menorrhagia
  - Hematomas over lower extremities

Diagnostic Evaluation

- In ITP, the platelet count is reduced to below 20,000 mm^3; tests that depend on platelet function, such as the tourniquet test, bleeding time, and clot retraction, are abnormal.
- Although there is no definitive test on which to establish a diagnosis of ITP, several are usually performed to rule out other disorders in which thrombocytopenia is a manifestation, such as systemic lupus erythematosus, lymphoma, or leukemia.

Treatment

- Treatment for acute presentation is symptomatic and has included prednisone, IV immune globulin (IVIG), and anti-D antibody. These are not curative therapies.

- Some experts suggest that no therapy is necessary for the a-symptomatic patient, with no difference in the recovery of platelet counts over time.
- Anti-D antibody is a relatively new therapy for ITP.
- Splenectomy is reserved for those patients in whom ITP has persisted for 1 year or longer.

Nursing Care Management
- Nursing care is largely supportive and should include teaching regarding possible side effects of therapy and limitation in activities while the child's platelet count is 50,000 to 100,000/mm^3.

Patient and Family Teaching
- Children with ITP should not participate in any contact sports, bike riding, skateboarding, in-line skating, gymnastics, climbing, or running.
- Parents are encouraged to engage their children in quiet activities and to prevent any injuries to the child's head.
- Children with low platelet counts should NOT receive aspirin and NSAIDs; only salicylate substitutes (such as acetaminophen) are used.
- As in any condition with an uncertain outcome, the family needs emotional support.

IMPETIGO
Description
Nonbullous impetigo is a skin lesion on the face, or extremity that starts as a small vesicle or pustule and progresses to a light brown crusted plaque. Impetigo often begins as an insect bite, abrasion, laceration, burn, chickenpox or scabies that becomes infected. The causative organism is predominantly *Staphylococcus aureaus* although *group A beta- hemolytic streptococci* may be found in young children. The infection may easily be spread to other parts of the body by hand contact, clothing or towels.

Pathophysiology
Staphylococcus aureus is a gram positive organism that frequently inhabits the skin and mucous membranes of healthy children; the nose, axillae, throat, vagina, perineum, and rectum are common sites of colonization. Small children are vulnerable to staphylococcal

infections as a result of decreased immune reactivity, decreased awareness of hygiene measures such as handwashing, and increased hand to mouth and nose activity. Insect bites or other small lesions may be particularly bothersome to small children who may scratch the bite until it becomes colonized with bacteria from other sites such as the nose and rectum.

Clinical Signs and Symptoms
- Erythematous vesicle or pustule commonly on face or an extremity
- Lesions may be oozing or crusted, or both.
- In general, absence of fever and only minimal pruritis

Diagnostic Evaluation
- Based on appearance of lesion, absence of generalized symptoms such as fever, anorexia
- Wound culture positive for bacteria

Treatment
- Topical antibiotic ointment (Mupirocin [Bactroban] or retapamulin [Altabax])
- Systemic antibiotics if widespread lesions present or if lesions not responsive to topical antibiotics
- Antipruritic medication if pruritis is present
- Systemic antibiotics may be required for Methicillin-resistant Staph aureus (MRSA).

Nursing Care Management
- Administer antibiotic—topical or systemic.
- Parent teaching (see Patient and Family Teaching)
- Apply dressings as required to prevent further contact and spread of organism in small child.

Patient and Family Teaching
- Medication application (topical) or administration (if oral)
- General hygiene such as handwashing, washing lesions with soap and water, washing child's clothing in hot water, and helping child avoid scratching lesions
- Avoiding contamination and spread to other body parts or other small children

INFLAMMATORY BOWEL DISEASE
Description
Inflammatory bowel disease (IBD) is a term that is used for two forms of chronic intestinal inflammation—*ulcerative colitis (UC)* and *Crohn disease (CD)*. GI symptoms, extraintestinal and systemic inflammatory responses, and exacerbations and remissions without complete resolution characterize these diseases. Growth failure, particularly common in CD, is an important problem unique to the pediatric population. CD is more disabling, has more serious complications, and has less effective medical and surgical treatment than UC. Because UC is confined to the colon, theoretically it may be cured with a colectomy.

Pathophysiology
Ulcerative Colitis
The inflammation is limited to the colon and rectum, with the distal colon and rectum the most severely affected. Inflammation affects the mucosa and submucosa and involves continuous segments along the length of the bowel with varying degrees of ulceration, bleeding, and edema.

Crohn Disease
The chronic inflammatory process of CD involves any part of the GI tract from the mouth to the anus but most often affects the terminal ileum. The disease involves all layers of the bowel wall (transmural) in a discontinuous fashion, meaning that between areas of intact mucosa, there are areas of affected mucosa (skip lesions).

Clinical Signs and Symptoms
Ulcerative Colitis
The presentation may be mild, moderate, or severe, depending on the extent of mucosal inflammation and systemic symptoms. Children with UC usually present with diarrhea, rectal bleeding, and abdominal pain, often associated with tenesmus and urgency.

Crohn Disease
The most common symptoms are abdominal pain, diarrhea, and decrease in appetite resulting in weight loss. Perianal disease, including skin tags, fistulae, and abscesses occur in CD. Fever,

growth delay, and delayed sexual development are common. Mild GI symptoms, poor growth, and extraintestinal manifestations may be present for several years before overt GI symptoms occur.

Diagnostic Evaluation

- CBC to evaluate anemia and an ESR or CRP to assess the systemic reaction to the inflammatory process
- Total protein, albumin, iron, zinc, magnesium, vitamin B_{12}, and fat-soluble vitamins (may be low in children with CD)
- Stools for the presence of blood, leukocytes, and infectious organisms
- Serologic panel is often used to diagnose IBD and to differentiate between CD and UC. In IBD, autoantibodies called antineutrophil cytoplasm antibodies (ANCA) may be detected in the blood. The perinuclear antineutrophil cytoplasm antibody (pANCA) is associated with UC.
- Anti–*Saccharomyces cerevisiae* antibodies (ASCA) and anti–outer membrane porin of *Escherichia coli* (ompC) have been found in up to 60% of children with CD.
- In patients with CD, an upper GI series with small bowel follow-through assists in assessing the existence, location, and extent of disease in patients with CD.
- Upper endoscopy and colonoscopy with biopsies. Endoscopy allows direct visualization of the surface of the gastrointestinal tract so that the extent of inflammation and narrowing can be evaluated.
- Computed tomography and ultrasound also may be used to identify bowel wall inflammation, intra-abdominal abscesses, and fistulas.

Treatment

- The goals of therapy are to (1) control the inflammatory process to reduce or eliminate the symptoms, (2) obtain long-term remission, (3) promote normal growth and development, and (4) allow as normal a lifestyle as possible.
- *5-Aminosalicylates* (5-ASAs) are effective in the induction and maintenance of remission in mild to moderate UC. Mesalamine, olsalazine, and balsalazide are now preferred over sulfasalazine because of reduced side effects.

- Corticosteroids, such as prednisone and prednisolone, are indicated in induction therapy for moderate to severe UC and CD.
- *Immunomodulators,* such as azathioprine and its metabolite 6-mercaptopurine (6-MP), are used to induce and maintain remission in children with IBD who are steroid resistant or steroid dependent and in treating chronic draining fistulae.
- Cyclosporine and tacrolimus have both been shown to be effective in inducing remission in severe steroid-dependent UC. 6-MP or azathioprine is then used to maintain remission.
- *Antibiotics,* such as metronidazole and ciprofloxacin, may be used as an adjunctive therapy to treat complications such as perianal disease or small bowel bacterial overgrowth in CD.
- Infliximab is approved for the treatment of fistulae in CD as well as systemic manifestations of IBD such as ankylosing spondylitis, pyoderma gangrenosum, and chronic uveitis. Recently Infliximab was approved by the FDA for the treatment of UC unresponsive to steroids. Many patients relapse if treatment is stopped; therefore, long-term maintenance therapy with inflixamab every 8 weeks may be required.
- Nutritional support is important in the treatment of IBD. Growth failure is a common serious complication, especially in CD. Goals of nutritional support include (1) correction of nutrient deficits and replacement of ongoing losses, (2) provision of adequate energy and protein for healing, and (3) provision of adequate nutrients to promote normal growth. Nutritional support includes both enteral and parenteral nutrition.
- Surgery is indicated for UC when medical and nutritional therapies fail to prevent complications. Surgical options include a **subtotal colectomy** and **ileostomy** that leaves a rectal stump as a blind pouch.

Nursing Care Management

- Nursing interventions involve continued guidance of families and children with (1) adhering to dietary and medical management, (2) coping with factors that increase stress and emotional lability, (3) adjusting to a disease of remissions and exacerbations, and (4) when indicated, preparing the child and parents for the possibility of diversionary bowel surgery.

■ Frequently, the nurse can help children to adjust to problems of growth retardation, delayed sexual maturation, dietary restrictions, feelings of being "different" or "sickly," inability to compete with peers, and necessary absence from school during exacerbations of the illness.

Patient and Family Teaching

■ If a permanent colectomy/ileostomy is required, the nurse can teach the child and family how to care for the ileostomy.

■ Because of the chronic and often lifelong nature of the disease, families benefit from the educational services provided by organizations such as the Crohn's and Colitis Foundation of America, Inc. (CCFA)*.

■ Wound Ostomy and Continence Nurses Society‡ are available to assist with ileostomy care and provide important psychologic support through their self-help groups. Adolescents often benefit by participating in peer-support groups, which are sponsored by the CCFA.

INTUSSUSCEPTION (MALABSORPTION SYNDROME)

Description

Intussusception is an acute intestinal obstruction that occurs when one portion of bowel invaginates into a more distant portion of the bowel pulling the mesentery with it. The peak age is 3 to 9 months of age.

Pathophysiology

Lymphatic and venous congestion and bowel wall edema can cause obstruction of the intestine and infarction and perforation of the bowel wall can occur. Venous engorgement also leads to leaking of blood and mucus into the intestinal lumen, forming the classic currant jelly–like stools. Most cases of intussusception do not have a pathologic lead point, such as a polyp, lymphoma, or Meckel

---

*386 Park Avenue South, 17th Floor, New York, NY 10016; (800) 932-2423; website: www. ccfa.org.

†UOAA P.O. Box 66, Fairview, TN 37062-0066; (800) 826-0826; website: www.uoaa.org.

‡1550 South Coast Highway, Suite 201, Laguna Beach, CA 92651; (888) 224-9626; website: www.wocn.org.

diverticulum. The idiopathic cases are most likely a result of hypertrophy of intestinal lymphoid tissue secondary to viral infection.

Clinical Signs and Symptoms
- Abdominal pain
- Abdominal distention
- Screaming, irritability, lethargy, vomiting, diarrhea or constipation, fever, dehydration, and shock
- Passage of red, currant jelly–like stools (stool mixed with blood and mucus)
- Palpable sausage-shaped mass in upper right quadrant
- Empty lower right quadrant (Dance sign)
- Child appears normal and comfortable during intervals between episodes of pain.

Diagnostic Evaluation
- Clinical manifestations
- Ultrasound

Treatment
- Pneumoenema (air enema) with or without water-soluble contrast, or ultrasound-guided hydrostatic (saline) enema (80% effective in reducing intestine)
- Surgical reduction of invaginated intestine

Nursing Care Management
- Identification of disorder
- Assist with diagnostic process.
- IV access, gastric decompression, and antibiotics
- Postoperative care includes pain management, vital signs monitoring, assessment for return of bowel function, and incision care.
- Parent support and information during diagnostic process or surgery

Patient and Family Teaching
- Signs of condition recurrence if surgery not performed
- Pain management in postoperative period
- Observation for complications, including wound infection or signs of obstruction (vomiting, abdominal distention, currant jelly–like stools)

KAWASAKI DISEASE (MUCOCUTANEOUS LYMPH NODE SYNDROME)

Description
Kawasaki disease (KD) is an acute systemic vasculitis of unknown cause. The etiology of KD is unknown. Although it is not spread by person-to-person contact, several factors support infectious etiologic factors. It is often seen in geographic and seasonal outbreaks, with most cases reported in the late winter and early spring.

Pathophysiology
The principal area of involvement is the cardiovascular system. During the initial stage of the illness, extensive inflammation of the arterioles, venules, and capillaries occurs. In addition, segmental damage to the medium-sized muscular arteries, mainly the coronary arteries, can occur, causing the formation of coronary artery aneurysms in some children.

Clinical Signs and Symptoms
Fever for >5 days along with 4/5 clinical criteria (diagnosis may be made on day 4 by an experienced clinician if child has all the clinical criteria).

- Changes in the extremities; in the acute phase edema, erythema of the palms and soles; in the subacute phase, periungual desquamation (peeling) of the hands and feet
- Bilateral conjunctival injection (inflammation) without exudation
- Changes in the oral mucous membranes, such as erythema of the lips, oropharyngeal reddening; or "strawberry tongue" (large papillae are exposed)
- Polymorphous rash
- Cervical lymphadenopathy (one lymph node >1.5 cm)

Note: KD can be diagnosed with less clinical criteria when coronary artery changes are noted.

KD manifests in three phases: acute, subacute, and convalescent.

- *Acute phase* begins with the abrupt onset of high fever that is unresponsive to antibiotics and antipyretics. The child then develops the remaining diagnostic symptoms described above. During this stage, the child is typically *very* irritable.

- ▪ *Subacute phase* begins with resolution of the fever and lasts until all clinical signs of KD have disappeared. During this phase, the child is at greatest risk for the development of coronary artery aneurysms. Irritability persists during this phase.
- ▪ *Convalescent phase* During this phase, all the clinical signs of KD have resolved, but the laboratory values have not returned to normal. This phase is complete when all blood values are normal (6 to 8 weeks after onset). At the end of this stage, the child has regained his or her usual temperament, energy, and appetite.

Diagnostic Evaluation
- ▪ Echocardiograms are used to monitor myocardial and coronary artery status. A baseline echocardiogram should be obtained at the time of diagnosis for comparison with future studies.
- ▪ CBC with differential, ESR, platelet count, C-reactive protein, liver transaminases, GGT, UA
- ▪ Blood, urine, CSF, and GABHS pharyngeal cultures

Treatment
- ▪ The current treatment of KD includes high-dose IV gamma globulin along with salicylate therapy.
- ▪ A single, large infusion of IV gamma globulin 2 g/kg over 10 to 12 hours is recommended. Retreatment with IVIG is indicated in patients who continue with fever after treatment.
- ▪ Aspirin is given initially in an antiinflammatory dose (80 to 100 mg/kg/day in divided doses every 6 hours) to control fever and symptoms of inflammation. After fever has subsided, aspirin is continued at an antiplatelet dose (3 to 5 mg/kg/day). Low-dose aspirin is continued in patients without echocardiographic evidence of coronary abnormalities until the platelet count has returned to normal (6 to 8 weeks).

Nursing Care Management
- ▪ Monitor the child's cardiac status carefully.
- ▪ Record strict intake and output and obtain daily weight measurements.
- ▪ Fluids need to be administered with care because of the usual finding of myocarditis.

- Assess frequently for signs of CHF, including decreased urine output, gallop rhythm (an additional heart sound), tachycardia, and respiratory distress.
- Focus nursing care on symptomatic relief. To minimize skin discomfort, cool cloths, unscented lotions, and soft, loose clothing are helpful. During the acute phase, mouth care, including lubricating ointment to the lips, is important for the mucosal inflammation.
- Administration of gamma globulin should follow the same guidelines as for any blood product, with frequent monitoring of vital signs.
- Patient irritability is perhaps the most challenging problem. These children need a quiet environment that promotes adequate rest.

Patient and Family Teaching
- Parents need accurate information about KD, including the importance of follow-up monitoring and when they should contact their practitioner.
- Educate parents on the common symptoms that may last for weeks to months.
  - Irritability is likely to persist for up to 2 months after the onset of symptoms. Parents need support in their efforts to comfort an often inconsolable child.
  - Peeling of the hands and feet is painless and occurs primarily in the second and third weeks.
  - Arthritis, especially of the larger weight-bearing joints, may persist for several weeks. Children are typically most stiff in the mornings, during cold weather, and after naps. Passive range of motion in the bathtub is often helpful in increasing flexibility.
- All parents should understand the unlikely but real possibility of myocardial infarction, as well as the signs and symptoms of cardiac ischemia, in a child.
  - Parents of children with known severe coronary artery sequelae may be taught cardiopulmonary resuscitation.
- Live immunizations (e.g., measles-mumps-rubella, varicella) should be deferred for 11 months after the administration of gamma globulin because the body might not produce the appropriate amount of antibodies.

LACTOSE INTOLERANCE
Description
Lactose intolerance refers to at least four different entities that involve a deficiency of the enzyme *lactase*, which is needed for the hydrolysis or digestion of lactose in the small intestine; lactose is hydrolyzed into glucose and galactose. (1) *Congenital lactase deficiency*, an inborn error of metabolism that involves the complete absence or severely reduced presence of lactase (extremely rare); (2) *Primary lactase deficiency*, or *late-onset lactase deficiency*, is the most common type of lactose intolerance and is manifested usually after 4 or 5 years of age, although the time of onset is variable; more common in certain ethnic groups; (3) *Secondary lactase deficiency* occurs secondary to damage of the intestinal lumen, which decreases or destroys the enzyme lactase; and (4) *Developmental lactase deficiency* refers to the relative lactase deficiency observed in preterm infants less than 34 weeks gestation. This discussion will focus on primary lactase deficiency.

Pathophysiology
In primary lactase deficiency, there is a gradual decrease of the enzyme lactase within the brush border of the intestine with increasing age; the enzyme lactase helps break down ingested lactose for eventual absorption. Without this digestive enzyme, lactose-containing products produce the typical symptoms of bloating, flatulence, and abdominal pain. This process is not considered to be a disease but a normal physiologic process.

Clinical Signs and Symptoms
After the ingestion of lactose:
- Abdominal pain
- Bloating
- Flatulence
- Diarrhea

Diagnostic Evaluation
- Diagnosed on the basis of the history and improvement with a lactose-reduced diet

- The breath hydrogen test is used to positively diagnose the condition.
- In infants, lactose malabsorption may be diagnosed by evaluating fecal pH and reducing substances; fecal pH in infants is usually lower than in older children, but an acidic pH may indicate malabsorption.

Treatment
- Elimination of offending dairy products; however, some advocate decreasing amounts of dairy products rather than total elimination, especially in small children.
- One concern is that dairy avoidance in children and adolescents with lactose intolerance will contribute to reduced bone mineral density and osteoporosis.
- *Probiotics* (food preparations containing microorganisms such as *Lactobacillus,* which alter the gastrointestinal microflora and thus are beneficial to the host) may improve lactose intolerance when live cultures are fermented in dairy products.
- Other remedies: lactase tablets with dairy consumption; fresh yogurt consumption; hard cheeses; and lactase-treated dairy products.

Nursing Care Management
- Identifying the condition
- Parent and child education (see Patient and Family Teaching)

Patient and Family Teaching
- Explain the dietary restrictions to the family.
- Identify alternate sources of calcium such as yogurt and calcium supplementation.
- Explain the importance of supplementation.
- Discuss sources of lactose, especially hidden sources such as its use as a bulk agent in certain medications, and ways of controlling the symptoms.

LARYNGOTRACHEOBRONCHITIS, ACUTE
Description
Acute inflammation of the tissues of the larynx and trachea with airway narrowing. Acute LTB is the most common croup syndrome and typically affects children less than 5 years of age.

Pathophysiology

The causative organisms are the parainfluenza virus types 2 and 3, human metapneumovirus, RSV, influenza A and B, and *Mycoplasma pneumoniae*. The disease is usually preceded by a URI, which gradually descends to adjacent structures. Inflammation of the mucosa lining of the larynx and trachea causes a narrowing of the airway. When the airway is significantly narrowed, the child struggles to inhale air past the obstruction and into the lungs, producing the characteristic inspiratory stridor and suprasternal retractions.

Clinical Signs and Symptoms

- Gradual onset of low-grade fever
- Barky, brassy cough
- Cough and hoarseness
- Respiratory distress in infants and toddlers may be manifested by nasal flaring, intercostal retractions, tachypnea, and continuous stridor.
- Classic barking or seal-like cough and acute stridor after several days of rhinitis

Diagnostic Evaluation

The diagnosis is primarily based on clinical manifestations and the history of the illness.

Treatment

- Maintaining an airway and providing for adequate respiratory exchange
- Cool humidified mist is traditionally used to decrease edema.
- Nebulized epinephrine (racemic epinephrine) may be used. The α-adrenergic effects cause mucosal vasoconstriction and subsequent decreased subglottic edema.
- Oral steroids have been proven effective in the treatment of croup; IM dexamethasone may be given to children who are unable to tolerate oral dosing.
- Nebulized budesonide may be administered in conjunction with IM dexamethasone.

Nursing Care Management

- Assessment of respiratory status and recognition of deteriorating respiratory condition

- Administration of cool humidified mist or nebulized racemic epinephrine
- Administration of medications such as oral corticosteroid
- Inform parents of child's status and allay anxiety.
- Encourage small amounts of oral fluids as tolerated once the child's status begins improving.

Patient and Family Teaching

- Teach parents to recognize signs and symptoms of respiratory distress.
- Teach parents how to place child in cooler air initially (such as in bathroom with hot shower as mist therapy) if respiratory distress is not evident.
- Teach parents how to administer oral corticosteroid and importance of adhering to prescribed dosage regimen to prevent adverse effects of drug.

LEAD POISONING

Description

Acute childhood lead poisoning is most commonly caused by ingestion of nonintact lead-based paint in an older home or lead-contaminated bare soil in the yard.

Pathophysiology

Lead can affect any part of the body, including the renal, hematologic, and neurologic systems. Of most concern for young children is the developing brain and nervous system, which is more vulnerable than that of an older child or adult. Lead in the body moves via an equilibration process between the blood, the soft tissues and organs, and the bones and teeth. Lead ultimately settles in the bones and teeth, where it remains inert and in storage.

Clinical Signs and Symptoms

- Mild and moderate lead poisoning cause cognitive and behavioral problems in young children, which may include aggression, hyperactivity, impulsivity, delinquency, disinterest, and withdrawal.
- Long-term neurocognitive signs of lead poisoning include developmental delays, lowered intelligence quotient, reading skill

deficits, visual-spatial problems, visual-motor problems, learning disabilities, and lower academic success.
■ Physical growth and reproductive efficiency may also be adversely affected by chronic lead toxicity.
■ Acute signs of lead poisoning include nausea, vomiting, constipation, anorexia, and abdominal pain.

Diagnostic Evaluation
■ Lead testing of a venous blood specimen from a venipuncture; an elevated blood lead level (BLL) of ≥10 mg/dL warrants further assessment and management.

Treatment
Treatment actions vary depending on the child's blood lead level (see Table 3-7).

TABLE 3-7
Treatment for Lead Levels

BLOOD LEAD LEVEL (Mg/dL)	ACTION
<10	Reassess or rescreen in 1 year. If exposure status changes, do this sooner.
10-14	Provide family with lead poisoning education, follow-up testing, and social service referral if necessary.
15-19	Provide family with lead poisoning education (dietary and environmental), follow-up testing, and social service referral as needed; if blood lead level persists, initiate actions for blood lead level of 20-44 microgram/dL.
20-44	Provide coordination of care, clinical management, environmental investigation, and lead hazard control.
45-69	Within 48 hours, provide coordination of care and clinical management, including treatment, environmental investigation, and lead hazard control. The child must not remain in a lead hazardous environment if resolution is to occur.
≥70	*Immediately* provide medical treatment and begin coordination of care, clinical management, environmental investigation, and lead hazard control.

Nursing Care Management

The primary nursing goal in lead poisoning is to prevent the child's initial or further exposure to lead.

- The following areas that should be discussed with the family of every child who has an elevated blood lead level(10 microgram/dL and above):
  - The child's blood lead level and what it means
  - Potential adverse health effects of an elevated blood lead level
  - Sources of lead exposure and suggestions on how to reduce exposure
  - Importance of wet cleaning to remove lead dust on floors, window sills, and other surfaces
  - Importance of good nutrition in reducing the absorption and effects of lead; for persons with poor nutritional patterns, adequate intake of calcium and iron and importance of regular meals
  - Need for follow-up testing to monitor the child's blood lead level
  - Results of an environmental investigation if applicable
  - Hazards of improper removal of lead paint (dry sanding, scraping, or open-flame burning)

Patient and Family Teaching

An important aspect of teaching is to assess children at risk for lead poisoning. These questions should be asked at well-child visits:

- Does your child live in or regularly visit a house that was built before 1950?
- Does your child live in or regularly visit a house built before 1978 with recent or ongoing renovations or remodeling within the past 6 months?
- Does your child have a sibling or playmate who has or did have lead poisoning?

LEGG-CALVÉ-PERTHES DISEASE

Description

Legg-Calvé-Perthes disease, also called *coxa plana* or *osteochondritis deformans juvenilis,* is a self-limited disorder in which there is aseptic necrosis of the femoral head. The disease affects children ages 2 to 12 years, but most cases occur in boys between 4 and 8 years of age as an isolated event.

Pathophysiology

The cause of the disease is unknown, but there is a disturbance of circulation to the femoral capital epiphysis that produces an ischemic aseptic necrosis of the femoral head. During middle childhood, circulation to the femoral epiphysis is more tenuous than at other ages and can become obstructed by trauma, inflammation, coagulation defects, and a variety of other causes.

Clinical Signs and Symptoms

- Limp on the affected side
- Hip soreness, ache, or stiffness

Diagnostic Evaluation

- Radiographic examination
- Magnetic resonance imaging demonstrates osteonecrosis is definitive diagnosis.

Treatment

- Varies according to the age of the child at the time of diagnosis and the appearance of the femoral head vasculature and position within the acetabulum
- Nonsurgical: Initial treatment is rest and non–weight bearing with abduction brace, leg casts, or a leather harness sling; abduction-ambulation braces may be used.
- Surgical: pelvic or femoral osteotomy to contain the femoral head

Nursing Care Management

- Assist with diagnostic procedures.
- Pain management
- Helping child cope with restricted mobility; diversional activities; school work
- Postoperative care; vital signs monitoring; pain management
- Child and family teaching

Patient and Family Teaching

- Care and management of the corrective appliance selected for therapy
- Cast care; brace care as applicable

LEUKEMIAS: ACUTE LYMPHOCYTIC AND ACUTE MYELOGENOUS

Description

Leukemia is a cancer of the blood-forming tissues. It is the most common form of childhood cancer.

In children, two forms are generally recognized: acute lymphoid leukemia (ALL) and acute myelogenous leukemia (AML). Synonyms for ALL include lymphatic, lymphocytic, lymphoblastic, and lymphoblastoid leukemia.

Pathophysiology

Leukemia is an unrestricted proliferation of immature white blood cells in the blood-forming tissues of the body. Leukemia cells depress bone marrow production of the formed elements of the blood by competing for and depriving the normal cells of the essential nutrients for metabolism. The three main consequences are (1) anemia from decreased erythrocytes, (2) infection from neutropenia, and (3) bleeding from decreased platelet production. Invasion of the bone marrow with leukemic cells gradually causes a weakening of the bone and a tendency toward fractures. As leukemic cells invade the periosteum, increasing pressure causes severe pain. Bone marrow examination reveals greatly elevated counts of immature cells or "blasts."

Clinical Signs and Symptoms

- Fever, pallor, fatigue, anorexia, hemorrhage (usually petechiae), and bone and joint pain are common.
- Spleen, liver, and lymph glands are enlarged. Hepatosplenomegaly is more common than lymphadenopathy.
- Leukemia cells can infiltrate the meninges causing increased intracranial pressure: severe headache, vomiting, papilledema, irritability, lethargy, and eventually coma.

Diagnostic Evaluation

- Leukemia is usually suspected from the history and physical symptoms.
- Peripheral blood smear contains immature forms of leukocytes, frequently in combination with low blood counts.

- Definitive diagnosis is based on bone marrow aspiration or biopsy. Cytogenetics, immunophenotyping, and special staining are performed on the bone marrow specimen. Typically the bone marrow is hypercellular with primarily blast cells.
- Once the diagnosis is confirmed, a lumbar puncture is performed to determine if there is any central nervous system involvement.

Treatment

Chemotherapeutic with or without cranial irradiation in four phases:
- Induction, which achieves a complete remission or disappearance of leukemic cells
- Intensification, or consolidation, therapy, which further decreases the tumor burden
- Central nervous system prophylactic therapy, which prevents leukemic cells from invading the central nervous system
- Maintenance, which serves to maintain the remission phase

Patient Outcomes

Prognostic factors in determining long-term survival for children with ALL are the initial white blood cell count, the patient's age at diagnosis, cytogenetics, the immunologic subtype, and the child's sex (see Table 3-8).

TABLE 3-8

Favorable prognostic factors for acute lymphoblastic leukemia

FACTOR	CRITERIA
Leukocyte count	<50,000/mm^3
Age	>2 and <10 years
Immunologic	CALLA-positive, early pre-B-cell
Subtype	L$_1$
FAB morphology Cytogenetics	Hyperdiploid (>50 chromosomes, DNA index >1.16); trisomies 4 and 10 and translocations t(12; 21) (p21; q22)
Sex	Female
Leukemia cell burden	Minimal

Nursing Care Management
Administer Treatment
- Review child's history related to previous tolerance to therapy.
- Determine appropriate premedication prior to therapy.
- Be aware of drug-specific interactions.
- Assess the child's laboratory findings prior to therapy administration.
- Ensure that the chemotherapy doses are correct by checking orders according to the institution's policies and procedures.
- Follow guidelines for chemotherapy administration.
- If the treatment is given intravenously, observe the IV site for signs of irritation or infiltration.
- Follow the institution's policy for safe handling chemotherapy wastes, including the patient's body fluids.
- Observe the child for signs of reaction during and following treatment.

Manage Common Side Effects of Cancer Treatment
- Assess for toxicities specific to the cancer treatment.
- Monitor for signs of infection, obtain cultures, and initiate antibiotics if indicated.
- Monitor nutrition and weight changes and alternative methods of nutrition if appropriate.
- Monitor fluid and electrolytes.
- Evaluate child's response to treatment.
- Manage central line care.

Monitor for Complications Related to Leukemia and Treatment
- Assess for symptoms related to leukemia and treatment.
- Review laboratory findings.
- Obtain a complete history evaluating the incidence and duration of symptoms.
- Perform a complete physical examination; assess for pallor, petechiae, bleedings, signs of infection, rash, lymphadenopathy, hepatosplenomegaly, and neurologic changes.

Provide Support for the Child and Family
- Communicate with the child and family in an appropriate style.
- Provide the child and family with honest answers.

▪ Provide emotional support.
▪ Offer age-appropriate interventions.
▪ Provide information on available resources for support for the child and family.

Patient and Family Teaching

▪ Prepare the child and family for diagnostic and operative procedures.
▪ Provide explanation of diagnostic tests and why each test is performed because many of them, such as bone marrow aspiration and lumbar puncture, are invasive procedures.
▪ Prepare the child prior to the invasive procedure. Remember that discussion is dependent upon the child's age and development.
▪ Use simple words to describe procedures, and answer all questions the child and family may have.

Educate the Child and Family

▪ Assess child's and family's level of knowledge regarding the leukemia and treatment.
▪ Assess child's and family's understanding of what they have heard about leukemia and treatment.
▪ Explain that chemotherapeutic reactions vary with the specific drug regimen. Most common side effects from chemotherapy include nausea and vomiting, body image changes, neuropathy, and mucosal ulceration.
▪ Educate the family regarding neutropenia, anemia, and thrombocytopenia, the signs and symptoms of infection, and fever precautions.
▪ Provide appropriate educational resources, and review materials with them.
▪ Clarify information presented by the health care team.

LYME DISEASE
Description
Lyme disease (LD) is the most common tick-borne disorder in the United States; caused by the spirochete *Borrelia burgdorferi,* which enters the skin and bloodstream through the saliva and feces of ticks, especially the deer tick. Most cases of Lyme disease are reported in the Northeast from southern Maine to northern Virginia.

Pathophysiology

The disease may present in any of three stages.

- *Stage 1* consists of the tick bite at the time of inoculation, followed in 3 to 31 days by the development of distinctive rash, ***erythema migrans*** at the site of the bite.
- *Stage 2,* the most serious stage of the disease, is characterized by systemic involvement of neurologic, cardiac, and musculoskeletal systems that appears several weeks after the cutaneous phase is completed.
- *Stage 3,* or the late stage, includes musculoskeletal pain that involves the tendons, bursae, muscles, and synovia. Arthritis may occur, and late neurologic problems include deafness and chronic encephalopathy.

Clinical Signs and Symptoms
Early manifestations

- Rash
- Fever
- Malaise
- Headache
- Mild neck stiffness
- Joint pain

Diagnostic Evaluation

- Early recognition of signs and symptoms and rash
- Serologic testing for antibodies by enzyme immunoassay (EIA) or immunofluorescent antibody assay (IFA)

Treatment

- Close monitoring for signs of illness if ticks removed (for 30 days)
- Antibiotics: oral doxycycline (14- to 21-day regimen) for child 8 years and older; amoxicillin (14- to 21-day regimen) for child younger than 8 years

Nursing Care Management

- Parent and child education for prevention of exposure to ticks; wear long-sleeve shirt or pants; wear boots or tuck pants leg inside socks; use a DEET-containing insecticide (diethyltoluamide) and permethrin on the child's clothing; check child for ticks following excursions into tick-infested areas.

■ Safe tick removal: Remove tick as soon as observed with tweezers—pull tick straight out—wash area with soap and water or alcohol; *do not use* match, petroleum jelly, nail polish, or other products to remove a tick.

Patient and Family Teaching
■ Medication administration: stress completion of regimen
■ Prevention of exposure: see previous page
■ Safe tick removal: see above

LYMPHOCYTIC THYROIDITIS
Description
Lymphocytic thyroiditis (Hashimoto disease, juvenile autoimmune thyroiditis) is the most common cause of thyroid disease in children and adolescents. It accounts for many of the enlarged thyroid glands formerly designated as *thyroid hyperplasia of adolescence* or *adolescent goiter.*

Pathophysiology
There is a strong genetic predisposition to the development of lymphocytic thyroiditis, although no mode of inheritance has been delineated and the basic stimulus or autoimmune defect is unknown. The disease is characterized by lymphocytic infiltration of the gland, germinal center inflammation, and, in many patients, replacement with fibrous tissue. In the early stages, there may be only hyperplasia. A defect in autoregulation allows the persistence of a T-cell clone, which induces a cell-mediated immune response. Several antithyroid antibodies have been recognized in patients with thyroiditis.

Clinical Signs and Symptoms
■ Presence of the enlarged thyroid gland is usually detected by the practitioner during a routine examination, although it may be noted by parents when the youngster swallows.
■ In most children the entire gland is enlarged symmetrically (but may be asymmetric) and is firm, freely movable, and nontender.
■ Moderate tracheal compression (sense of fullness, hoarseness, and dysphagia), but it is extremely rare for a nontoxic diffuse goiter to enlarge to the extent that it causes mechanical

obstruction. Most children are euthyroid, but some display symptoms of hypothyroidism.

Diagnostic Evaluation
- Thyroid function tests are usually normal, although TSH levels may be slightly or moderately elevated.
- With progressive disease, the T4 decreases, followed by a decrease in T3 levels and an increase in TSH.
- A variety of abnormalities in radioactive iodine uptake may be noted.
- The majority of children have serum antibody titers to thyroid antigens, but fewer children have a positive red blood cell hemagglutination test result. When both tests are used, almost all children with thyroid autoimmunity are detected.

Treatment
- In many cases, the goiter is transient and asymptomatic and regresses spontaneously within a year or two.
- Therapy of a nontoxic diffuse goiter is usually simple, uncomplicated, and effective. Oral administration of thyroid hormone decreases the size of the gland significantly and provides the feedback needed to suppress TSH stimulation, and the hyperplastic thyroid gland gradually regresses in size.
- Surgery is contraindicated in this disorder.
- Untreated patients should be evaluated periodically.

Nursing Care Management
- Careful assessment to help identify the child with thyroid enlargement
- Provide reassurance to the child and family that the condition is usually temporary.

Patient and Family Teaching
- Reinforce instructions for thyroid therapy if on medication.

MECKEL DIVERTICULUM
Description
Meckel diverticulum is a remnant of the fetal omphalomesenteric duct that connects the yolk sac with the primitive midgut during fetal life.

Pathophysiology

Meckel diverticulum is a true diverticulum because it arises from the anti-mesenteric border of the small intestine and contains all layers of the intestinal wall with a separate blood supply from the vitelline artery. Normally this structure is obliterated by the fifth to seventh week of gestation when the placenta replaces the yolk sac as the source of nutrition for the fetus. Failure of obliteration may result in an omphalomesenteric fistula (a fibrous band connecting the small intestine to the umbilicus). The symptomatic complications of Meckel diverticulum are ulceration, bleeding, intussusception, intestinal obstruction, diverticulitis, and perforation. Bleeding is caused by peptic ulceration or perforation because of the unbuffered acidic gastric secretion. Several mechanisms can cause obstruction. Intussusception may be led by the diverticulum. Obstruction may also be caused by entanglement of the small intestine around a fibrous cord, trapping of a loop of intestine under the band, incarceration within a hernia sac, or volvulus of the intestinal segment containing the diverticulum. Diverticulitis occurs when peptic ulceration or obstruction leads to inflammation.

Clinical Signs and Symptoms

- Painless rectal bleeding; currant jelly–like stools
- Abdominal pain
- Anemia
- Signs of intestinal obstruction: colicky abdominal pain, abdominal distention, vomiting (may be bilious), constipation and obstipation, dehydration, rigid and boardlike abdomen, decreased or absent bowel sounds, with increasing distention; respiratory distress, shock

Diagnostic Evaluation

- Based on the history, physical examination, and radiographic study (technetium-99m pertecnate scan), which detects presence of gastric mucosa

Treatment

- Surgical removal of the diverticulum
- Preoperative blood replacement, IV fluids, and oxygen, as required

- Antibiotics may be used preoperatively to control infection.
- With obstruction, GI decompression, NPO, IV fluids

Nursing Care Management
- Identification of disorder; test stool for occult blood.
- Assist with diagnostic tests.
- IV access, gastric decompression, and antibiotics
- Observe for signs of anemia; if severe, hypovolemic shock.
- Postoperative care includes pain management, vital signs monitoring, assessment for return of bowel function, and incision care.
- Parent support and information during diagnostic process and surgery; provide reassurance.

Patient and Family Teaching
- Encourage physical care of child as condition allows.
- Postoperative care of incision
- Pain management

MENINGITIS, BACTERIAL
Description
Bacterial meningitis is an acute inflammation of the meninges and CSF. Bacterial meningitis remains a significant cause of illness in the pediatric age-groups because of the residual damage caused by undiagnosed and untreated or inadequately treated cases. The majority of reported cases occur in children between 1 month and 5 years of age, with an increased mortality risk in the adolescent and young adult.

Meningococcal meningitis occurs in epidemic form and is the only type readily transmitted by droplet infection from nasopharyngeal secretions. This condition may develop at any age, but the risk of meningococcal infection increases with the number of contacts; therefore it occurs predominantly in school-age children and adolescents.

Pathophysiology
Bacterial meningitis can be caused by a variety of bacterial agents, among which are *H. influenzae* type b, *S. pneumoniae,* and *Neisseria meningitidis* (meningococcus), which are responsible for bacterial meningitis in 95% of children older than 2 months.

Other organisms are β-hemolytic streptococci, *Staphylococcus aureus*, and *Escherichia coli*. The leading causes of neonatal meningitis are group B streptococci, *E. coli*, and *Listeria monocytogenes*. The most common route of infection is vascular dissemination from a focus of infection elsewhere. Organisms from the nasopharynx invade the underlying blood vessels and enter the cerebral blood supply or form local thromboemboli that release septic emboli into the bloodstream. Organisms also gain entry by direct implantation after penetrating wounds, skull fractures that provide an opening into the skin or sinuses, lumbar puncture or surgical procedures, anatomic abnormalities such as spina bifida, or foreign bodies such as an internal ventricular shunt or an external ventricular device. Once implanted, the organisms spread into the CSF, by which the infection spreads throughout the subarachnoid space.

The infective process in bacterial meningitis includes inflammation, exudation, white blood cell accumulation, and varying degrees of tissue damage. The brain becomes hyperemic and edematous, and the entire surface of the brain is covered by a layer of purulent exudate that varies with the type of organism. As infection extends to the ventricles, thick pus, fibrin, or adhesions may occlude the narrow passages and obstruct the flow of CSF.

Clinical Signs and Symptoms
Signs and symptoms vary according to type of organism, age of child, effectiveness of therapy in treating for antecedent illness, and whether it occurs as an isolated entity or as a complication of another illness or injury. The onset of illness is likely to be abrupt, with fever, chills, headache, and vomiting that are associated with or quickly followed by alterations in sensorium. Additional clinical manifestations include:

Children and Adolescents
- Seizures (often the initial sign)
- Irritability
- Agitation
- May develop:
  - Photophobia
  - Delirium

- - Hallucinations
  - Aggressive behavior
  - Drowsiness
  - Stupor
  - Coma
  - Nuchal rigidity
- May progress to opisthotonos
- Positive Kernig and Brudzinski signs
- Hyperactive but variable reflex responses
- Petechial or purpuric rashes (meningococcal infection), especially when associated with a shocklike state
- Joint involvement (meningococcal and *H. influenzae* infection)
- Chronically draining ear (pneumococcal meningitis)

Infants and Young Children
- Classic picture (above) rarely seen in children between 3 months and 2 years of age
- Fever
- Poor feeding
- Vomiting
- Marked irritability
- Frequent seizures (often accompanied by a high-pitched cry)
- Bulging fontanel
- Nuchal rigidity may or may not be present.
- Brudzinski and Kernig signs are not helpful in diagnosis.
- Difficult to elicit and evaluate in this age-group
- Subdural empyema (*H. influenzae* infection)

Neonates: Specific Signs
- Manifestations vague and nonspecific
- Refuses feedings
- Poor sucking ability
- Vomiting or diarrhea
- Poor tone
- Lack of movement
- Weak cry
- Full, tense, and bulging fontanel may appear late in course of illness.
- Neck usually supple

Neonates: Nonspecific Signs that May Be Present
■ Hypothermia or fever (depending on the maturity of the infant [in weeks/months])
■ Jaundice
■ Irritability
■ Drowsiness
■ Seizures
■ Apnea or other respiratory irregularities
■ Cyanosis
■ Weight loss

Diagnostic Evaluation
■ Lumbar puncture: gram stain; culture and sensitivity (to determine organism); blood cell count; and glucose (reduced) and protein (increased); possibly elevated CSF pressure, but this alone is not diagnostic
■ White blood cells are elevated with predominant polymorphonuclear lymphocytes.
■ Blood culture
■ Nose and throat cultures may provide helpful information in some cases.

Treatment
■ Isolation precautions
■ Initiation of antimicrobial therapy
■ Maintenance of hydration
■ Maintenance of ventilation
■ Reduction of increased ICP
■ Management of systemic shock
■ Control of seizures
■ Control of temperature
■ Treatment of complications

Nursing Care Management
■ Intensive care
■ Decrease environmental stimuli.
■ Comfort measures including analgesics
■ Observation and monitoring of neurologic signs and vital signs
■ Monitor ICP, LOC, urinary output, central venous pressure.

- Monitor fluid intake (intravenous) carefully to prevent ICP.
- Prevent complications in immobile, sedated, or unconscious child (skin care, pain management, prevent contractures).
- Medication administration: antibiotics; analgesics; sedatives; volume expanders; possibly mannitol; antipyretics; antiepileptics
- Provide family support and information about child's condition.

Patient and Family Teaching
- Involve in care of child as feasible to prevent helplessness.
- Provide information about disease, treatments, and child's progress.
- Communication with sedated child

MENINGITIS, NONBACTERIAL (ASEPTIC)
Description
Acute inflammation of the meninges, brain tissue, and CSF; caused by a number of agents, primarily viruses, often associated with other diseases such as measles, mumps, herpes, and leukemia; enteroviruses and mumps account for a large number of cases. The onset may be gradual or abrupt.

Pathophysiology
Direct invasion of meningeal and brain tissue by actively multiplying viruses, which may result in neuronal destruction, meningeal congestion, and edema. Usually acquired by person-to-person contact.

Clinical Signs and Symptoms
- Infants: irritability and lethargy
- Older children: headache, fever, malaise, nuchal rigidity, nausea and vomiting
- Photophobia
- Seizure activity
- Variability in clinical symptoms from mild illness to severe meningoencephalitis, depending on the viral agent

Diagnostic Evaluation
- Clinical presentation
- Examination of CSF (lumbar puncture)

- EEG
- CT or MRI

Treatment
- Isolation until viral agent identified
- Administration of antibiotics until virus is isolated
- Primarily supportive
- Herpes: administer acyclovir.

Nursing Care Management
- Assist with diagnostic procedures.
- Decrease environmental stimuli.
- Isolation
- IV access; monitor for fluid and electrolyte imbalance.
- Monitor for elevated intracranial pressure.
- Monitor for progression of neurologic symptoms including seizures.
- Seizure precautions
- Pain management
- Fever, headache, and GI symptom management with medications (acetaminophen, ondansetron, morphine)
- Prevention through routine childhood immunization against polio, mumps, measles, and varicella
- Provide family support.
- Support and communication with mechanically ventilated child (as applicable)

Patient and Family Teaching
- Involvement in care of child
- Immunizations for prevention
- Medication administration after discharge home
- Seizure management as applicable

MONONUCLEOSIS, INFECTIOUS
Description
Infectious mononucleosis is an acute, self-limiting infectious disease that is common among older school-aged children and adolescents. The herpes-like Epstein-Barr virus (EBV) is the principal cause of infectious mononucleosis.

Pathophysiology

Mononucleosis is believed to be transmitted in saliva by direct intimate contact; it is mildly contagious, but the period of communicability is unknown. There is an increase in the mononuclear elements of the blood, and symptoms may vary from mild to moderately serious complications. Sexual transmission of mononucleosis has been documented.

Clinical Signs and Symptoms

- Fever
- Sore throat
- Swollen lymph nodes
- Fatigue
- Anorexia
- Macular eruption on trunk
- Exudative pharyngitis/tonsillitis

Diagnostic Evaluation

- Complete blood count may show lymphocytic leukocytosis.
- Increase in atypical leukocytes in the peripheral blood smear
- Leukocyte count low or normal
- Heterophil antibody test: positive for IgM (also called the Mono spot test)
- Serologic antibody test against viral capsid antigen (VCA)

Treatment

- Supportive: aimed at decreasing symptoms
- Rest, analgesic, fluids
- Corticosteroids may be used if respiratory distress from significant tonsillar inflammation, hemolytic anemia, thrombocytopenia, and neurologic complications occur.
- Avoidance of contact sports to prevent splenic rupture

Nursing Care Management

- Supportive care and comfort measures
- Pain management
- Encourage fluid intake.
- Warm saline gargles for sore throat may be helpful.

- Identification of deteriorating condition (dysphagia, respiratory distress)

Patient and Family Teaching
- Avoidance of close, intimate contact with infected person
- Avoidance of contact sports until spleen is nonpalpable and person is symptom free
- Measures to reduce contamination of household members—handwashing, avoid sharing eating utensils
- Comfort measures during acute phase
- Recognition of respiratory distress or of extreme tonsillar inflammation

MUSCULAR ATROPHIES, SPINAL
Description
Spinal muscular atrophies are degenerative diseases characterized by progressive weakness and wasting of skeletal muscles caused by degeneration of anterior horn cells. SMA begins in fetal life and progresses in infancy and childhood. SMA type 1, or Werdnig-Hoffman disease, is inherited as an autosomal-recessive trait and is the most common paralytic form of the floppy infant syndrome (congenital hypotonia). Infants often do not live more than a year or so as a result of severe respiratory insufficiency. SMA type 2 appears late in infancy and is slower in progression than type 1. SMA type 3, or Kugelberg-Welander disease, is considered a chronic form of the disease; appearance of symptoms may appear late in childhood with gradual loss of ambulation ability 8 or 9 years after onset of symptoms, but child may live into adulthood.

Pathophysiology
Neuronal cell degeneration occurs in the anterior horn cells of the spinal cord and the motor nuclei of the brainstem, but the primary effect is atrophy of skeletal muscles. Neuronal cell death continues after embryonic development due to the lack of survivor motor neuron gene 1 usually located on chromosome 5q13; the remaining survivor motor neuron gene 2 produces limited quantities of SMN protein necessary for muscle strength. The age of onset is variable, but the earlier the onset, the more disseminated and severe the motor weakness.

Clinical Signs and Symptoms
Type 1 (Werdnig-Hoffmann Disease)
- Clinical manifestations within first few weeks or months of life
- Onset within 6 months of life
- Inactivity: most prominent feature
- Infant lying in a frog-leg position with legs externally rotated, abducted, and flexed at knees
- Generalized weakness
- Absent deep tendon reflexes
- Limited movements of shoulder and arm muscles
- Active movement usually limited to fingers and toes
- Diaphragmatic breathing with sternal retractions (diaphragmatic paralysis may occur)
- Abnormal tongue movements (at rest)
- Weak cry and cough
- Poor suck reflex
- Tires quickly during feedings (if breast-fed, may lose weight before noticeable)
- Growth failure (nutritional)
- Alert facies
- Normal sensation and intellect
- Affected infants not able to sit alone, roll over, or walk

Type 2 (Intermediate SMA)
- Onset before age 18 months
- Early: weakness confined to arms and legs
- Later: generalized
- Legs usually involved to greater extent than arms
- Prominent pectus excavatum
- Movements absent during complete relaxation or sleep
- Some infants able to sit if placed in position, but few can ambulate

Type 3 (Kugelberg-Welander Syndrome; Mild SMA)
- Onset of symptoms after 18 months of age
- Normal head control and ability to sit unassisted by 6 to 8 months of age
- Thigh and hip muscles weak
- Scoliosis common
- Failure to walk a common presentation

- In those who manage to walk:
  - Waddling gait
  - Genu recurvatum
  - Protuberant abdomen
  - Ambulation becoming increasingly difficult
- Confined to a wheelchair by second decade
- Deep tendon reflexes may be present early but disappear.

Diagnostic Evaluation
- Based on the molecular genetic marker for the SMN (survival motor neuron) gene
- Prenatal diagnosis: genetic analysis of circulating fetal cells in maternal blood
- Muscle electromyography (EMG)
- SMA type 1 is often mistaken as infant botulism due to similarities in clinical presentation.
- CK levels slightly elevated or normal

Treatment
- Early recognition and diagnosis
- Respiratory support: sleep-disordered breathing is common; use of noninvasive ventilation methods such as bilevel positive airway pressure (BIPAP)
- Antibiotics: Treat upper respiratory infections.
- Nutritional growth failure: supplemental feedings; gastrostomy feedings
- Prevent muscle and joint contractures: physical therapy; orthoses.
- Orthopedic care: Scoliosis may occur.

Nursing Care Management
- Early detection of symptoms
- Assist with diagnostic tests.
- Maintain oxygenation: supplemental oxygen; monitor respirations; removal of secretions from airway; management of noninvasive mechanical ventilation devices; tracheostomy care as applicable.
- Support family and child with chronic and terminal illness in types 1 and 2.
- Encourage family to care for infant and child as any other child.
- Promote child's growth and development and performance of ADLs.

Patient and Family Teaching

- Respiratory monitoring and support: removal of secretions; care of tracheostomy
- Feeding methods: gastrostomy for infants too weak to breast feed or bottle feed
- Prevention of infections: childhood immunizations; special precautions during winter months for URIs
- Prevention of muscle and joint contractures and special mobilization devices as applicable to severity of muscle weakness
- Encourage child to engage in ADLS to capability, including school as applicable.
- Involvement in support group

MUSCULAR DYSTROPHY
Description
A group of unrelated muscle diseases of childhood that has a genetic origin in which there is gradual degeneration of muscle fibers, characterized by progressive weakness and wasting of symmetric groups of skeletal muscles, with increasing disability and deformity. In all forms of MD, there is insidious loss of strength, but each type differs in regard to muscle groups affected, age of onset, rate of progression, and inheritance pattern. Facioscapulohumeral (Landouzy-Déjérine) muscular dystrophy is characterized by difficulty in raising the arms over the head, lack of facial mobility, and a forward slope of the shoulders. Limb-girdle muscular dystrophy is characterized by weakness of proximal muscles of the pelvic and shoulder girdles. Duchenne muscular dystrophy (DMD), or pseudohypertrophic muscular dystrophy, is the most severe and the most common muscular dystrophy of childhood; the muscles initially affected primarily involve the shoulders and legs, whereas later the respiratory, oropharyngeal, and facial muscles are affected. Becker muscular dystrophy is similar to DMD, but the onset of symptoms occurs later and severity is less than observed in DMD.

Pathophysiology
At the genetic level, both DMD and Becker MD result from mutations of the gene that encodes dystrophin, a protein product in skeletal muscle. Dystrophin is absent from the muscle of children

with DMD and is reduced or abnormal in children with Becker MD. Pseudohypertrophy is muscular enlargement caused by fatty infiltration. Profound muscular atrophy occurs in later stages, and as the disease progresses, contractures and deformities involving large and small joints are common complications. Ambulation usually becomes impossible by 12 years of age. Ultimately the disease process involves the diaphragm and auxiliary muscles of respiration, and cardiovascular involvement (cardiomyopathy, dysrhythmias, and heart failure) is common.

Clinical Signs and Symptoms
Duchenne Muscular Dystrophy
- Relentless progression of muscle weakness; possible death from respiratory or cardiac failure
- Waddling gait
- Lordosis
- Frequent falls
- *Gower sign* (child turns onto side or abdomen, flexes knees to assume a kneeling position, then with knees extended gradually pushes torso to an upright position by "walking" the hands up the legs)
- Enlarged (hypertrophied) muscles (especially calves, thighs, and upper arms)
  - Feel unusually firm or woody on palpation
  - Later stages: profound muscular atrophy
- Mental deficit present in 25% to 30% of patients
- Complications
  - Contracture deformities of hips, knees, and ankles
  - Disuse atrophy
  - Cardiomyopathy
  - Obesity, and at times undernutrition
  - Respiratory compromise and cardiac failure

Diagnostic Evaluation
- DNA analysis (molecular genetic diagnosis) of peripheral blood or tissue cells obtained by muscle biopsy
- Electromyography (EMG)
- Muscle biopsy in some cases (unless child has diagnosed brother and typical features of DMD)
- Serum CK levels extremely high

Treatment
- Supportive
- Prevent muscle contractures and maintain muscle function; orthoses; physical therapy.
- Medication: corticosteroids
- Respiratory support: noninvasive mechanical ventilation (Bi-PAP); removal of secretions
- Prevention of URIs; immunizations
- Assess for complication such as cardiomyopathy.

Nursing Care Management
- Assist with diagnostic evaluation.
- Support child and family at time of diagnosis.
- Promote ADLs and optimal development.
- Prevent muscle contractures: physical therapy; range of motion.
- Promote optimal nutrition and encourage exercise.
- Promote mobilization with orthoses and wheelchair as applicable.
- Involve parents in support group; locate and identify resources for assistance with child with chronic and terminal illness.

Patient and Family Teaching
- Respiratory care; noninvasive mechanical ventilation management and secretions removal; prevention of URIs; childhood immunizations including influenza and pneumococcal
- Prevention of muscle contractures; exercises; orthoses
- Involvement in ADLs
- Support child with chronic and often terminal illness; child may have anger in adolescence as a result of helplessness and prognosis.
- Medication administration and observation for complications

NASOPHARYNGITIS, ACUTE VIRAL
Description
Acute nasopharyngitis or the equivalent of the "common cold" is caused by the rhinovirus, RSV, adenovirus, influenza virus, and the parainfluenza virus. Symptoms are more severe in infants and children than in adults.

Pathophysiology

Viral agents are easily spread among young children when they cough and sneeze when close to each other. Young children often lack immunity to the viruses that cause nasopharyngitis. Nasal inflammation may lead to obstruction of passages, producing open-mouth breathing. In infants, this often causes a decrease in oral intake when the infant is in a semi-reclining position. The body reacts to the viral infection by increasing the body temperature, and thus a fever. Neonates and younger infants may not be able to mount an immune response and therefore may only have a low grade fever if at all. Nasal discharge is caused by the body's response to the virus; postnasal discharge often causes a cough. Otitis media may ocur secondary to the cold in infants. The disease is self-limited and usually resolves within 4 to 10 days.

Clinical Signs and Symptoms
- Nasal congestion and discharge
- Watery, itchy eyes
- Cough
- Fever
- Sore throat
- Malaise
- Vomiting and diarrhea
- Muscle aches
- Anorexia
- Dry, scratchy throat

Diagnostic Evaluation

Diagnosis is based on clinical symptoms.

Treatment
- Primarily symptomatic. There are no specific medications to "treat" a cold, especially in young infants and toddlers.
- Medication: for fever (acetaminophen); possibly decongestants for children over 6 months to shrink swollen nasal passages
- Cough suppressants containing dextromethorphan for a dry, hacking cough in children over 2 years of age; however, most literature suggests this does not help children and may be harmful.

- Nasal saline irrigation in small infants and toddlers who are unable to blow nose and expel mucous
- Rest and oral fluids are encouraged.

Nursing Care Management
- Medication administration
- Assist family in managing child's symptoms.
- Emotional support

Patient and Family Teaching
- Primary prevention: avoiding children with colds; discarding tissues; covering mouth when coughing or sneezing; avoiding taking sick child to church, school, daycare and other areas where there are children and elderly who may catch the cold
- Handwashing; avoiding placing hands to mouth, eyes, and nose
- Medication administration
- Comfort measures: rest, quiet activities, nasal saline irrigation in infants before feeding and sleeping
- Cool-mist vaporizer may provide some relief from dry mucous membranes.

NEPHROTIC SYNDROME
Description
Nephrotic syndrome is a clinical state that includes massive proteinuria, hypoalbuminemia, hyperlipidemia, and edema. The disorder can occur as (1) a primary disease known as *idiopathic nephrosis, childhood nephrosis*, or *minimal-change nephrotic syndrome (MCNS)*; (2) a secondary disorder that occurs as a clinical manifestation after or in association with glomerular damage of known or presumed etiology; or (3) a congenital form inherited as an autosomal recessive disorder.

Pathophysiology
There may be a metabolic, biochemical, physiochemical, or immune-mediated disturbance that causes the basement membrane of the glomeruli to become increasingly permeable to protein, but the cause and mechanisms are only speculative. The glomerular membrane, normally impermeable to albumin and other proteins, becomes permeable to proteins, especially albumin, which

leak through the membrane and are lost in urine (**hyperalbumin-uria**). This reduces the serum albumin level (**hypoalbuminemia**), decreasing the colloidal osmotic pressure in the capillaries. As a result, the vascular hydrostatic pressure exceeds the pull of the colloidal osmotic pressure, causing fluid to accumulate in the interstitial spaces (**edema**) and body cavities, particularly in the abdominal cavity (**ascites**). The shift of fluid from the plasma to the interstitial spaces reduces the vascular fluid volume (**hypo-volemia**), which in turn stimulates the renin-angiotensin system and the secretion of antidiuretic hormone and aldosterone. Tubular reabsorption of sodium and water is increased in an attempt to increase intravascular volume. The elevation of serum lipids is not fully understood.

Clinical Signs and Symptoms
- Periorbital, gonadal, or lower extremity edema
- Weight gain over that expected based on previous pattern
- Decreased urine output
- Pallor, fatigue

Diagnostic Evaluation
- The diagnosis of MCNS is suspected on the basis of the history and clinical manifestations (edema, proteinuria, hypoalbuminemia, and hypercholesterolemia in the absence of hematuria and hypertension) in children between the ages of 2 and 8 years.
- The hallmark of MCNS is massive proteinuria (higher than 3+ on urine dipstick). Hyaline casts, oval fat bodies, and a few red blood cells can be found in the urine of some affected children, although there is seldom gross hematuria.
- Total serum protein concentration is low, with the serum albumin significantly reduced and plasma lipids elevated.
- Hemoglobin and hematocrit are usually normal or elevated as a result of hemoconcentration. The platelet count may be elevated.
- Serum sodium concentration may be low.
- If the patient does not respond to a 4- to 8-week course of steroids, a renal biopsy may be needed to distinguish between other types of nephrotic syndrome. The biopsy results of children with MCNS are remarkable for effacement of the foot

processes of the epithelial cells lining the basement membrane, but otherwise the kidney tissue is normal.

Treatment

- Treatment includes (1) reducing excretion of urinary protein, (2) reducing fluid retention in the tissues, (3) preventing infection, and (4) minimizing complications related to therapies.
- Corticosteroids are the first line of therapy. The starting dose for prednisone is usually 2 mg/kg body weight per day, in one or more divided doses. In most children this response occurs within 7 to 21 days. The medication is then tapered over a period of several months and eventually stopped if the child remains asymptomatic.
- Dietary restrictions include a low-salt diet and, in more severe cases, fluid restriction.
- If complications of edema develop, diuretic therapy may be initiated to provide temporary relief from edema.
- Sometimes infusions of 25% albumin are used.
- Acute infections are treated with appropriate antibiotics.

Nursing Care Management

- Monitor fluid retention or excretion by maintaining strict intake and output.
- Other methods of monitoring progress include urine examination for albumin, daily weight, and measurement of abdominal girth.
- Assess for edema (e.g., increased or decreased swelling around the eyes and dependent areas), the degree of pitting, and the color and texture of skin.
- Monitor vital signs to detect any early signs of complications such as shock or an infective process.
- Infection is a constant source of danger to edematous children and those on corticosteroids. Children are vulnerable to upper respiratory infection; they must be kept warm and dry, active, and protected from contact with infected individuals (i.e., roommates, visitors, and personnel).
- Consult with dietitian, parents, and the child to formulate a nutritionally adequate and attractive diet.
- Salt is usually restricted (but not eliminated) during the edema phase and while on steroid therapy. Fluid restriction (if prescribed) is limited to short-term use during massive edema.

Patient and Family Teaching
- Parents are taught to detect signs of relapse and to call for changes in treatment at the earliest indications (edema, weight gain, fatigue, decreased urine output and pallor).
- Teach parents to test urine for albumin, administer medications, and to provide general care.
- Stress importance of avoiding contact with infected playmates; however, allow the child to attend school.

NEURAL TUBE DEFECTS (SPINA BIFIDA, MENINGOCELE, MYELOMENINGOCELE)
Description
Neural tube defects include defects of the spinal cord that occur as a result of failure of neural tube closure in embryonic development. They may involve the entire length of the neural tube or may be restricted to a small area. Defects involving failure of the osseous (bony) spine to close are called *spina bifida (SB)*; SB occulta occurs in lumbosacral area (L5 and S1), and there is no obvious external opening; SB cystica refers to a visible defect with an external saclike protrusion. The two major forms of SB cystica are meningocele, which encases meninges and spinal fluid but no neural elements and myelomeningocele (or meningomyelocele), which contains meninges, spinal fluid, and nerves. Meningocele is not associated with neurologic deficit, which occurs in varying degrees in myelomeningocele. With myelomeningocele, the degree of neurologic dysfunction depends on where the sac protrudes through the vertebrae, the anatomic level of the defect, and the amount of nerve tissue involved. Most myelomeningoceles involve the lumbar or lumbosacral area. Hydrocephalus is a frequently associated anomaly in 80% to 90% of children.

Pathophysiology
Most authorities believe that the primary defect in NTDs is a failure of neural tube closure during early development (the first 3 to 5 weeks) of the embryo. There is evidence implicating a multifactorial etiology including drugs, radiation, maternal malnutrition, chemicals, and possibly a genetic mutation in folate pathways in some cases, which may result in abnormal development. A genetic component in the development of SB is seen in some cases; myelomeningocele may occur in association with syndromes such as

trisomy 18, PHAVER syndrome and Meckel-Gruber syndrome. Myelomeningocele may result in musculoskeletal problems of the lower extremities affecting ambulation; in addition, neurologic deficits may be evident in bowel and bladder function. Cognitive function is normal in such children.

Clinical Signs and Symptoms
- SB occulta: no defect noted except by palpation of vertebra
- Meningocele: visible evidence of protruding sac on spinal cord (lumbar)
- Myelomeningocele: visible sac protruding on lumbar or lumbosacral area

Diagnostic Evaluation
- MRI, CT scan, and myelography
- Bladder function studies may be performed.

Treatment
- Meningocele and myelomeningocele: protection of sac; moist saline gauze; avoid laying on sac; early surgical closure in most cases
- Evaluation of lower extremity involvement, urinary function, bowel function and interventions to preserve function, enhance mobilization, and prevent complications
- Long-term care involves promotion of optimal functioning in regards to ambulation and mobilization, and urinary and bowel continence.
- Physical therapy

Nursing Care Management
- Focused on myelomeningocele
- Identification of defect
- Protect sac: moist saline gauze; avoid laying on sac.
- Assist parents and support; encourage close contact; explain treatments.
- Pre- and postoperative care; monitoring vital signs; protection and care of incision; prevent infection.
- Routine newborn care: temperature maintenance; may be fed postoperatively
- Observe for development of hydrocephalus postoperatively: increasing head circumference.

■ Physical therapy to prevent lower extremity contractures and muscle atrophy
■ Observe for complications such as urinary stasis and UTI; perianal skin care for stool incontinence.
■ Discharge teaching

Patient and Family Teaching
■ Holding and feeding (postop)
■ Newborn care
■ Observation for complications: urinary stasis (may require clean intermittent catheterization at home); head circumference growth; poor feeding; perianal skin care for loose stools
■ Encourage follow-up visits with specialists (urologist, orthopedist, neurosurgeon, primary practitioner).
■ Access to multidisciplinary team (spina bifida clinic) as applicable to promote optimal development

NEUROBLASTOMA
Description
Neuroloblastoma is a malignant tumor that develops from neural crest cells.

Pathophysiology
These tumors originate from embryonic neural crest cells that normally give rise to the adrenal medulla and the sympathetic nervous system. Consequently, the majority of the tumors arise from the adrenal gland or from the retroperitoneal sympathetic chain. Therefore, the primary site is within the abdomen. Other sites may be within the head, neck, chest, or pelvis.

Clinical Signs and Symptoms
■ Most presenting signs are caused by compression of adjacent structures.
■ With abdominal tumors, the most common presenting sign is a firm, nontender, irregular mass in the abdomen that crosses the midline.
■ Compression of the kidney, ureter, or bladder may cause urinary frequency or retention.

- Distant metastasis frequently causes supraorbital ecchymosis, periorbital edema, and proptosis (exophthalmos) from invasion of retrobulbar soft tissue.
- Lymphadenopathy, especially in the cervical and supraclavicular areas, may also be an early presenting sign.
- Bone pain may or may not be present with skeletal involvement.
- Vague symptoms of widespread metastasis include pallor, weakness, irritability, anorexia, and weight loss.

Diagnostic Evaluation
- Skeletal survey; skull, neck, chest, abdominal, bone scan; CT scans
- Bilateral bone marrow aspirate and biopsies
- Neuroblastomas, particularly those arising on the adrenal glands or from a sympathetic chain, excrete the catecholamines epinephrine and norepinephrine. Urinary excretion of catecholamines is detected in approximately 95% of children with adrenal or sympathetic tumors. Analyzing the breakdown products that are normally excreted in the urine, namely, vanillylmandelic acid (VMA), homovanillic acid (HVA), dopamine, and norepinephrine, permits detection of a suspected tumor both before and after medical/surgical intervention.
- Amplification of the N-myc gene and abnormalities in chromosomes are associated with a poorer prognosis.
- Increased ferritin, neuron-specific enolase (NSE), and ganglioside (GD2) are associated with neuroblastoma.

Treatment
Accurate clinical staging is important for establishing initial treatment. Therefore, surgery is employed both to remove as much of the tumor as possible and to obtain biopsies. In stages I and II, complete surgical removal of the tumor is the treatment of choice. If the tumors are large, partial resection is attempted, with a course of irradiation postoperatively to shrink the tumor in the hope of complete removal at a later date. Surgery is usually limited to biopsy in stages III and IV because of the extensive metastasis, although the use of additional surgery to assess tumor regression or remove a regressed tumor is not unlikely.

The precise role of radiotherapy is unclear. It does not appear to be of any benefit in children with stage I and II disease; it is commonly used with stage III disease, although it may not improve survival expectancy, and it may make a large tumor operable. Radiotherapy provides emergency management of a massive neuroblastoma causing spinal cord compression. It also offers palliation for metastatic lesions in bones, lungs, liver, or brain. Chemotherapy is the mainstay of therapy for extensive local or disseminated disease.

Neuroblastoma is a "silent" tumor. Diagnosis is often made after metastasis occurs, with the first signs caused by involvement in the nonprimary site, usually the lymph nodes, bone marrow, skeletal system, skin, or liver. Because of the frequency of invasiveness, the prognosis for neuroblastoma is poor.

Nursing Care Management

Because this tumor carries a poor prognosis for many children, every consideration must be given to the family in terms of coping with a life-threatening illness. Because of the high degree of metastasis at the time of diagnosis, many parents suffer much guilt for not having recognized signs earlier. Often the guilt is expressed as anger toward professionals for not diagnosing it sooner. Parents need much support in dealing with these feelings and expressing them to the appropriate people.

Nursing care for the child with neuroblastoma involves (1) preparing the child and family for diagnostic and operative procedures, (2) administering therapy, (3) managing treatment side effects, (4) monitoring to prevent complications related to leukemia and treatment, (5) educating the child and family, and (6) providing child and family support.

Prepare the Child and Family for Diagnostic and Operative Procedures

- Once a diagnosis of neuroblastoma is suspected, a battery of diagnostic tests is ordered. The family needs an explanation of why each test is performed because many of them, such as bone marrow aspiration and biopsy, are invasive procedures.
- Appropriate preparation for the child prior to the invasive procedure is dependent upon the child's age and development. Use simple words to describe procedures, and answer all questions the child and family may have.

Administer Therapy
- Review child's history related to previous tolerance to therapy.
- Determine appropriate premedication prior to therapy.
- Be aware of drug-specific interactions.
- Assess the child's laboratory findings prior to therapy administration.
- Ensure that the chemotherapy doses are correct by checking orders according to the institution's policies and procedures.
- Follow the guidelines for chemotherapy administration.
- If the treatment is given intravenously, observe the IV site for signs of irritation or infiltration.
- Follow the institution's policy for safe handling chemotherapy wastes, including the patient's bodily fluids.
- Observe the child for signs of reaction during and following treatment.

Manage Common Side Effects of Cancer Treatment
- Assess for toxicities specific to the cancer treatment.
- Monitor for signs of infection, and obtain cultures and initiate antibiotics if indicated.
- Monitor nutrition and weight changes and alternative methods of nutrition if appropriate.
- Monitor fluid and electrolytes.
- Evaluate child's response to treatment.
- Manage central line care.

Monitor for Complications Related to Neuroblastoma and Treatment
- Assess for symptoms related to neuroblastoma and treatment.
- Review laboratory findings.
- Obtain a complete history evaluating the incidence and duration of symptoms.
- Perform a complete physical examination; assess for fever, night sweats, weight loss, pallor, signs of infection, lymphadenopathy.

Patient and Family Teaching
Educate the Child and Family
- Assess child's and family's level of knowledge regarding the neuroblastoma and treatment.

- Assess child's and family's understanding of what they have heard about neuroblastoma and treatment.
- Explain that chemotherapeutic reactions vary with the specific drug regimen. Explain that the most common side effects from chemotherapy include nausea and vomiting, body image changes, neuropathy, and mucosal ulceration.
- If the child is to receive radiation therapy, review the common side effects associated with radiation therapy and precautions that should be followed during treatment.
- Educate the family regarding neutropenia, anemia, and thrombocytopenia, the signs and symptoms of infection, and fever precautions.
- Provide appropriate educational resources, and review materials with them.
- Clarify information presented by the health care team.

Provide Support for the Child and Family
- Communicate with the child and family in an appropriate style.
- Provide the child and family with honest answers.
- Provide emotional support.
- Offer age-appropriate interventions.
- Provide information on available resources for support for the child and family.

NON-HODGKIN LYMPHOMA
Description
Non-Hodgkin lymphoma (NHL) is a neoplastic disease that arises from the lymphoid and hemopoietic systems. Most pediatric lymphomas are classified as NHL.

Pathophysiology
NHL is heterogeneous, exhibiting a variety of morphologic, cytochemical, and immunologic features, not unlike the diversity seen in leukemia. Classification is based on the pattern of histologic presentation: (1) lymphoblastic, (2) Burkitt or non-Burkitt, or (3) large cell (Reiter and others, 1995). Immunologically these cells are also classified as T-cells, B-cells (an example of which is Burkitt lymphoma), or non-T–non-B–cells, which lack specific immunologic properties.

Clinical Signs and Symptoms

▪ Clinical signs and symptoms depend on the anatomic site and extent of involvement.

▪ Metastasis to the bone marrow or central nervous system may produce signs and symptoms typical of leukemia.

▪ Lymphoid tumors compressing various organs may cause intestinal or airway obstruction, cranial nerve palsies, or spinal paralysis.

▪ The exception to the usual presentation of NHL is Burkitt's lymphoma, a type of cancer that is rare in the United States but endemic in parts of Africa. It is a rapidly growing neoplasm that is most commonly seen as a mass in the jaw, abdomen, or orbit.

Diagnostic Evaluation

▪ Surgical biopsy for histopathologic confirmation of disease with immunophenotyping and cytogenetic evaluation

▪ Bone marrow aspiration and biopsy

▪ Radiologic studies, especially CT scans of the lungs and gastrointestinal organs

▪ Lumbar puncture

A favorable prognosis is defined by:

▪ Lymph node involvement only and limited to one or two adjacent lymphatic regions (excluding the mediastinum)

▪ An extranodal site in the nasopharynx, oropharynx, or other isolated extranodal site, with or without regional lymphadenopathy

▪ Gastrointestinal involvement, with or without regional lymphadenopathy, limited to the mesentery

Treatment

The present treatment protocols for NHL include an aggressive approach using irradiation and chemotherapy. Similar to leukemic therapy, the protocols include induction, consolidation, and maintenance phases, some with intrathecal chemotherapy. At present, the differentiation between lymphoblastic lymphoma and all other lymphomas is widely used as a way to categorize patients for specific treatment regimens.

Nursing Care Management and Patient and Family Teaching

Nursing care of the child with NHL and patient and family teaching is very similar to the care discussed in the care of the child with leukemia (p. 243). Because of the intensive chemotherapy protocol, nursing care is primarily directed toward managing the side effects of these agents.

OMPHALOCELE AND GASTROSCHISIS
Description

Omphalocele: Protrusion of intraabdominal viscera into base of umbilical cord; sac is covered with peritoneum without skin. Omphalocele often is associated with other anomalies, including cardiac, neurologic, skeletal, and GU anomalies; imperforate anus; ileal atresia; and bladder exstrophy. Omphalocele is also associated with trisomies 13, 18, and 21 (Down syndrome).

Gastroschisis: Protrusion of intra-abdominal contents through defect in abdominal wall lateral to umbilical ring; there is no peritoneal sac.

Pathophysiology

Omphalocele is related to a true failure of embryonic development. It occurs when there is failure of the caudal or lateral infolding of the abdominal wall at approximately the third week of gestation. With the deficiency in the abdominal wall, the bowel is unable to complete its return to the abdomen between the tenth and twelfth week of gestation.

Controversy exists regarding the etiology of gastroschisis. It has been suggested that at some point between the bowel's stay in the umbilical cord and the completion of fixation, a tear occurs at the base of the umbilical cord, allowing the intestine to herniate. The gap between the cord and the tear is filled in by skin, giving the appearance of a defect in the abdominal wall to the right of the umbilical cord. The base of the defect is narrow, and the lack of membranes results in thickening and foreshortening of the bowel. Gastroschisis is usually not associated with other major congenital anomalies; however, jejunoileal atresia, ischemic enteritis, and malrotation may occur as a result of the defect itself.

Clinical Signs and Symptoms

- Obvious abdominal wall defect noted on visual inspection
- Omphalocele may appear to be a large hematoma in umbilical cord in some cases.

Diagnostic Evaluation
- Visual inspection of defect

Treatment
Omphalocele
- Cover the exposed abdominal contents and membranes with a bowel bag or saline-soaked pads and a plastic drape to prevent excessive fluid loss, drying, and temperature instability.
- IV fluids and antibiotics are administered, and a further evaluation for other associated anomalies is completed.
- Placement of a Silastic double-lumen catheter (NG-OG) is performed to accomplish gastric bowel decompression.
- Surgical repair involves replacement of bowel in abdominal cavity; may be delayed to allow increased weight gain or may be performed in early neonatal period; a staged repair may be necessary.

Gastroschisis
- Same as for omphalocele; prevent drying of exposed bowel; prevent compression and necrosis of exposed bowel; staged silo may be used if bowel does not fit into abdominal cavity.
- Requires close management of fluid and electrolytes as fluids are easily lost through unprotected bowel; third spacing may occur.

Nursing Care Management
- Essentially same for both defects with some minor differences depending on size of defect and bowel function pre- and postoperatively
- Identification of defect at birth (although prenatal US may identify defect before birth)
- Protection of exposed bowel or viscera with moist saline dressing or bowel bag
- Maintain fluid and electrolyte balance; IV access; NPO.
- Bowel decompression
- Temperature regulation for neonate
- Explain defect to parents; encourage and allow parent contact.
- Pre- and postoperative care including monitoring vital signs, pain management, bowel decompression, observation for complications; monitor return of bowel function.

- Incision care postoperatively
- Provide parental support.
- Individualized developmental care

Patient and Family Teaching
Discharge Teaching
- Feeding after surgical repair; gastrostomy may be required in some cases; gastrostomy feedings
- Encouraging care of neonate in acute care center and discussion of special feeding needs at home (as applicable)

OSTEOGENESIS IMPERFECTA
Description
Osteogenesis imperfecta (OI) is a heterogeneous, autosomal dominant disorder characterized by fractures and bone deformity. There are at least five types of OI, which accounts for significant disease variability.

Pathophysiology
Most types of OI have defects in the COL1A1 or COL1A2 genes, which code for polypeptide chains in type 1 procollagen, a precursor of type 1 collagen, a major structural component of bone. The error results in faulty bone mineralization, abnormal bone architecture, and increased susceptibility to fracture. Inheritance follows an autosomal dominant pattern in most cases; rare autosomal recessive inheritance exists.

Clinical Signs and Symptoms
- Varying degrees of bone fragility, deformity, and fracture
- Blue sclerae
- Hearing loss
- Dentinogenesis imperfecta (hypoplastic discolored teeth)

Diagnostic Evaluation
OI is a differential diagnosis that must be ruled out in the event of multiple fractures that may be attributed to nonaccidental injury. A detailed history, no evidence of associated soft-tissue injury, and the presence of other symptoms related to OI help to determine the diagnosis.

Treatment
- Primarily supportive
- Bone marrow transplant (considered experimental)
- Bisphosphonate therapy with intravenous pamidronate to promote increased bone density and prevent fractures
- Lightweight braces and splints help support limbs, prevent fractures, and aid in ambulation.
- Physical therapy to prevent disuse osteoporosis and strengthen muscles
- Surgical: correction of orthopedic deformities that prevent bracing, standing, or walking; at times, insertion of intramedullary rod to provide stability to bones
- Genetic counseling

Nursing Care Management
- Careful handling to prevent fractures
- Helping family plan care for the child's activities
- Medication administration
- Pre- and postoperative nursing care
- Physical therapy
- Skin care

Patient and Family Teaching
- Planning suitable activities that promote optimal development and protect the child from harm
- Care of braces, splints; skin care
- Medication administration
- Realistic occupational planning and genetic counseling
- Medical evaluations and follow-up visits; physical therapy

OSTEOGENIC SARCOMA
Description
Osteogenic sarcoma (osteosarcoma) is the most common bone cancer in children. Its peak incidence is between 10 and 25 years of age.

Pathophysiology
It presumably arises from bone-forming mesenchyme, which gives rise to malignant osteoid tissue. Most primary tumor sites are in the metaphysis (wider part of the shaft, adjacent to the epiphyseal

growth plate) of long bones, especially in the lower extremities. More than half occur in the femur, particularly the distal portion, with the rest involving the humerus, tibia, pelvis, jaw, and phalanges.

Clinical Signs and Symptoms

■ Most malignant bone tumors produce localized pain in the affected site, which may be severe or dull and may be attributed to trauma or the vague complaint of "growing pains."

■ Bone pain is often relieved by a flexed position, which relaxes the muscles overlying the stretched periosteum. Frequently it draws attention when the child limps, curtails physical activity, or is unable to hold heavy objects.

Diagnostic Evaluation

■ Definitive diagnosis is based on radiologic studies, such as CT to determine the extent of the lesion.

■ MRI to assess soft tissue, tumor boundaries, nerve and vessel involvement; radioisotope bone scans to evaluate metastasis; and either needle or surgical bone biopsy to determine the histologic pattern.

■ Radiologic findings are characteristic for each type of tumor. In osteogenic sarcoma, needlelike new bone formation growing at right angles to the diaphysis (shaft) produces a "sunburst" appearance.

■ At present, there is no reliable biochemical test for bone cancers. Elevated alkaline phosphatase levels may occur in osteoid tumors.

■ Lung tomography is usually a standard procedure, because pulmonary metastasis is the most common complication of primary bone tumors.

Treatment

Optimum treatment of osteosarcoma is surgery and chemotherapy. The surgical approach consists of surgical biopsy followed by either limb salvage or amputation. Depending on the tumor site, surgery includes amputation of the affected extremity at least 7.5 cm (3 inches) above the proximal tumor margin or above the joint proximal to the involved bone. With tumors of the distal femur, preservation of the hip joint may be possible. Other procedures include an above-the-knee amputation for tumors of the tibia or fibula, a hemipelvectomy for tumors of the innominate (hip) bone, and a forequarter amputation (removal of arm, scapula, and portion of the clavicle on the affected side) for tumors of the upper humerus. The other surgical approach for selected patients is the limb salvage procedure, which involves en bloc resection of the primary tumor with prosthetic replacement of the involved bone. For example, with osteosarcoma of the distal femur, a total femur and joint replacement is performed. Frequently children undergoing a limb salvage procedure will receive preoperative chemotherapy in an attempt to decrease the tumor size and make surgery more manageable.

Chemotherapy plays a vital role in treatment of osteosarcoma. When pulmonary metastasis is found, thoracotomy and chemotherapy have resulted in prolonged survival and potential cure.

Nursing Care Management

- Preparing the child and family for diagnostic and operative procedures
- Administering therapy
- Managing treatment side effects
- Monitoring to prevent complications related to osteogenic sarcoma and treatment
- Educating the child and family
- Providing child and family support

Prepare the Child and Family for Diagnostic and Operative Procedures

- Nursing care depends on the type of surgical approach. Obviously the family may have more difficulty adjusting to an amputation than a limb salvage procedure. In either instance, preparation of the child and family is critical. Straightforward honesty is essential in gaining the cooperation and trust of the child. The diagnosis of cancer should not be disguised with falsehoods such as "infection." To accept the need for radical surgery, the child must be aware of the lack of alternatives for treatment.
- Sometimes children have many questions about the prosthesis, limitations on physical ability, and prognosis in terms of cure. At other times, they react with silence or with a calm manner that belies their concern and fear. Either response must be accepted, because it is part of the grieving process of a loss.

- If an amputation is performed, the child is usually fitted with a temporary prosthesis immediately after surgery, which permits early functioning and fosters psychologic adjustment. If this is not done, the child requires stump care, which is the same as for any amputee. A permanent prosthesis is usually fitted within 6 to 8 weeks. During hospitalization the child begins physical therapy to become proficient in the use and care of the device.
- Phantom limb pain may develop following amputation. This symptom is characterized by sensations such as tingling, itching and, more frequently, pain felt in the amputated limb. The child and family need to know that the sensations are real, not imagined. Amitriptyline (Elavil) has been used successfully in children to decrease the pain.

Administer Therapy
- Review child's history related to previous tolerance to therapy.
- Determine appropriate premedication prior to therapy.
- Be aware of drug-specific interactions.
- Assess the child's laboratory findings prior to therapy administration.
- Ensure that the chemotherapy doses are correct by checking orders according to the institution's policies and procedures.
- Follow the guidelines for chemotherapy administration.
- If the treatment is given intravenously, observe the IV site for signs of irritation or infiltration.
- Follow the institution's policy for safe handling chemotherapy wastes, including the patient's bodily fluids.
- Observe the child for signs of reaction during and following treatment.

Manage Common Side Effects of Cancer Treatment
- Assess for toxicities specific to the cancer treatment.
- Monitor for signs of infection, and obtain cultures and initiate antibiotics if indicated.
- Monitor nutrition and weight changes and alternative methods of nutrition if appropriate.
- Monitor fluid and electrolytes.
- Evaluate child's response to treatment.
- Manage central line care.

Monitor for Complications Related to Osteogenic Sarcoma and Treatment
- Assess for symptoms related to osteogenic sarcoma and treatment.
- Review laboratory findings.
- Obtain a complete history evaluating the incidence and duration of symptoms.
- Perform a complete physical examination; assess for fever, fatigue, pallor, signs of infection.

Patient and Family Teaching
Educate the Child and Family
- Assess child's and family's level of knowledge regarding the osteogenic sarcoma and treatment.
- Assess child's and family's understanding of what they have heard about osteogenic sarcoma and treatment.
- Explain that chemotherapeutic reactions vary with the specific drug regimen. Explain that the most common side effects from chemotherapy include nausea and vomiting, body image changes, neuropathy, and mucosal ulceration.
- Educate the family regarding neutropenia, anemia, and thrombocytopenia, the signs and symptoms of infection, and fever precautions.
- Provide appropriate educational resources, and review materials with them.
- Clarify information presented by the health care team.

Provide Support for the Child and Family
- Communicate with the child and family in an appropriate style.
- Provide the child and family with honest answers.
- Provide emotional support.
- Offer age-appropriate interventions.
- Provide information on available resources for support for the child and family.

OSTEOMYELITIS
Description
Osteomyelitis, an infectious process in the bone, can occur at any age but most frequently is seen in children 10 years of age or younger. *S. aureus* is the most common causative organism.

Pathophysiology

Osteomyelitis can be acquired exogenously by direct inoculation of bone during trauma, puncture, or surgery; the hand and foot are common sites. Hematogenous osteomyelitis is seeded by organisms from a preexisting infection such as tonsillitis or impetigo or from a contiguous source such as an adjacent infected bone or joint. Hematogenous osteomyelitis usually occurs in the metaphyses of long bones, the femur, or tibia. The infecting organism travels from the site of infection to the small end-artery capillary loops in the bone metaphyses, causing obstruction and initiating infection, with complications of bone destruction and abscess formation. Most cases involve the femur or tibia. Generally healthy bone is not likely to become infected. Factors that contribute to infection include inoculation with a large number of organisms, presence of a foreign body, bone injury, high virulence of an organism, immunosuppression, and malnutrition; certain types and locations of bone are also more vulnerable to infection.

Clinical Signs and Symptoms
General
- History of trauma to affected bone (frequent)
- Child appears very ill.
- Irritability
- Restlessness
- Elevated temperature
- Rapid pulse
- Dehydration

Local
- Tenderness
- Increased warmth
- Diffuse swelling over involved bone.
- Involved extremity painful, especially on movement
- Involved extremity held in semiflexion
- Surrounding muscles tense and resist passive movement.

Diagnostic Evaluation
- Physical examination of extremity
- Radiograph
- CT, MRI may be helpful.
- Blood cultures

- Aspiration of joint fluid or wound tissue
- In some cases, bone biopsy

Treatment
- Long-term IV antibiotics
- Surgical intervention if no response to specific antibiotic therapy, persistent soft tissue abscess is seen, or the infection spreads to the joint

Nursing Care Management
- Assist with diagnostic evaluation.
- Comfort—pain management; positioning
- Child and family support
- Keep family informed of treatment plan.
- Medication administration
- Wound care as applicable; handwashing, standard precautions

Patient and Family Teaching
- Comfort measures; pain management; positioning
- Wound care and prevention of infection; handwashing
- Medication administration: Parents may have to administer the antibiotics in the home.
- Importance of follow-up medical care

OTITIS EXTERNA
Description
Otitis externa (or swimmer's ear) is an infection of the external ear that results from normal ear flora (*Staphylococcus epidermidis* and *Corynebacterium* organisms) that assume pathogenic characteristics under certain conditions, primarily excessive wetness or dryness.

Pathophysiology
Ordinarily the external ear canal is protected by a waxy, water-repellent coating composed of highly viscid secretions of the sebaceous glands and the watery, pigmented secretions of apocrine glands in combination with exfoliated surface cells. Inflammation occurs when this environment is altered by swimming, bathing, or increased environmental humidity; by infection, dermatoses, or insufficient cerumen; or by trauma from a foreign body (FB) or a finger. Secondary invasion of foreign pathogens may also occur; the offending agents can be *Pseudomonas aeruginosa* (most common),

Enterobacter aerogenes, Proteus mirabilis, Klebsiella pneumoniae, streptococci, and fungi such as *Candida* and *Aspergillus* organisms. The ear canal becomes irritated, and maceration takes place.

Clinical Signs and Symptoms
- Ear pain accentuated by manipulation of the pinna, especially pressure on the tragus
- Conductive hearing loss as a result of the edema, secretions, and accumulation of debris within the canal
- Edema, erythema, a cheesy green-blue-gray discharge, and tenderness as the infection progresses
- External canal may be so tender and swollen that visualization is difficult.
- Fever
- Jaw pain with advanced cases

Diagnostic Evaluation
- Diagnosis is made by visualization of external ear.

Treatment
- Analgesics for pain
- Otic preparations containing neomycin with either colistin or polymyxin and corticosteroids are instilled in the canal.
- Gauze wick may be inserted if edema is present to facilitate the medication reaching the site of inflammation.
- Removal of debris with gentle suction

Nursing Care Management
- Medication administration
- At times, removal of ear debris
- Child and parent teaching

Patient and Family Teaching
- Keeping ear dry: Limit their stay in the water to less than an hour, if possible, and ears should dry completely (1 to 2 hours) before entering the water again.
- Place a combination of white vinegar and rubbing alcohol (50:50) in both ear canals on arising, at bedtime, and at the end of each swim to prevent recurrence.
- A 2% acetic acid solution may also be used.

- Avoid picking at the ears with a pencil, cotton swab, bobby pin, or other object, which can injure or infect the ear canal.

OTITIS MEDIA
Description
Otitis media (OM) is an inflammation of the middle ear without reference to etiology or pathogenesis. The incidence of OM is highest in the winter months; bacterial otitis media is often preceded by a viral respiratory infection. Viruses most likely to precipitate otitis media are respiratory syncytial virus and influenza. Acute otitis media (AOM) is an inflammation of the middle ear space with a rapid onset of the signs and symptoms of acute infection, namely, fever and otalgia (ear pain). Otitis media with effusion (OME) describes fluid in the middle ear space without symptoms of acute infection.

Pathophysiology
OM is primarily a result of a dysfunctioning Eustachian tube. Mechanical or functional obstruction of the eustachian tube causes accumulation of secretions in the middle ear. Intrinsic obstruction can be caused by infection or allergy; extrinsic obstruction is usually a result of enlarged adenoids or nasopharyngeal tumors. Eustachian tube obstruction results in negative middle ear pressure and, if persistent, produces a transudative middle ear effusion. Drainage is inhibited by sustained negative pressure and impaired ciliary transport within the tube. When the passage is not totally obstructed, contamination of the middle ear can take place by reflux, aspiration, or insufflation during crying, sneezing, nose blowing, and swallowing when the nose is obstructed.

Clinical Signs and Symptoms
- Acute ear pain
- Fever
- Infants may refuse to nurse or bottle feed or may decrease intake.
- Irritability and fussiness

Diagnostic Evaluation
Assessment of tympanic membrane mobility with a pneumatic otoscope reveals purulent, discolored effusion and a bulging or full, opacified, or very reddened immobile membrane. Tympanometry may be used to test TM mobility.

Treatment
- Analgesics for ear pain (acetaminophen and ibuprofen)
- Topical drops with benzocaine
- Antibiotics—oral amoxicillin (first line); second line includes amoxicillin-clavulanate; azithromycin; and cephalosporins such as cefdinir, cefuroxime, and cefpodoxime
- IM ceftriaxone (Rocephin) is used when the causative organism is a highly resistant pneumococcus, or when the parents are noncompliant with the therapy.
- Myringotomy: surgical incision of the eardrum to alleviate the severe pain of AOM
- Tympanostomy: Tube placement and adenoidectomy may be performed to treat recurrent OM.

Nursing Care Management
- Identification of symptoms
- Pain and fever management; medications; instillation of drops (topical anesthetic)
- Parent and child teaching
- Administration of IM antibiotics in some cases
- Providing emotional support to family
- Nursing care of child following myringotomy, tympanostomy tube placement, and adenoidectomy

Patient and Family Teaching
- Avoid risk factors: exposure to secondhand smoke, bottle propping, bedtime milk bottle; avoid known allergens.
- Childhood immunizations to prevent OM
- Anticipatory guidance for hearing testing
- Medication administration: analgesics and antibiotics; stress completion of antibiotics
- Follow-up for evaluation after antibiotics.

PATENT DUCTUS ARTERIOSUS
Description
Failure of the fetal ductus arteriosus (artery connecting the aorta and pulmonary artery) to close within the first weeks of life. The continued patency of this vessel allows blood to flow from the higher-pressure aorta to the lower-pressure pulmonary artery, which causes a left-to-right shunt.

Pathophysiology

The hemodynamic consequences of patent ductus arteriosus (PDA) depend on the size of the ductus and the pulmonary vascular resistance. At birth, the resistance in the pulmonary and systemic circulations is almost identical, so that the resistance in the aorta and pulmonary artery is equalized. As the systemic pressure comes to exceed the pulmonary pressure, blood begins to shunt from the aorta across the duct to the pulmonary artery (left-to-right shunt). The additional blood is recirculated through the lungs and returned to the left atrium and left ventricle. The effect of this altered circulation is increased workload on the left side of the heart, increased pulmonary vascular congestion and possibly resistance, and potentially increased right ventricular pressure and hypertrophy. If the pulmonary and systemic vascular resistance is the same, bidirectional shunting may be present.

Clinical Signs and Symptoms

Patients may be asymptomatic or show signs of CHF (see Box 3-1). There is a characteristic machinery-like murmur. A widened pulse pressure and bounding pulses result from runoff of blood from the aorta to the pulmonary artery. Patients are at risk for bacterial endocarditis and pulmonary vascular obstructive disease in later life from chronic excessive pulmonary blood flow.

Diagnostic Evaluation

See Tables 3-1 and 3-2.

Treatment

- Medical management: Administration of indomethacin (prostaglandin inhibitor) has proved successful in closing a patent ductus in premature infants and some newborns.
- Surgical management: Surgical division or ligation of the patent vessel is performed via a left thoracotomy. In a newer technique, video-assisted thoracoscopic surgery, a thoracoscope and instruments are inserted through three small incisions on the left side of the chest to place a clip on the ductus. The technique is used in some centers and eliminates the need for a thoracotomy, thereby speeding postoperative recovery.

■ Nonsurgical treatment: Coils to occlude the PDA are placed in the catheterization laboratory in many centers. Premature or small infants (with small-diameter femoral arteries) and patients with large or unusual PDAs may require surgery.

Nursing Care Management
Assist in Measures to Assess and Improve Cardiac Function
Monitor Cardiac Function
■ Vital signs monitoring
■ Respiratory assessment
■ Cardiac assessment
   ■ Cardiac output (color, pulses, perfusion, capillary refill, renal function, and neurologic function)
   ■ Heart sounds
■ Keep accurate record of intake and output.
■ Weigh child or infant on same scale at same time of day.
■ Monitor for any difficulty feeding or swallowing after surgery.

Administer Medications
■ Review child's history related to cardiac management.
■ Administer medications on schedule.
■ Assess effectiveness of medications and any side effects noted.
■ Be aware of drug-drug and drug-food interactions.
■ Follow guidelines for medication administration.

Manage Common Side Effects of Cardiac Defects
■ Prevent fatigue during feeding; offer small frequent feedings to infant's or child's tolerance.
■ Organize nursing care to allow child/infant uninterrupted rest.
■ Promote activities that do not cause fatigue.

Provide Support for the Child and Family
■ Communicate with the child and family in an appropriate style.
■ Provide the child and family with honest answers.
■ Provide emotional support.
■ Offer age-appropriate interventions.
■ Provide information on available resources for support for the child and family.

Patient and Family Teaching
Prepare the Child and Family for Diagnostic and Operative Procedures

- Provide explanation of diagnostic tests and why each test is performed because many of them are invasive procedures.
- Prepare the child prior to the invasive procedure. Remember discussion is dependent upon the child's age and development.
- Use simple words or pictures to describe procedures, and answer all questions the child and family may have.
- Postoperative wound care teaching as needed
- Postcardiac catheterization wound care teaching as needed
- Assess and record results of teaching and family's participation in care.

Educate the Child and Family

- Assess child's and family's level of knowledge regarding the PDA.
- Assess child's and family's understanding of what they have heard about PDA.
- Assess child's and family's understanding of the surgery and/or cardiac catheterization.
- Teach the child and/or family at least four characteristics of congestive heart failure that may occur because of the PDA such as:
  - Fatigue after exertion
  - Fast heart rate
  - Fast breathing, shortness of breath, dyspnea
  - Retractions
  - Nasal flaring
  - Cool extremities
  - Diaphoresis
  - Decreased urine output
  - Puffiness (edema)
  - Fussiness
  - Decreased appetite
- Educate child and family about care such as medication preparation and administration.
- Assess child's and family's access to appropriate pharmacy for any special preparation medications.
- Educate child and family about when to notify their physician of any clinical changes.

- Assess and record results and family's participation in care.
- Provide appropriate educational resources, and review materials with them.
- Clarify information presented by the health care team including appointment for follow-up visit.
- Discuss SBE (subacute bacterial endocarditis) prophylaxis with your pediatric cardiologist.

PEDICULOSIS CAPITIS
Description
Pediculosis capitis (head lice) is an infestation of the scalp by *Pediculus humanus capitis,* a common parasite in school-age children.

Pathophysiology
The adult louse lives only about 48 hours when away from a human host, and the lifespan of the average female is 1 month. The female lays her eggs at night at the junction of a hair shaft and close to the skin because the eggs need a warm environment. The **nits,** or eggs, hatch in approximately 7 to 10 days.

Clinical Signs and Symptoms
- Itching is usually the only symptom.
- Common areas involved are the occipital area, behind the ears, and the nape of the neck.
- Scratch marks or inflammatory papules, caused by secondary infection, may also be found on the scalp in the vulnerable areas.

Diagnostic Evaluation
- Diagnosis is made by observation of the white eggs (nits) firmly attached to the hair shafts.
- Lice are small and grayish tan, have no wings, and are visible to the naked eye. The nits, or eggs, appear as tiny whitish oval specks adhering to the hair shaft about ¼ inch from the scalp. The adherent nature of the nits distinguishes them from dandruff, which falls off readily.
- Empty nit cases, indicating hatched lice, are translucent rather than white and are located more than ¼ inch from the scalp.

BOX 3-8

Preventing the Spread and Recurrence of Pediculosis

- Machine-wash all washable clothing, towels, and bed linens in hot water, and dry in a hot dryer for at least 20 minutes. Dry clean nonwashable items.
- Thoroughly vacuum carpets, car seats, pillows, stuffed animals, rugs, mattresses, and upholstered furniture.
- Seal nonwashable items in plastic bags for 14 days if unable to dry clean or vacuum.
- Soak combs, brushes, and hair accessories in lice-killing products for 1 hour or in boiling water for 10 minutes.
- In day care centers, store children's clothing items such as hats and scarves and other headgear in separate cubicles.
- Discourage the sharing of items such as hats, scarves, hair accessories, combs, and brushes among children in group settings such as day care centers.
- Avoid physical contact with infested individuals and their belongings, especially clothing and bedding.
- Inspect children in a group setting regularly for head lice.
- Provide educational programs on the transmission of pediculosis, its detection, and treatment.

Modified from Chin J, ed: *Control of communicable diseases manual*, Washington, DC, 2000, American Public Health Association.

Treatment

- Treatment consists of the application of pediculicides and manual removal of nit cases.
- The drug of choice for infants and children is permethrin 1% creme rinse (Nix), which kills adult lice and nits. This product and preparations of pyrethrin with piperonyl butoxide (RID or A-200 Pyrinate) can be obtained without a prescription and are more effective and safer than lindane.
- Daily removal of nits from the child's hair with a metal nit comb for at least 2- 3 days is a control measure following treatment with a pediculicide.

Nursing Care Management

- An important nursing role is providing the parents with education about pediculosis. Nurses should emphasize that anyone can get pediculosis; it has no respect for age, socio-economic level, or cleanliness.

- Nurses or parents should carefully inspect children who scratch their head more than usual for bite marks, redness, and nits. The hair is systematically spread with two flat-sided sticks or tongue depressors, and the scalp is observed for any movement that indicates a louse. Nurses should wear gloves when examining the hair.

Patient and Family Teaching
- Families should be taught how to prevent the spread and recurrence (see Box 3-8).
- Families should also be advised that the pediculicide is relatively expensive, especially when several members of the household require treatment.

PEPTIC ULCER DISEASE
Description
Peptic ulcers may be classified as acute or chronic, and peptic ulcer disease (PUD) is a chronic condition that affects the stomach or duodenum. Ulcers are described as gastric or duodenal and as primary or secondary. A *gastric ulcer* involves the mucosa of the stomach; a *duodenal ulcer* involves the pylorus or duodenum. Most *primary ulcers* occur in the absence of a predisposing factor and tend to be chronic, occurring more frequently in the duodenum. *Stress ulcers* result from the stress of a severe underlying disease or injury (e.g., severe burns, sepsis, increased intracranial pressure, severe trauma, multisystem organ failure) and are more frequently acute and gastric.

Pathophysiology
There is a significant relationship between the bacterium *Helicobacter pylori* (*H. pylori*) and ulcers. *H. pylori* is a microaerophilic, Gram-negative, slow-growing, spiral-shaped, and flagellated bacterium known to colonize the gastric mucosa in about half of the population of the world. There is no conclusive evidence to implicate particular foods, such as caffeine-containing beverages or spicy foods, but polyunsaturated fats and fiber may play a role in ulcer formation. Psychologic factors may play a role in the development of PUD, and stressful life events, dependency, passiveness, and hostility have all been implicated as contributing factors.

Clinical Signs and Symptoms
▪ Epigastric abdominal pain, nocturnal pain, oral regurgitation, heartburn, weight loss, hematemesis, and melena
▪ History should include questions relating to the use of potentially causative medications such as NSAIDS, corticosteroids, alcohol, and tobacco.

Diagnostic Evaluation
▪ CBC to detect anemia, stool analysis for occult blood, liver function tests, sedimentation rate, or CRP to evaluate inflammatory bowel disease, amylase and lipase to evaluate pancreatitis, and gastric acid measurements to identify hypersecretion
▪ A lactose breath test may be performed to detect lactose intolerance. An upper endoscopy is the most reliable procedure to diagnose PUD.
▪ A biopsy is taken to determine the presence of *H. pylori*. It can also be diagnosed by a blood test that identifies the presence of the antigen to this organism.
▪ The C urea breath test measures bacterial colonization in the gastric mucosa. This test is used to screen for *H. pylori* in adults and children.
▪ Polyclonal and monoclonal stool antigen tests are accurate noninvasive methods for the initial diagnosis of *H. pylori*.

Treatment
▪ The major goals of therapy for children with PUD are to relieve discomfort, promote healing, prevent complications, and prevent recurrence. Management is primarily medical and consists of administration of medications to treat the infection and to reduce or neutralize gastric acid secretion.
▪ Antacids are beneficial medications to neutralize gastric acid.
▪ Histamine (H2) receptor antagonists (antisecretory drugs) act to suppress gastric acid production. Cimetidine (Tagamet), ranitidine (Zantac), and famotidine (Pepcid) are examples of these medications. These medications have few side effects.
▪ Proton pump inhibitors (PPI), such as omeprazole and lansoprazole, act to inhibit the hydrogen ion pump in the parietal cells, thus blocking the production of acid.
▪ Mucosal protective agents, such as sucralfate and bismuth-containing preparations, may be prescribed for PUD.

- Triple drug therapy is the recommended treatment regimen for *H. pylori*. Examples of drug combinations used in triple therapy are: (1) bismuth, clarithromycin, and metronidazole; (2) lansoprazole, amoxicillin, and clarithromycin; and (3) metronidazole, clarithromycin, and omeprazole.
- In addition to medications, the child with PUD should be given a nutritious diet and be advised to avoid caffeine. Adolescents are warned about gastric irritation associated with alcohol use and smoking.
- Children with an acute ulcer who have developed complications, such as massive hemorrhage, require emergency care. The administration of IV fluids, blood, or plasma depends on the amount of blood loss. Replacement with whole blood or packed cells may be necessary for significant loss.
- Surgical intervention may be required for complications such as hemorrhage, perforation, or gastric outlet obstruction.

Nursing Care Management
- Promote healing of the ulcer through compliance with the medication regimen.
- If an analgesic/antipyretic is needed, use acetaminophen, not aspirin or NSAIDs.
- Critically ill neonates, infants, and children in intensive care units should receive H2 blockers to prevent stress ulcers. Critically ill children receiving IV H2 blockers should have their gastric pH values checked at frequent intervals.

Patient and Family Teaching
- The role of stress in ulcer formation should be considered for nonhospitalized children with chronic illnesses.
- In children, many ulcers occur secondarily to other conditions, and the nurse should be aware of family and environmental conditions that may aggravate or precipitate ulcers.
- Children may benefit from psychologic counseling and from learning how to cope constructively with stress.

PNEUMONIA, VIRAL AND BACTERIAL
Description
Pneumonia is an inflammation of the pulmonary parenchyma that may occur either as a primary disease or as a complication of another illness. Pneumonia occurs more frequently in infancy and early

childhood. The classification of pneumonia is often based on the etiologic agent (e.g., viral, bacterial, mycoplasmal, or aspiration of foreign substances). *Streptococcus pneumoniae* is the most common bacterial pathogen responsible for community-acquired pneumonia in both children and adults. Other bacteria that cause pneumonia in children are group A streptococcus, *Staphylococcus aureus, M. catarrhalis, Mycoplasma pneumoniae,* and *Chlamydia pneumoniae.*

Pneumonitis is a localized acute inflammation of the lung without the toxemia associated with lobar pneumonia. *Atypical pneumonia* refers to pneumonia that is caused by pathogens other than the traditionally most common and readily cultured bacteria. *Mycoplasma pneumoniae* and *Chlamydia pneumoniae* are the most common causes of community-acquired pneumonia in children 5 years old or older. It occurs in the fall and winter months and is more prevalent in crowded living conditions.

Viral pneumonia, which occurs more frequently than bacterial pneumonia, is seen in children of all ages and is often associated with viral URIs. Viruses that cause pneumonia include RSV in infants, and parainfluenza, influenza, human metapneumovirus, and adenovirus in older children.

Pathophysiology

The inflammation process caused by the bacteria or viral agent initiates in the terminal bronchioles, which become clogged with mucopurulent exudate to form consolidated patches in nearby lobules; this is called *lobular pneumonia.* With interstitial pneumonia, the inflammatory process is more or less confined within the alveolar walls (interstitium) and the peribronchial and interlobular tissues. The clinical manifestations of the disease vary depending on the etiologic agent, the child's age, the child's systemic reaction to the infection, the extent of the lesions, and the degree of bronchial and bronchiolar obstruction.

Differentiation among viruses is usually made by clinical features such as child's age, past medical history, season of the year, and radiographic and laboratory examination. Viral infections of the respiratory tract render the affected child more susceptible to secondary bacterial invasion, especially when there is denuded bronchial mucosa.

Bacterial pneumonias display distinct clinical patterns. The onset of illness is abrupt and generally follows a viral infection that disturbs the natural defense mechanisms of the upper respiratory tract. The child with bacterial pneumonia usually appears ill.

Clinical Signs and Symptoms
General Signs
- Fever: usually high
- Respiratory
  - Cough: unproductive to productive with white sputum
  - Tachypnea
  - Breath sounds: crackles, decreased breath sounds, rales
  - Dullness with percussion
  - Chest pain
  - Retractions
  - Nasal flaring
  - Pallor to cyanosis (depends on severity)
- Chest radiograph: diffuse or patchy infiltration with peribronchial distribution
- Behavior: irritable, restless, malaise, lethargy
- Gastrointestinal: anorexia, vomiting, diarrhea, abdominal pain

Diagnostic Evaluation
- Diagnosis is based in part on the physical findings and history as well as the chest radiograph.
- Bacterial pneumonia: complete blood count, elevated WBCs

Treatment
- Bacterial: antibiotics; oxygenation; fluids; rest; antipyretic for fever; cool mist; chest physiotherapy; hospitalization if hydration and compliance with treatment regimen is impossible at home, toxic appearing, or if pleural effusion or empyema accompanies the disease; infants less than 1 month old may require hospitalization.
- Viral: symptomatic; oxygenation; fluids; rest; antipyretics; cool mist; chest physiotherapy; antibiotics may be administered to reduce or prevent secondary bacterial infection.

Nursing Care Management
- Identify illness and interventions to promote adequate oxygenation.
- Assist with diagnostic procedures.
- Medication administration: antipyretics; antibiotics; bronchodilators in some cases; nebulized or inhalation medications
- Maintain oxygenation; monitor respiratory status.

- Maintain adequate hydration; oral or IV.
- Prevention of bacterial pneumonia by encouraging childhood immunizations; prevention of viral by teaching parents and child about contagion spread
- Monitor for complications such as pneumothorax, empyema, and sepsis.

Patient and Family Teaching
- Importance of administering medications to completion
- Medication administration methods including nebulization or inhalation
- Comfort measures including antipyretic administration
- Oral fluid administration in child with anorexia
- Prevention: teaching parents and child about contagion spread
- Instilling normal saline and suctioning nasopharynx of infants

PRECOCIOUS PUBERTY
Description
Precocious puberty occurs when the physical changes of puberty begin before age 8 for girls and before age 9 for boys. An uncommon condition, precocious puberty occurs more often in girls than in boys.

Pathophysiology
Normally the hypothalamic-releasing factors stimulate secretion of the gonadotropic hormones from the anterior pituitary at the time of puberty. In the male, interstitial cell-stimulating hormone stimulates Leydig cells of the testes to secrete testosterone; in the female, follicle-stimulating hormone and luteinizing hormone stimulate the ovarian follicles to secrete estrogens. This sequence of events is known as the *hypothalamic-pituitary-gonadal axis*. If for some reason the cycle undergoes premature activation, the child will display evidence of advanced or precocious puberty.

Clinical Signs and Symptoms
Girls
- Breast growth
- First period (menstruation)

Boys
- Enlarged testicles and penis
- Facial hair (usually grows first on the upper lip)
- Deepening voice

Both Girls and Boys
- Pubic or underarm hair
- Rapid growth
- Acne
- Adult body odor

Diagnostic Evaluation
Based on recent research findings, precocious puberty evaluation for a pathologic etiology should be performed for Caucasian girls 7 years of age and younger or for African-American girls younger than 6 years of age. Boys should be evaluated if physical changes occur before 9 years of age.
- Detailed history and physical examination
- Radiographic studies including wrist X-ray for bone age, CT or MRI to assess for central cause
- Estradiol (female) or testosterone (male), LH and FSH, basal or GnRH stimulation test; adrenal androgens, serum hCG (male), ACTH stimulation test, T4, TSH, prolactin

Treatment
Treatment of precocious puberty is directed toward the specific cause when known.
- Precocious puberty of central (hypothalamic-pituitary) origin is managed with monthly injections of a synthetic analog of luteinizing hormone–releasing hormone, which regulates pituitary secretions.
- The available preparation, leuprolide acetate (Lupron Depot), is given in a dose of 0.2 to 0.3 mg/kg intramuscularly once every 4 weeks. Breast development regresses or does not advance, and growth returns to normal rates, enhancing predicted height.
- Treatment is discontinued at a chronologically appropriate time, allowing pubertal changes to resume.

Nursing Care Management
- Identification of early changes in physical development is important; evaluation of the child's Tanner stage of development should occur during every well-child visit.
- If the child is on medication, provide family education concerning medication preparation and storage, injection sites, injection technique, and syringe disposal.

Patient and Family Teaching
Children who begin puberty early may feel different from their peers, which can cause social and emotional problems.
- Psychologic support and guidance of the child and family are the most important aspects of management.
- Discuss with family that dress and activities for the physically precocious child should be appropriate to the chronologic age.
- Emphasize to parents that the child is fertile.

PULMONIC STENOSIS
Description
Narrowing at the entrance to the pulmonary artery. Resistance to blood flow causes right ventricular hypertrophy and decreased pulmonary blood flow. Pulmonary atresia is the extreme form of pulmonic stenosis (PS) in that there is total fusion of the commissures and no blood flows to the lungs. The right ventricle may be hypoplastic.

Pathophysiology
When PS is present, resistance to blood flow causes right ventricular hypertrophy. If right ventricular failure develops, right atrial pressure will increase, and this may result in reopening of the foramen ovale, shunting of unoxygenated blood into the left atrium, and systemic cyanosis. If PS is severe, CHF occurs, and systemic venous engorgement will be noted. An associated defect such as a patent ductus arteriosus partially compensates for the obstruction by shunting blood from the aorta to the pulmonary artery and into the lungs.

Clinical Signs and Symptoms
Patients may be asymptomatic; some have mild cyanosis. CHF is rare, but may be observed in severe pulmonary stenosis (see Box 3-1).

Progressive narrowing causes increased symptoms. Newborns with severe narrowing will be cyanotic. There is a characteristic murmur with a high-pitched ejection click heard best along the left upper sternal border. Cardiomegaly is evident on chest radiographic films. Patients are at risk for bacterial endocarditis.

Diagnostic Evaluation
See Tables 3-1 and 3-2.

Treatment
Surgical Treatment
Transventricular (closed) valvotomy (Brock procedure) or pulmonary valvotomy with cardiopulmonary bypass. Need for surgical treatment is rare with widespread use of balloon angioplasty techniques.

Nonsurgical Treatment
Balloon angioplasty in the cardiac catheterization laboratory to dilate the valve. A catheter is inserted across the stenotic pulmonic valve into the pulmonary artery, and a balloon at the end of the catheter is inflated and rapidly passed through the narrowed opening. The procedure is associated with few complications and has proved to be highly effective. It is the treatment of choice for discrete PS in most centers and can be done safely in neonates.

Nursing Care Management
Assist in Measures to Assess and Improve Cardiac Function
Monitor Cardiac Function
- Vital signs monitoring
- Respiratory assessment
- Cardiac assessment
  - Cardiac output (color, pulses, perfusion, capillary refill, renal function, and neurologic function)
  - Heart sounds
- Keep accurate record of intake and output.
- Weigh child or infant on same scale at same time of day.

Administer Medications
- Review child's history related to cardiac management.
- Administer medications on schedule.

- Assess effectiveness of medications and any side effects noted.
- Be aware of drug-drug and drug-food interactions.
- Follow guidelines for medication administration.

Manage Common Side Effects of Cardiac Defects
- Prevent fatigue during feeding; offer small frequent feedings to infant's or child's tolerance.
- Organize nursing care to allow child/infant uninterrupted rest.
- Promote activities that do not cause fatigue.

Provide Support for the Child and Family
- Communicate with the child and family in an appropriate style.
- Provide the child and family with honest answers.
- Provide emotional support.
- Offer age-appropriate interventions.
- Provide information on available resources for support for the child and family.

Patient and Family Teaching
Prepare the Child and Family for Diagnostic and Operative Procedures
- Provide explanation of diagnostic tests and why each test is performed because many of them are invasive procedures.
- Prepare the child prior to the invasive procedure. Remember that discussion is dependent upon the child's age and development.
- Use simple words or pictures to describe procedures, and answer all questions the child and family may have.
- Postoperative wound care teaching as needed
- Post-cardiac catheterization wound care teaching as needed
- Assess and record results of teaching and family's participation in care.

Educate the Child and Family
- Assess child's and family's level of knowledge regarding pulmonary stenosis.
- Assess child's and family's understanding of what they have heard about pulmonary stenosis.

- Assess child's and family's understanding of the surgery and/or cardiac catheterization.
- Educate child and family about care such as medication preparation and administration.
- Assess child's and family's access to appropriate pharmacy for any special preparation medications.
- Educate child and family about when to notify their physician of any clinical changes.
- Assess and record results and family's participation in care.
- Provide appropriate educational resources and review materials with them.
- Clarify information presented by the health care team including appointment for follow-up visit.
- Discuss SBE (subacute bacterial endocarditis) prophylaxis with your pediatric cardiologist.

RABIES

Description

Rabies is an acute infection of the nervous system caused by a virus that is almost invariably fatal if left untreated. It is transmitted to humans by the saliva of an infected mammal and is introduced through a bite or skin abrasion.

Pathophysiology

After entry into a new host, the virus multiplies in muscle cells and is spread through neural pathways without stimulating a protective host immune response. Carnivorous wild animals (skunks, raccoons, and bats) are the animals most often infected with rabies and the cause of most indigenous cases of human rabies in the United States. Although rabies is common among wildlife species, human rabies is rarely acquired. Modern-day prophylaxis is nearly 100% successful. The highest incidence occurs in children under age 15 years. The incubation period usually ranges from 1 to 3 months but may be as short as 10 days or as long as 8 months. Only 10% to 15% of persons bitten develop the disease, but once symptoms are present, rabies progresses to a fatal outcome. Human fatalities associated with rabies occur in people who fail to seek medical attention, usually because they are unaware of their exposure.

Clinical Signs and Symptoms
Initial Signs
- General malaise
- Fever
- Sore throat

Excitement Phase
- Hypersensitivity
- Increased reaction to external stimuli
- Seizures
- Maniacal behavior
- Choking

Severe Spasm of Respiratory Muscles
- Apnea
- Cyanosis
- Anoxia

Diagnostic Evaluation
- Based on history and clinical features
- Animal brain tissue should be examined for presence of virus-specific fluorescent antigen.
- An unprovoked bite is more likely to transmit rabies than a provoked bite; a provoked bite typically occurs when an animal is feeding and the child interferes with feeding process.
- Virus may be detected in saliva of victim, detection of antibody in CSF, or serum of nonimmunized person.

Treatment
- Once symptoms appear in human, neither rabies vaccine nor Rabies Immune Globulin (RIG) provide improvement.
- Thorough cleansing of the wound and passive immunization with human rabies immunoglobulin (RIG, 20 IU/kg) as soon as possible after exposure to provide rapid, short-term passive immunity; RIG is infiltrated into and around the wound and the remainder of the dosage is given IM; consider tetanus prophylaxis.
- Inactivated rabies vaccine administration on day of treatment (wound cleaning and RIG administration), followed by injections at 3, 7, 14, and 28 days after the first dose; vaccine is administered IM.

- World Health Organization recommends additional dose at day 90.

Nursing Care Management
- Cleansing of wound
- Administration of rabies vaccine and rabies immune globulin
- Monitoring child's status post-vaccination

Patient and Family Teaching
- Explain necessity of rabies treatment.
- Avoid animals likely to transmit rabies.
- Avoid interfering with animals during feeding.
- Wound care as appropriate

RECURRENT ABDOMINAL PAIN
Description
Recurrent abdominal pain (RAP) is a complaint of childhood that is often attributed to psychogenic causes, although it can be a symptom of either psychosomatic or organic disease. RAP is traditionally defined as three or more separate episodes of abdominal pain during a 3-month period that interferes with functioning. The disorder affects mostly school-age children and is rarely seen in children younger than 5 years of age. Girls are affected slightly more often than boys.

Pathophysiology
Only a minority of youngsters with RAP have an organic basis for their pain. Organic causes include inflammatory bowel disease, peptic ulcer disease, lactose intolerance, pelvic inflammatory disease, urinary bladder infection, and pancreatitis. Psychogenic causes of abdominal pain, such as school phobia, depression, acute reactive anxiety, and conversion reaction, account for a small number of cases. The bulk of children with RAP suffer from functional abdominal pain. Functional conditions causing RAP include constipation, chronic stool retention, overeating, irritable colon, and intestinal gas with heightened awareness of intestinal motility or dysmotility. Normally, intestinal contents arrive at the distal portion of the intestine with a relatively high fluid content, and fluid is extracted in the distal colon and rectum. If the normally relaxed distal intestine fails to relax and prevents the flow of its contents

toward the rectum, the resulting excessive distention and spasms of the distal intestinal musculature produce pressure on nerve endings, causing pain.

Clinical Signs and Symptoms
- Children with RAP have real pain that is usually located in the periumbilical and/or epigastric area.
- On palpation the pain is more likely to be experienced in the epigastric area or in the lower right or left quadrant and is accompanied by vague tenderness without muscle guarding. The pain is irregular in time, duration, and intensity and is associated with either loose or pellet-formed stools.
- Symptoms that may accompany abdominal pain are headache, flushing, pallor, dizziness, and fatigue. Nausea, vomiting, diarrhea, and dysuria are sometimes part of the syndrome.

Diagnostic Evaluation
- Diagnosis is based on a complete family history, the child's health history, physical examination, and laboratory tests.
- The family history may provide evidence of a hereditary disorder or mimicry of adult symptoms.
- Pain is assessed for location, quality, frequency, duration, any associated symptoms, alleviating factors, and exacerbating factors.

Treatment
- Treatment involves providing reassurance and reducing or eliminating symptoms.
- Hospitalization may be necessary, and the child frequently shows improvement in the hospital environment.
- Initial efforts are directed toward ruling out organic causes of the pain, relieving discomfort, and attempting to determine the situations that precipitate attacks.
- A high-fiber diet, psyllium bulk agents, lubricants such as mineral oil, and bowel training are emphasized for pain associated with bowel patterns.
- Treatment may also include acid-reduction therapy for pain associated with dyspepsia; antispasmodic agents, smooth muscle relaxants, or low doses of psychotropic agents for pain.
- Other treatments include cognitive-behavioral therapy and biofeedback.

Nursing Care Management
- Careful assessment to help identify factors that contribute to the child's symptoms
- Evaluate the child's social and psychologic adjustment.
- Obtain details of the pain directly from the child.
- Discuss a high-fiber diet with the child and family and teach bowel training.
- Encourage the child to establish a pattern of sitting on the toilet for 10 to 15 minutes immediately after breakfast to take advantage of the increased colonic activity following meals.
- If necessary, stimulatory suppositories can be used to induce early morning defecation.
- The simple measure of having the child rest in a peaceful, quiet environment and providing comfort will often relieve the symptoms in a short time.
- Application of a heating pad may also ease the discomfort.
- If pain is not relieved by these simple measures, administer antispasmodics, if prescribed. For example, if pain is precipitated by meals, having the child take the medication 20 to 30 minutes before mealtime may prevent an episode.

Patient and Family Teaching
- Once the diagnosis has been established, the parents and the child need an explanation of the pain, which can be compared to a skeletal muscle cramp, "charley horse," or headache for easier comprehension.
- The most valuable assistance that the nurse can provide is support and reassurance to the family.
- Follow-up care and continued support are essential because the symptoms tend to remit and exacerbate; therefore, the availability of a supportive health professional can be a source of comfort to the child and family.

RENAL FAILURE, ACUTE
Description
Acute renal failure (ARF) is said to exist when the kidneys suddenly are unable to regulate the volume and composition of urine appropriately in response to food and fluid intake and the

needs of the organism. The principal feature of ARF is oliguria*
associated with azotemia, metabolic acidosis, and diverse electrolyte disturbances.

Pathophysiology

The pathologic conditions that produce ARF caused by glomerulonephritis and hemolytic-uremic syndrome have been discussed in relation to those disorders. ARF can also develop
as a result of a large number of related or unrelated clinical
conditions: poor renal perfusion, urinary tract obstruction,
acute renal injury, or the final expression of chronic, irreversible
renal disease. The most common cause in children is transient
renal failure resulting from severe dehydration or other causes
of poor perfusion that may respond to restoration of fluid
volume.

Clinical Signs and Symptoms

- Diminished urine output and lethargy in a child who is dehydrated, in shock, or recently postoperative should be evaluated
  for possible acute kidney failure.
- Nausea and vomiting, edema, and hypertension can occur.
  Manifestations of an underlying disorder or pathologic condition may be present.
- Fluid overload and electrolyte disturbances can precipitate cardiovascular complications such as hypertension and cardiac
  failure.
- Fluid and electrolyte imbalances, acidosis, and accumulation
  of nitrogenous waste products can produce neurologic involvement manifested by coma, seizures, or alterations in
  sensorium.

Diagnostic Evaluation

- Bladder tap or catheterization to evaluate inadequate urine
  output, urinalysis, urine osmolarity, urine sodium and potassium
- Serum electrolytes
- Complete blood count

---

*The definition of *oliguria* varies extensively in the literature, from 1.8 to 4 dL/m2/24 hr.

Treatment

- Treatment of ARF is directed toward:
  - Treatment of the underlying cause
  - Management of the complications of renal failure
  - Provision of supportive therapy within the constraints imposed by the renal failure
- Treatment of poor perfusion resulting from dehydration consists of volume restoration.
- Regular measurement of plasma electrolyte, pH, blood urea nitrogen, and creatinine levels is required to assess the adequacy of fluid therapy and to anticipate complications that require specific treatment.
- The amount of exogenous water provided should not exceed the amount needed to maintain zero water balance. It is calculated on the basis of estimated endogenous water formation and losses from sensible (primarily gastrointestinal) and insensible sources. No allotment is calculated for urine as long as oliguria persists.
- When the output begins to increase, either spontaneously or in response to diuretic therapy, the intake of fluid, potassium, and sodium must be monitored and adequate replacement provided to prevent depletion and its consequences. Some patients pass enormous amounts of electrolyte-rich urine.
- The child with ARF has a tendency to develop water intoxication and hyponatremia, which makes it difficult to provide calories in sufficient amounts to meet the needs of the child and reduce the tissue catabolism, metabolic acidosis, hyperkalemia, and uremia.

Nursing Care Management

- Control water balance in these patients by careful monitoring of feedback information, such as accurate intake and output, body weight, and electrolyte measurements.
- Meticulous attention to fluid intake and output is mandatory and includes all of the physical measurements discussed previously in relation to problems of fluid balance.
- Limiting fluid intake requires ingenuity on the part of caregivers to cope with the child who is thirsty. Rationing the daily intake in small amounts of fluid served in containers that give the impression of larger volumes is one strategy.

- Meet nutritional needs; the child may be nauseated, and encouraging foods without fluids may be difficult.
- When nourishment is provided by the IV route, carefully monitor to prevent fluid overload.
- Maintain an optimal thermal environment, reducing any elevation of body temperature.
- Reduce restlessness and anxiety to decrease the rate of tissue catabolism.

Patient and Family Teaching
- The seriousness of ARF and its emergency nature are stressful to parents, and most feel some degree of guilt regarding the child's condition, especially when the illness is a result of ingestion of a toxic substance, dehydration, or a genetic disease.
- Provide parents reassurance and be a sympathetic listener.
- Keep parents informed of the child's progress, and provided explanations regarding the therapeutic regimen.

RESPIRATORY DISTRESS SYNDROME, NEWBORN
Description
Respiratory distress syndrome (RDS) refers to a severe lung disorder that is found almost exclusively in preterm infants but may also be associated with multifetal pregnancies, infants of diabetic mothers, cesarean section delivery, delivery before 37 weeks' gestation, precipitous delivery, cold stress, asphyxia, and a history of previous RDS. The terms *respiratory distress syndrome* and *hyaline membrane disease* are most often applied to this condition.

Pathophysiology
Preterm infants are born before the lungs are fully prepared to serve as efficient organs for gas exchange. RDS results from a combination of structural and functional immaturity of the lungs. Because the final unfolding of the alveolar septa (which increases the surface area of the lungs) occurs during the last trimester of pregnancy, premature infants are born with numerous underdeveloped and many uninflatable alveoli. In addition, the fetal chest wall is highly compliant because of the predominance of cartilage rather than bone; and the diaphragm, the dominant respiratory muscle, is prone to fatigue.

Functionally, the fetal lungs are deficient in surfactant. Surfactant is a surface-active phospholipid secreted by type II cells in the alveolar epithelium. Acting much like a detergent, this substance reduces the surface tension of fluids that line the alveoli and respiratory passages, resulting in uniform expansion and maintenance of lung expansion at low intraalveolar pressure. Deficient surfactant production causes unequal inflation of alveoli on inspiration and the collapse of alveoli on end expiration. Without surfactant, infants are unable to keep their lungs inflated and therefore exert a great deal of effort to reexpand the alveoli with each breath. It has been estimated that each breath requires as much negative pressure (60 to 75 cm H_2O) as the initial lung expansion at birth. With increasing exhaustion, they are able to open fewer and fewer alveoli. This inability to maintain lung expansion produces widespread atelectasis.

In the absence of alveolar stability (normal functional residual capacity) and with progressive atelectasis, pulmonary vascular resistance (PVR) increases, whereas with normal lung expansion it would decrease. Consequently, there is hypoperfusion to the lung tissue, with a decrease in effective pulmonary blood flow. The increase in PVR causes partial reversion to the fetal circulation, with a right-to-left shunting of blood through the persisting fetal communications—the ductus arteriosus and foramen ovale. Inadequate pulmonary perfusion and ventilation produce hypoxemia and hypercapnia. Pulmonary arterioles are markedly reactive to diminished oxygen concentration and a decrease in oxygen tension causes vasospasm in the pulmonary arterioles that is further enhanced by a decrease in blood pH. This vasoconstriction contributes to a marked increase in PVR. Prolonged hypoxemia activates anaerobic glycolysis, which produces increased amounts of lactic acid. An increase in lactic acid causes metabolic acidosis; inability of the atelectatic lungs to blow off excess carbon dioxide produces respiratory acidosis. Lowered pH causes further vasoconstriction. With deficient pulmonary circulation and alveolar perfusion, PaO_2 continues to fall, pH falls, and the materials needed for surfactant production are not circulated to the alveoli.

Clinical Signs and Symptoms
- Rapid breathing
- Retractions-suprasternal or substernal, supracostal, subcostal or intercostals
- Labored breathing

Diagnostic Evaluation
- Chest radiographs show a diffuse granular pattern over both lung fields that resembles ground glass and represents alveolar atelectasis and dark streaks, or air bronchograms, within the ground glass areas that represent dilated, air-filled bronchioles.
- Neonatal tracheal aspirate measure of phosphatidylglycerol (PG), a key surfactant stabilizer
- Fetal lung maturity can be evaluated by measuring lecithin/sphingomyelin (L/S) ratio.

Treatment
- The goals of treatment are to:
    - Maintain adequate ventilation and oxygenation with supplemental oxygen via nasal cannula; oxygen hood; continuous positive airway pressure (CPAP [noninvasive]); endotracheal intubation and mechanical ventilation; exogenous surfactant administration; high-frequency oscillation or high-frequency jet ventilation.
    - Maintain acid-base balance by maintaining adequate oxygenation.
    - Maintain a neutral thermal environment: radiant warmer or incubator.
    - Maintain adequate tissue perfusion and oxygenation.
    - Prevent hypotension.
    - Maintain adequate hydration and electrolyte status: intravenous fluids and electrolytes in acute phase.
    - Prevent infection: standard precautions; handwashing; minimal invasive procedures and exposure to viral and bacterial infections.
    - Prevent and treat complications of prematurity—bronchopulmonary dysplasia, retinopathy of prematurity, necrotizing enterocolitis.

Nursing Care Management
- Identify signs and symptoms and institute treatment: oxygen administration.
- Monitor vital signs; monitor oxygenation: pulse oximetry; arterial blood gases; respiratory status; provide care for mechanically ventilated infant, and prevent complications of same (hypoxia, pneumothorax).

- Monitor fluid and electrolyte balance: monitor renal function, urine output.
- Skin care: skin is prone to damage as a result of immature stratus corneum and potential toxins such as cleansers, invasive procedures; handwashing.
- Provide nutrition: enteral feedings; monitor tolerance of feedings; encourage breastfeeding in infants who can tolerate and save expressed breast milk for later in acutely ill.
- Encourage parent participation in infant's care: encourage maternal infant contact, skin-to-skin contact, and holding.
- Prevent infection: handwashing; skin care.
- Maintain thermoregulation: incubator; radiant warmer; skin-to-skin maternal contact.
- Provide neurodevelopmental care.
- Discharge teaching: See Patient and Family Teaching.

Patient and Family Teaching
- Discharge teaching: infant care—feeding, bathing, diapering, immunizations, follow-up health care visits, car seat safety, cord care (as applicable), jaundice information (as applicable), infant CPR, prevention of RSV (including pharmacologic prophylaxis)
- Special needs such as gavage or gastrostomy feeding; colostomy care; special formula preparation
- Medication administration: caffeine citrate; supplements such as vitamin D, multivitamins, GER medications

RETINOBLASTOMA
Description
Retinoblastoma, which arises from the retina, is the most common intraocular malignancy of childhood.

Pathophysiology
Retinoblastoma may be caused by (1) a somatic mutation, (2) a germinal mutation, or (3) a chromosome aberration. Somatic mutations (those occurring in the general body cells, as opposed to the germ cells or gametes) are a sporadic, nonhereditary event. They result in unilateral tumors. Germinal mutations are passed to future generations. Almost all bilateral retinoblastomas are considered hereditary, and 15% of individuals with unilateral disease have the hereditary form.

Retinoblastoma has also been associated with partial deletion of the long arm of a group D chromosome 13 and polyploidy (excessive number of chromosomes), such as trisomy 21. In children who have chromosome aberrations and retinoblastoma, there is often an increased incidence of mental retardation and congenital malformations, although the vast majority of children with retinoblastomas apparently have normal chromosomes and intelligence.

Clinical Signs and Symptoms

- Typically it is the parent who first observes a whitish "glow" in the pupil, known as the cat's eye reflex or *leukokoria*. The reflex represents visualization of the tumor as the light momentarily falls on the mass. It is best observed when a bright light is shining toward the child as the child looks forward. It is sometimes accidentally discovered by parents when taking a photograph of their child using a flash attachment.
- The next most common sign is strabismus resulting from poor fixation of the visually impaired eye, particularly if the tumor develops in the macula, the area of sharpest visual acuity.
- Blindness is usually a late sign, but it frequently is not obvious unless the parent consciously observes for behaviors indicating loss of sight, such as bumping into objects, slowed motor development, or turning of the head to see objects lateral to the affected eye.

Diagnostic Evaluation

- The first step in diagnosis is carefully listening to and recognizing the significance of reports from family members regarding suspected abnormalities within the eye. Children suspected of having this disorder are referred to an ophthalmologist.
- Definitive diagnosis is usually based on indirect ophthalmoscopy employing scleral indentation, which is done with the patient under general anesthesia and with maximum dilation of the pupils.
- Metastatic disease at time of retinoblastoma diagnosis is rare. Therefore staging procedures such as bone marrow aspiration, bone survey, and lumbar puncture are not performed.
- Staging of retinoblastomas is done under indirect ophthalmoscopy before surgery to determine accurately the tumor size

(measured in disc diameters [DD]) and location (according to an imaginary line called the *equator* drawn on the midplane of the eye.

Treatment

Treatment of retinoblastoma depends chiefly on the stage of the tumor at diagnosis. In general, unilateral retinoblastomas in stages I, II, and III are treated with irradiation. The aim of radiotherapy is to preserve useful vision in the affected eye and eradicate the tumor.

Other approaches toward treating small, localized tumors involve (1) plaque brachytherapy (surgical implantation of an iodine-125 applicator on the sclera until the maximum radiation dose has been delivered to the tumor), (2) photocoagulation (use of a laser beam to destroy retinal blood vessels that supply nutrition to the tumor), and (3) cryotherapy (freezing of the tumor, which destroys the microcirculation to the tumor and the cells themselves through microcrystal formation). One of the reasons for investigating treatments other than radiotherapy is to minimize the risk of radiation-induced malignancies later in life.

With advanced tumor growth, especially optic nerve involvement, enucleation of the affected eye is the treatment of choice. The use of chemotherapy in advanced disease, even in group V, is controversial and has not shown improved survival. With bilateral disease, every attempt is made to preserve useful vision in the less affected eye with enucleation of the severely diseased eye. When bilateral tumors are found very early, enucleation may be prevented with the use of radiotherapy to both eyes.

Nursing Care Management

- ▪ Nursing care for the child with retinoblastoma involves:
  - ▪ Preparing the child and family for diagnostic and operative procedures
  - ▪ Administering therapy
  - ▪ Managing treatment side-effects
  - ▪ Monitoring to prevent complications related to leukemia and treatment
  - ▪ Educating the child and family
  - ▪ Providing child and family support

Prepare the Child and Family for Diagnostic and Operative Procedures

- Because the tumor is usually diagnosed in infants or very young children, most of the preparation for diagnostic tests and treatment involves parents. After indirect ophthalmoscopy, the child may not see very clearly, or the eyes may be sensitive to light because of pupillary dilation. Parents are made aware of these normal reactions before the procedure.

- After surgery, the parents need to be prepared for the child's facial appearance. An eye patch is in place, and the child's face may be edematous or ecchymotic. Parents often fear seeing the surgical site because they imagine a cavity in the skull. On the contrary, the lids are usually closed, and the area does not appear sunken because a surgically implanted sphere maintains the shape of the eyeball. The implant is covered with conjunctiva, and when the lids are open, the exposed area resembles the mucosal lining of the mouth. Once the child is fitted for a prosthesis, usually within 3 weeks, the facial appearance returns to normal.

- Initial instructions for care of the prosthesis are given by the ocularist, who fits and manufactures the device. The prosthesis is cleaned by placing it in hot water and soaking it for several minutes. Reinsertion is easier if the prosthesis remains wet. To reinsert the prosthesis, the lids are separated, and with the prosthesis held in the correct position (it should be marked to indicate the nasal side), it is pushed up under the upper lid, allowing the lower lid to cover its lower edge.

Monitor for Complications Related to Retinoblastoma and Treatment

- Assess for symptoms related to retinoblastoma and treatment.
- Review laboratory findings.
- Obtain a complete history evaluating the incidence and duration of symptoms.
- Perform a complete physical examination; assess for fever, weight loss, pallor, signs of infection.

Patient and Family Teaching
Educate the Child and Family

- Assess child's and family's level of knowledge regarding the treatment.

- Assess child's and family's understanding of what they have heard about retinoblastoma and treatment.
- If the child is to receive radiation therapy, review the common side effects associated with radiation therapy and precautions that should be followed during treatment: high-dose radiotherapy often causes a skin reaction of dry or moist desquamation followed by hyperpigmentation. Because of increased sensitivity, the area is protected from sunlight and sudden changes in temperature, such as from heating pads or ice packs.
- Educate the family regarding the signs and symptoms of infection and fever precautions.
- Provide appropriate educational resources, and review materials with them.
- Clarify information presented by the health care team.

Provide Support for the Child and Family
The diagnosis of retinoblastoma presents some special concerns in addition to those created by any type of cancer. Families with a history of the disorder may feel great guilt for transmitting the defect to their offspring, especially if they knowingly "played the odds" and parented an affected child. Conversely, when parents are aware of the probability and have an affected child, early treatment results in such favorable outcomes that parental adjustment may be rapid. In families with no history of retinoblastoma, the discovery of the diagnosis is a shock, frequently complicated by guilt for not having discovered it sooner.

REYE SYNDROME
Description
Reye Syndrome (RS) is defined as toxic encephalopathy associated with other characteristic organ involvement and is characterized by fever, profoundly impaired consciousness, and disordered hepatic function.

Pathophysiology
The etiology of RS is not well understood, but most cases follow a common viral illness, most commonly influenza or varicella. The condition is characterized pathologically by cerebral edema and fatty changes of the liver. The onset of RS is notable for profuse vomiting and varying degrees of neurologic impairment, including

personality changes and deterioration in consciousness. The cause of RS is a mitochondrial insult induced by different viruses, drugs, exogenous toxins, and genetic factors. The potential association between aspirin therapy for the treatment of fever in children with varicella or influenza and the development of RS precludes its use in these patients.

Clinical Signs and Symptoms
Staging Criteria for Reye Syndrome
Stage I:—Vomiting, lethargy, and drowsiness; liver dysfunction; type I electroencephalogram (EEG); follows commands; pupillary reaction brisk

Stage II:—Disorientation, combativeness, delirium, hyperventilation, hyperactive reflexes, appropriate responses to painful stimuli; evidence of liver dysfunction; type I EEG; sluggish pupillary reaction

Stage III:—Obtunded, coma, hyperventilation, decorticate rigidity, preservation of pupillary light reaction and oculovestibular reflexes (although sluggish); type II EEG

Stage IV:—Deepening coma, decerebrate rigidity, loss of oculocephalic reflexes, large and fixed pupils, loss of doll's eye reflex, loss of corneal reflexes; minimal liver dysfunction; type III or IV EEG; evidence of brainstem dysfunction

Stage V:—Seizures, loss of deep tendon reflexes, respiratory arrest, flaccidity; type IV EEG; usually no evidence of liver dysfunction

Diagnostic Evaluation
Definitive diagnosis is established by liver biopsy. The staging criteria for RS are based on liver dysfunction and on neurologic signs that range from lethargy to coma.

Treatment
▪ Early diagnosis and aggressive intervention to prevent progression

Nursing Care Management
▪ Monitor vital signs; provide intensive care; monitor central venous pressure; administer medications to decrease or prevent elevation of ICP.

- Assist with diagnostic exams.
- Monitor neurologic signs.
- Monitor and maintain fluid and electrolyte balance.
- Care for central lines including Swan-Ganz catheter
- Care for child who is unconscious and immobile as a result of illness, sedation, or both
- Seizure care: monitor; describe seizure activity; seizure precautions.
- Provide parent and family support.

Patient and Family Teaching
- Provide information regarding intensive care; treatment regimen; equipment used.
- Provide information and education about communicating and care of unconscious, sedated child.
- Encourage involvement in child's care.

RHABDOMYOSARCOMA
Description
Rhabdomyosarcoma (rhabdo—striated) is the most common soft tissue sarcoma in children.

Pathophysiology
These malignant neoplasms originate from undifferentiated mesenchymal cells in muscles, tendons, bursae, and fascia, or in fibrous, connective, lymphatic, or vascular tissue. They derive their name from the specific tissue(s) of origin, such as myosarcoma (myo—muscle). Because striated (skeletal) muscle is found almost anywhere in the body, these tumors occur in many sites, the most common of which are the head and neck, especially the orbit.

Clinical Signs and Symptoms
- Initial signs and symptoms are related to the site of the tumor and compression of adjacent organs (see Table 3-9).
- Some tumor locations, particularly the orbit, produce symptoms early in the course of the illness and contribute to rapid diagnosis and an improved prognosis.
- Other tumors, such as those of the retroperitoneal area, produce no symptoms until they are large, invasive, and widely metastasized.

TABLE 3-9

Clinical Signs and Symptoms of Rhabdomyosarcoma According to Tumor Site

LOCATION	SIGNS AND SYMPTOMS
Orbit	Rapidly developing unilateral proptosis Ecchymosis of conjunctiva Loss of extraocular movements (strabismsus)
Nasopharynx	Stuffy nose (earliest sign) Nasal obstruction: dyphagia, nasal voice (obstruction of posterior nasal conchae), serous otitis media (obstruction of Eustachian tube) Pain (sore throat and ear) Epistaxis Palpable neck nodes Visible mass in oropharynx (late sign)
Paranasal sinuses	Nasal obstruction Local pain Discharge Sinusitis Swelling
Middle ear	Signs of chronic serous otitis media ■ Pain ■ Sanguinopurulent drainage ■ Facial nerve palsy
Retroperitoneal area (usually a "silent" tumor)	Abdominal mass Pain Signs of intestinal or genitourinary obstruction
Perineum	Visible superficial mass Bowel or bladder dysfunction (from tumor compression)

■ Unfortunately, many of the signs and symptoms attributable to rhabdomyosarcoma are vague and frequently suggest a common childhood illness, such as "earache" or "runny nose."

■ In some instances, a primary tumor site is never identified.

Diagnostic Evaluation

■ Diagnosis begins with a careful examination of the head and neck area, particularly palpation of a nontender, firm, hard mass. The nasopharynx and oropharynx are inspected for any evidence of a visible mass.

- CT, MRI, bone surveys, and chest x-ray
- Bone marrow aspiration and biopsy to rule out metastasis
- Lumbar puncture is indicated for head and neck tumors to examine the cerebrospinal fluid for malignant cells.
- An excisional biopsy is done to confirm the histologic type.

Treatment

Because this tumor is highly malignant, with metastasis frequently occurring at the time of diagnosis, aggressive multimodal therapy is recommended. In the past, radical surgical removal of the tumor was the treatment of choice, but with improved survival from combined chemotherapy and irradiation, surgery plays a lesser role. Complete removal of the primary tumor is advocated whenever possible. However, only biopsy is required in certain tumor locations, such as those of the orbit, when followed by irradiation and chemotherapy. This is a fortunate change, because it avoids the devastating effects of enucleation, amputation, or pelvic exenteration. High-dose irradiation to the primary tumor is recommended, except in group I tumors. Chemotherapy plays a major role in treatment of all groups.

Nursing Care Management

Nursing care for the child with rhabdomyosarcoma involves:

- Preparing the child and family for diagnostic and operative procedures
- Administering therapy
- Managing treatment side-effects
- Monitoring to prevent complications related to leukemia and treatment
- Educating the child and family
- Providing child and family support

Prepare the Child and Family for Diagnostic and Operative Procedures

- Once a diagnosis of rhabdomyosarcoma is suspected, a battery of diagnostic tests is ordered. The family needs an explanation of why each test is performed because many of them, such as bone marrow aspiration and biopsy, are invasive procedures.

■ Appropriate preparation for the child prior to the invasive procedure is dependent upon the child's age and development. Use simple words to describe procedures, and answer all questions the child and family may have.

Administer Therapy
■ Review child's history related to previous tolerance to therapy.
■ Determine appropriate premedication prior to therapy.
■ Be aware of drug-specific interactions.
■ Assess the child's laboratory findings prior to therapy administration.
■ Ensure that the chemotherapy doses are correct by checking orders according to the institution's policies and procedures.
■ Follow the guidelines for chemotherapy administration.
■ If the treatment is given intravenously, observe the IV site for signs of irritation or infiltration.
■ Follow the institution's policy for safe handling of chemotherapy wastes, including the patient's bodily fluids.
■ Observe the child for signs of reaction during and following treatment.

Manage Common Side Effects of Cancer Treatment
■ Assess for toxicities specific to the cancer treatment.
■ Monitor for signs of infection, and obtain cultures and initiate antibiotics if indicated.
■ Monitor nutrition and weight changes and alternative methods of nutrition if appropriate.
■ Monitor fluid and electrolytes.
■ Evaluate child's response to treatment.
■ Manage central line care.

Monitor for Complications Related to Rhabdomyosarcoma and Treatment
■ Assess for symptoms related to rhabdomyosarcoma and treatment.
■ Review laboratory findings.
■ Obtain a complete history evaluating the incidence and duration of symptoms.
■ Perform a complete physical examination; assess for fever, night sweats, weight loss, pallor, signs of infection, lymphadenopathy.

Patient and Family Teaching
Educate the Child and Family
- Assess child's and family's level of knowledge regarding the rhabdomyosarcoma and treatment.
- Assess child's and family's understanding of what they have heard about rhabdomyosarcoma and treatment.
- Explain that chemotherapeutic reactions vary with the specific drug regimen. Explain that the most common side effects from chemotherapy include nausea and vomiting, body image changes, neuropathy, and mucosal ulceration.
- If the child is to receive radiation therapy, review the common side effects associated with radiation therapy and precautions that should be followed during treatment: high-dose radiotherapy often causes a skin reaction of dry or moist desquamation followed by hyperpigmentation. The child should wear loose-fitting clothes over the irradiated area to minimize additional skin irritation. Because of increased sensitivity, the area is protected from sunlight and sudden changes in temperature, such as from heating pads or ice packs. The child is encouraged to use the extremity as tolerated. Occasionally an active exercise program may be planned by the physical therapist to preserve maximum function.
- Educate the family regarding neutropenia, anemia, and thrombocytopenia, the signs and symptoms of infection, and fever precautions.
- Provide appropriate educational resources, and review materials with them.
- Clarify information presented by the health care team.

Provide Support for the Child and Family
- Communicate with the child and family in an appropriate style.
- Provide the child and family with honest answers.
- Provide emotional support.
- Offer age-appropriate interventions.
- Provide information on available resources for support for the child and family.

RHEUMATIC FEVER
Description
Rheumatic fever (RF) is a poorly understood inflammatory disease that occurs after infection with group A β-hemolytic streptococcal pharyngitis.

Pathophysiology
Strong evidence supports a relationship between upper respiratory infection with group A streptococci and subsequent development of RF (usually within 2 to 6 weeks). Acute RF is the result of an exaggerated immune response to a bacterium in a susceptible host. It occurs most often in late school-age children or adolescents and is rare in adults. It is a self-limited illness that involves the joints, skin, brain, serous surfaces, and heart. Cardiac valve damage (referred to as *rheumatic heart disease*) is the most significant complication of RF. The mitral valve is most often affected.

Clinical Signs and Symptoms
Major Manifestations
- Carditis
  - Tachycardia out of proportion to degree of fever
  - Cardiomegaly
  - New murmurs or change in preexisting murmurs
  - Muffled heart sounds
  - Pericardial friction rub
  - Chest pain
  - Changes in ECG (especially prolonged P-R interval)
- Polyarthritis
  - Swollen, hot, red, painful joint(s)
  - After 1 to 2 days affects different joint(s)
  - Favors large joints: knees, elbows, hips, shoulders, wrists
- Erythema Marginatum
  - Erythematous macules with clear center and wavy, well-demarcated border
  - Transitory
  - Nonpruritic
  - Primarily affects trunk and extremities (inner surfaces)

- Chorea (St. Vitus Dance, Sydenham chorea)
  - Sudden aimless, irregular movements of extremities
  - Involuntary facial grimaces
  - Speech disturbances
  - Emotional lability
  - Muscle weakness (can be profound)
  - Muscle movements exaggerated by anxiety and attempts at fine-motor activity; relieved by rest
- Subcutaneous Nodes
  - Nontender swelling
  - Located over bony prominences
  - May persist for some time, then gradually resolve

Minor Manifestations*
- Clinical findings
- Arthralgia
- Fever

Supporting Evidence of Antecedent Group AA Streptococcal Infection
- Positive throat culture or rapid streptococcal antigen test
- Elevated or rising streptococcal antibody titer

Diagnostic Evaluation
- Elevated acute-phase reactants
- Erythrocyte sedimentation rate
- C-reactive protein

Treatment
The goals of medical management are (1) eradication of hemolytic streptococci, (2) prevention of permanent cardiac damage, (3) palliation of the other symptoms, and (4) prevention of recurrences of RF.
- Penicillin is the drug of choice, with erythromycin as a substitute in penicillin-sensitive children.

---

*From Special Writing Group of the Committee on Rheumatic Fever, Endocarditis, and Kawasaki Disease of the Council on Cardiovascular Disease in the Young of the American Heart Association: Guidelines for the diagnosis of rheumatic fever: Jones criteria, 1992 (update), *JAMA* 268:2069-2073, 1992.

- Salicylates are used to control the inflammatory process, especially in the joints, and reduce the fever and discomfort.
- Bed rest is recommended during the acute febrile phase but need not be strict.
- Prophylactic treatment against recurrence of RF is started after the acute therapy and involves monthly intramuscular injections of benzathine penicillin G (1.2 million U), two daily oral doses of penicillin (200,000 U), or one daily dose of sulfadiazine (1 g). The duration of long-term prophylaxis is uncertain, but 5 years since the last episode or age 18 is suggested by the World Health Organization (longer with cardiac involvement).

Nursing Care Management
- The objectives of nursing care for the child with RF are to (1) encourage compliance with drug regimens, (2) facilitate recovery from the illness, (3) provide emotional support, and (4) prevent the disease.

Patient and Family Teaching
- Parents are instructed to provide rest and adequate nutrition during the early period of the illness.
- Usually, after the febrile stage is over, children can resume moderate activity.
- If carditis is present, the family must be aware of any activity restrictions and may need help in choosing less strenuous activities for the child.
- Compliance with the prophylactic treatment program is a major teaching focus.

SCABIES
Description
Scabies is an endemic infestation caused by the scabies mite, *Sarcoptes scabiei*.

Pathophysiology
Lesions are created as the impregnated female burrows into the stratum corneum of the epidermis (never into living tissue) to deposit her eggs and feces. The inflammatory response and intense itching occur after the host becomes sensitized to the mite,

approximately 30 to 60 days after initial contact. If the person has been previously sensitized to the mite, the response occurs within 48 hours after exposure.

Clinical Signs and Symptoms

There is great variability in the type of lesions, as described in Box 3-9.

Diagnostic Evaluation

- Diagnosis is made by observation of the lesion and distribution.

Treatment

- The treatment of scabies is the application of a scabicide. Currently, permethrin 5% cream (Elimite) is the drug of choice.
- Alternative drugs are 1% lindane cream or lotion and 10% crotamiton.
- Permethrin is preferred because it is safer, it avoids the risk of neurotoxicity, and it is more effective than lindane.
- Another prescription drug used to treat scabies is ivermectin. Ivermectin is administered orally in a single dose for treatment of severe or crusted scabies. It should be considered for patients whose infestation is refractory or those who cannot tolerate topical scabicides. However, the safety and efficacy of ivermectin for pediatric patients younger than 5 years of age or children weighing less than 15 kg (33 lb) is not established.

BOX 3-9

Clinical Manifestations of Scabies

LESION
Children: minute grayish-brown, threadlike (mite burrows), pruritic
Black dot at end of burrow (mite)
Infants: eczematous eruption, pruritic

DISTRIBUTION
Generally in intertriginous areas: interdigital, axillary-cubital, popliteal, inguinal
Children older than 2 years of age: primarily hands and wrists
Children younger than 2 years: primarily feet and ankles

Nursing Care Management
- Permethrin is applied to all skin surfaces from the neck down to the toes (not just areas with rash, but also areas between the fingers and toes, the umbilicus, and the cleft of the buttocks).
- The cream should remain on the skin for 8 to 14 hours and then be removed by bathing.
- A second treatment with the same lotion may be required 7 to 10 days later.
- Soothing ointments or lotions can be applied for itching.
- Antibiotics may be given for secondary infection.

Patient and Family Teaching
- Families need to know that although the mite that causes scabies will be killed with these treatments, the rash and the itch will not be eliminated until the stratum corneum is replaced in approximately 2 to 3 weeks.

SCOLIOSIS, IDIOPATHIC
Description
Scoliosis is a complex spinal deformity in three planes, usually involving lateral curvature, spinal rotation causing rib asymmetry, and thoracic hypokyphosis. The condition can be further classified according to age of onset. It can develop at birth or up to 3 years of age (***infantile***), or it can develop during childhood (***juvenile***), but it is most common during the growth spurt of early adolescence (***adolescent***).

Pathophysiology
- Cause of idiopathic scoliosis is unknown; occurs more commonly in females.
- Some neuromuscular conditions may cause scoliosis in younger children; e.g., cerebral palsy, spinal cord tumor, Duchenne muscular dystrophy.
- Other conditions: spina bifida; hemivertebrae (failure of vertebral development)

Clinical Signs and Symptoms
- Clothes that do not fit right
- Back pain in some cases
- Walks with a slight limp
- Asymmetric shoulders, waistline

Diagnostic Evaluation
- Physical examination of the spine; Adams test
- Radiographic evaluation

Treatment
- Bracing: Boston, Wilmington, Milwaukee; TLSO (thoracolumbosacral orthosis)
- Surgical: usually for curvatures of 40 degrees or more; realignment and straightening with internal fixation and instrumentation combined with bony fusion (arthrodesis) of the realigned spine; instrumentation systems: Harrington, Dwyer, Zielke, Luque, Cotrel-Dubousset, Isola, TSRH (Texas Scottish Rite Hospital), and Moss-Miami

Nursing Care Management
- Primary screening
- Assist with diagnostic tests.
- Brace care; skin care
- Emotional support for adolescent is imperative.
- Preoperative and postoperative care including vital signs monitoring, skin care, maintenance of spinal alignment, assessing neurologic function in extremities distal to instrumentation, ambulation, pain management, renal function, chest tube management as applicable, peer socialization, preoperative teaching, fluid and electrolyte balance, resumption of bowel function, and prevention of constipation

Patient and Family Teaching
- Care of brace; skin care; body image issues; ADLs; involvement in peer socialization and school
- Preoperative teaching regarding postoperative expectations: immobilization, pain management, resumption of self-care and ADLs, function of equipment used, expected course of recovery, living with a chronic condition as an adolescent

SEPTIC SHOCK
Description
Shock is a complex clinical syndrome characterized by inadequate tissue perfusion to meet the metabolic demands of the body, resulting in cellular dysfunction and eventual organ

failure. Although the causes are different, the physiologic consequences are the same: hypotension, tissue hypoxia, and metabolic acidosis. *Septic shock* is defined as sepsis with organ dysfunction and hypotension. Sepsis and septic shock are caused by an infectious organism. Normally an infection triggers an inflammatory response in a local area, which results in vasodilation, increased capillary permeability, and eventually elimination of the infectious agent. The widespread activation and systemic release of inflammatory mediators is called the *systemic inflammatory response syndrome* (SIRS).

Pathophysiology
Most of the physiologic effects of shock occur because the exaggerated immune response triggers more than 30 different mediators that results in diffuse vasodilation, increased capillary permeability, and maldistribution of blood flow. This impairs oxygen and nutrient delivery to the cells, resulting in cellular dysfunction. If the process continues, multiple organ dysfunction occurs and may result in death.

Clinical Signs and Symptoms
Three stages have been identified in septic shock:

- Early stage: The patient has chills, fever, and vasodilation with increased cardiac output, which results in warm, flushed skin that reflects vascular tone abnormalities and hyperdynamic, warm, or hyperdynamic-compensated responses. BP and urinary output are normal.
- Normodynamic, cool, or hyperdynamic-decompensated stage: Lasts only a few hours. The skin is cool, but pulses and BP are still normal. Urinary output diminishes, and the mental state becomes depressed. With advancing disease, certain signs of circulatory decompensation that deteriorate to signs of circulatory collapse are indistinguishable from late shock of any cause.
- Hypodynamic, or cold, stage: Cardiovascular function progressively deteriorates, even with aggressive therapy. The patient has hypothermia, cold extremities, weak pulses, hypotension, and oliguria or anuria. Patients are severely lethargic or comatose. Multiorgan failure.

Diagnostic Evaluation
- Early identification of the symptoms of septic shock
- Blood cultures and isolation of pathogenic organism

Treatment
- Provide hemodynamic stability: fluid volume resuscitation and inotropic agents.
- Provide adequate oxygenation to the tissues: intubation and mechanical ventilation, supplemental oxygen, sedation, and paralysis to decrease the work of breathing.
- Antimicrobials to treat the infectious organism; removal of infection source (if treatment-related; e.g., central line)
- Monitor for and treat associated complications of disseminated intravascular coagulation and multiorgan dysfunction.

Nursing Care Management
- High index of suspicion in patient at risk for infection or who has an identified infection
- Support patient and family and keep informed of treatments.
- Monitor hemodynamic status: vital signs; central venous pressure.
- Maintain adequate oxygenation; supplemental oxygenation; monitor respiratory status; evaluate function of mechanical ventilation and oxygenation.
- Maintain adequate circulation/cardiac output: fluids and inotropic medications.
- Medication administration and evaluation of effectiveness of same: antibiotics; inotropes; sedation
- Pain management
- Monitor for associated complications such as DIC: oozing, bleeding, bruising, petechiae, hypotension, early signs of organ dysfunction.
- Prevention of infection: handwashing; aseptic technique handling central lines and other invasive therapies; standard precautions
- Maintain and promote family contact; avoid unnecessary separation from child.
- Involve family in care of child to extent allowable to prevent sense of helplessness and loss of role as caregiver.

Patient and Family Teaching
- Information about treatments and required care
- Support systems for family support
- Care of child in acute and recuperative phase

SEVERE COMBINED IMMUNODEFICIENCY DISEASE

Description
Severe combined immunodeficiency disease (SCID) is a defect characterized by the absence of both humoral and cell-mediated immunity. The terms *Swiss-type lymphopenic agammaglobulinemia,* which refers to the autosomal recessive form of the disease, and *X-linked lymphopenic agammaglobulinemia* have been used to describe this disorder, which, as the names imply, can follow either mode of inheritance.

Pathophysiology
The exact cause of SCID is unknown. The theories include (1) a defective stem cell that is incapable of differentiating into B or T cells; (2) defects in the organs responsible for the differentiating process, primarily the thymus and lymphoid complex; or (3) an enzymatic defect that suppresses lymphocytic cell function.

Clinical Signs and Symptoms
- Most common manifestation is susceptibility to infection early in life, most often in the first month. Specifically, the disorder in children is characterized by chronic infection, failure to completely recover from an infection, frequent reinfection, and infection with unusual agents. In addition, the history reveals no logical source of infection.
- Failure to thrive is a consequence of the persistent illness. If the child should receive a foreign tissue (e.g., blood supplements), signs of graft-versus-host reaction, such as fever, skin rash, alopecia, hepatosplenomegaly, and diarrhea, are expected.
- Because tissue damage does not become evident in the reaction for 7 to 20 days, the symptoms may be mistaken for an infection. However, the presence of a graft-versus-host reaction increases the child's susceptibility to overwhelming infection and therefore is a grave complication.

Diagnostic Evaluation
- History of recurrent, severe infections from early infancy; a familial history of the disorder
- Specific laboratory findings, which include lymphopenia, lack of lymphocyte response to antigens, and absence of plasma cells in the bone marrow
- Documentation of immunoglobulin deficiency is difficult during infancy because of the normally delayed response of infants in producing their own immunoglobulins and maternal transfer of IgG.

Treatment
- The definitive treatment is a histocompatible HSCT.
- Other approaches to the management of SCID include providing passive immunity with IVIG and maintaining the child in a sterile environment. The latter is effective only if the measure is instituted before any infectious process takes hold in the infant, and it represents an extreme effort to prevent life-threatening infections.

Nursing Care Management
- Nursing care depends on the type of therapy used. If bone marrow transplantation is attempted, the care is consistent with that needed by patients undergoing bone marrow transplantation for any condition.
- To prevent infection, all interventions aimed at protecting the immunocompromised child are implemented. However, even with exacting environmental control, these children are prone to opportunistic infection.
- Chronic fungal infections of the mouth and nails with *Candida albicans* are frequent problems despite vigorous efforts at prevention or treatment.
- A hoarse voice may result from repeated esophageal and vocal cord erosions from the fungus.
- Parents should be encouraged to immediately notify a physician regarding any evidence of a worsening infection.

Patient and Family Teaching
- Because the prognosis for a child with SCID is very poor if a compatible bone marrow donor is not available, nursing care is

directed at supporting the family in caring for a child with a life-threatening illness.
- It is important to stress to parents that such conditions are not a result of laxity on their part in preventing them but are a result of the severe immunologic disorder.
- Genetic counseling is essential because of the modes of transmission in either form of the disorder.

SICKLE CELL ANEMIA
Description
Sickle cell anemia (SCA) is one of a group of diseases collectively termed *hemoglobinopathies*, in which normal adult hemoglobin (hemoglobin A [HbA]) is partly or completely replaced by abnormal sickle hemoglobin (HbS). *Sickle cell disease (SCD)* includes all those hereditary disorders whose clinical, hematologic, and pathologic features are related to the presence of HbS. Even though SCD is sometimes used to refer to SCA, this use is incorrect. Other correct terms for SCA are *SS* and *homozygous sickle cell disease* (see Box 3-10).

Pathophysiology
The clinical features of SCA are primarily the result of (1) *obstruction* caused by the sickled RBCs and (2) increased RBC *destruction*. The abnormal adhesion, entanglement and enmeshing of rigid

---

▌ BOX 3-10
Terms for Sickle Cell Anemia

SICKLE CELL ANEMIA
The homozygous form of the disease (HbSS or SS).

SICKLE CELL–C DISEASE
A heterozygous variant of SCD including both HbS and HbC (SC).

SICKLE CELL–HEMOGLOBIN E DISEASE
A variant of SCD in which glutamic acid has been substituted for lysine in the number-26 position of the β-chain (SE).

SICKLE THALASSEMIA DISEASE
A combination of sickle cell trait and β-thalassemia trait (Sβthal). β^+ refers to the ability to still produce some normal HbA. β^0 indicates that there is no ability to produce HbA.

sickle-shaped cells with one another intermittently block the micro-circulation, causing vaso-occlusion. The resultant absence of blood flow to adjacent tissues causes local hypoxia, leading to tissue ischemia and infarction (cellular death).

Clinical Signs and Symptoms
■ The most acute symptoms of the disease occur during periods of exacerbation called *crises*.
■ There are several types of episodic crises: vaso-occlusive, acute splenic sequestration, aplastic, hyperhemolytic, cerebrovascular accident (stroke), chest syndrome, and infection. The crises may occur individually or concomitantly with one or more other crises.
■ The episode may be a *vaso-occlusive crisis* (VOC), preferably called a "painful episode," characterized by distal ischemia and pain; *sequestration crisis*, a pooling of blood in the liver and spleen with decreased blood volume and shock; *aplastic crisis*, diminished RBC production resulting in profound anemia; or *hyperhemolytic crisis*, an accelerated rate of RBC destruction characterized by anemia, jaundice, and reticulocytosis.
■ Another serious complication is *acute chest syndrome* (ACS), which is clinically similar to pneumonia. It is the presence of a new pulmonary infiltrate and is associated with chest pain, fever, cough, tachypnea, wheezing, and hypoxia.
■ A *cerebrovascular accident* (CVA, stroke) is a sudden and severe complication, often with no related illnesses. Sickled cells block the major blood vessels in the brain, resulting in cerebral infarction, which causes variable degrees of neurologic impairment.

Diagnostic Evaluation
■ *Hemoglobin electrophoresis* ("finger printing" of the protein) is an accurate, rapid, and specific test for detecting the homozygous and heterozygous forms of the disease, as well as the percentages of the various types of Hgb.

Treatment
The aims of therapy are (1) to prevent the sickling phenomena, which are responsible for the pathologic sequelae; and (2) to treat the medical emergencies of sickle cell crisis. The successful achievement

of the aims depends on prompt nursing interventions, medical therapies, patient and family preventive measures, and use of innovative
treatments.

Medical management of a crisis is usually directed at supportive
and symptomatic treatment. The main objectives are to provide
(1) rest to minimize energy expenditure and oxygen use; (2) hydration through oral and IV therapy; (3) electrolyte replacement, because hypoxia results in metabolic acidosis, which also promotes
sickling; (4) analgesics for the severe pain from vaso-occlusion;
(5) blood replacement to treat anemia and hydration to reduce the
viscosity of the sickled blood; and (6) antibiotics to treat any existing infection.

Nursing Care Management

- Allow families to discuss feelings regarding transmitting a potentially fatal, chronic illness to their child.
- Emphasize the importance of adequate hydration to prevent
  sickling and to delay the adhesion-stasis-thrombosis-ischemia
  cycle in a crisis. It is not sufficient to advise parents to "force
  fluids" or "encourage drinking." They need specific instructions
  on how many daily glasses or bottles of fluid are required.
- Pain management is a difficult problem and often involves ex-
  perimenting with various analgesics, including opioids, and
  schedules before relief is achieved.
- Administer pneumococcal and meningococcal vaccines because
  of their susceptibility to infection as a result of a functional as-
  plenia. In addition to routine immunizations, the child with
  SCD should receive a yearly influenza vaccination. Oral penicillin prophylaxis is also recommended by 2 months of age to reduce the chance of pneumococcal sepsis.
- Be aware of the signs of splenic sequestions, acute chest syndrome, and CVA.

Patient and Family Teaching

- The most important issues to teach the family are to (1) seek
  early intervention for problems, such as fever of 38.5° C
  (101.5° F) or greater; (2) give penicillin as ordered; (3) recognize signs and symptoms of splenic sequestration, as well as
  respiratory problems that can lead to hypoxia; and (4) treat
  the child normally.

- Advise parents to be particularly alert to situations in which dehydration may be a possibility, such as hot weather, and to recognize early signs of reduced intake, such as decreased urine output (e.g., fewer wet diapers) and increased thirst.
- Avoid low-oxygen environment (e.g., high altitudes, nonpressurized airplane flights).

SLIPPED CAPITAL FEMORAL EPIPHYSIS
Description
Slipped femoral capital epiphysis (SFCE), or coxa vara, refers to the spontaneous displacement of the proximal femoral epiphysis in a posterior and inferior direction. It develops most frequently shortly before or during accelerated growth and the onset of puberty (children between the ages of 10 and 16 years: median age, 13 for boys, 12 for girls) and is most frequently observed in males and obese children.

Pathophysiology
SCFE can be associated with endocrine disorders, growth hormone therapy, renal osteodystrophy, and radiation therapy. The cause of idiopathic SFCE is multifactorial and includes obesity, physeal architecture and orientation, and pubertal hormone changes that affect physeal strength. Although obesity stresses the physeal plate, SFCE can also occur in children who are not obese. Radiographs show medial displacement of the epiphysis and uncovered upper portion of the femoral neck adjacent to the physis. There is a widened growth plate and irregular metaphysis. The capital femoral epiphysis remains in the acetabulum, but the femoral neck slips, deforming the femoral head and stretching blood vessels to the epiphysis.

Clinical Signs and Symptoms
- Limp on affected side
- Pain in hip
- Continuous or intermittent
- Frequently referred to groin, anteromedial aspect of thigh, or knee
- Restricted internal rotation on adduction with external rotation deformity
- Loss of abduction and internal rotation as severity increases

- Shortening of lower extremity
- Child may be overweight.

Diagnostic Evaluation
- Anterioposterior and frog-leg radiographic examination

Treatment
- Bed rest to prevent further slippage
- Traction before surgery may be used but is less common.
- Surgical pinning with possible osteotomy

Nursing Care Management
- Identification of condition
- Assist with diagnostic exams.
- Keep child and family informed of procedures for diagnosis.
- Preoperative care: traction care as applicable; if on prolonged bed rest, general nursing care related to health maintenance and promotion—activity, nutrition, skin and hygiene care; relief from boredom; socialization with peers; school work to avoid losing ground in school from treatment
- Postoperative care: monitoring vital signs; pain management; cast care including neurovascular status and monitoring of affected limb in cast; skin care; nutrition; school work as above
- Provide child and family support to cope with temporary disability.

Patient and Family Teaching
- Information about condition, treatment, and expected activity limitations and allowances
- Medication administration for pain
- Activities, socialization, and school work

STREPTOCOCCAL PHARYNGITIS, ACUTE
Description
Pharyngitis, or sore throat, is a common occurrence in children. The sore throat is commonly caused by the bacteria group A β-hemolytic streptococci (GABHS). GABHS is generally a relatively brief illness that varies in severity from subclinical (no symptoms) to severe toxicity infection of the upper airway (***strep throat***).

Pathophysiology

Children may be exposed to strep throat by GABHS in the home, school, or day care setting. The infection is spread by respiratory tract secretions from contact with an infected person. The tonsils and pharynx may be inflamed and covered with exudates, and the child may have difficulty swallowing. Children who experience group A β-hemolytic streptococci (GABHS) infection of the upper airway (*strep throat*) are at risk for *rheumatic fever* (RF), an inflammatory disease of the heart, joints, and central nervous system, and *acute glomerulonephritis*, an acute kidney infection. Permanent damage can result from these sequelae, especially RF.

Clinical Signs and Symptoms

- Sore throat with sudden onset. Pain can be relatively mild to severe enough to make swallowing difficult.
- Fever may or may not be present.
- Headache
- Stomachache
- Tongue may appear edematous and red (strawberry tongue).
- Characteristic erythematous fine sandpaper rash on the trunk, axillae, elbows, and groin
- Uvula is edematous and red.
- Anterior cervical lymphadenopathy in about 30% to 50% of cases

Diagnostic Evaluation

- Examination of throat
- Confirmation with throat culture positive for GABHS
- Rapid-strep test (rapid antigen detection test)

Treatment

- Penicillin: can be given by mouth or IM benzathine penicillin G (as one-time dose)
- Supportive care: acetaminophen or ibuprofen for throat pain; warm saline gargles
- Ensure adequate fluid intake during acute phase.

Nursing Care Management

- Assist with diagnosis by performing throat swab for culture and rapid strep test.
- Medication administration

Patient and Family Teaching

- Pain management: warm gargles
- Medication administration: take all of prescribed oral antibiotics.
- Prevention of exposure of others: avoid direct contact such as sneezing, coughing, drinking from same glass, or eating from same utensils; handwashing; disposal of soiled tissues.
- Prevention of reinfection: wash toothbrush in hot water dishwasher to kill bacteria, or obtain new toothbrush.
- Recognition of sequelae such as acute glomerulonephritis

SUDDEN INFANT DEATH SYNDROME

Description

Sudden infant death syndrome (*SIDS*) is the sudden death of an infant younger than 1 year of age that remains unexplained after a complete postmortem examination, including an investigation of the death scene and a review of the case history (see Box 3-11).

BOX 3-11

Epidemiology of SIDS

Factors	Occurrence
Incidence	0.57:1000 live births (2002)
Peak age	2 to 3 months; 95% occur by 6 months; infants born preterm died from SIDS at mean age of 6 weeks after mean age of death from SIDS for term infants
Sex	Higher percentage of males affected
Time of death	During sleep
Time of year	Increased incidence in winter
Racial	Greater incidence in African Americans, Native Americans, and hispanics. In 2001, SIDS in African Americans was 2.5 times higher than in caucasians; prone positioning rates were also higher in African Americans in 2001 (21% in African Americans vs 11 % in caucasians).
Socioeconomic	Increased occurrence in lower socioeconomic class

Continued

■ BOX 3-11—cont'd

Epidemiology of SIDS

Factors	Occurrence
Birth	Higher incidence in ■ Preterm infants, especially infants of extremely and very low birth weight ■ Multiple births* ■ Neonates with low Apgar scores ■ Infants with central nervous system disturbances and respiratory disorders such as bronchopulmonary dysplasia ■ Increasing birth order (subsequent siblings as opposed to firstborn child) ■ Infants with a recent history of illness
Sleep habits	Highest risk associated with prone position; use of soft bedding; overheating (thermal stress); cosleeping with adult, especially on sofa, or noninfant bed. Infants cosleeping with adult at higher risk if less than 11 weeks old
Feeding habits	Lower incidence in breast-fed infants
Pacifier	Lower incidence in infants put to sleep with pacifier
Siblings	May have greater incidence
Maternal	Young age; cigarette smoking, especially during pregnancy; poor prenatal care; substance abuse (heroin, methadone, cocaine); a few studies have shown an increased risk in infants exposed to second-hand environmental tobacco smoke.

*Although a rare event, simultaneous death of twins from sudden infant death syndrome can occur.

Pathophysiology

A number of theories have been proposed for the cause of SIDS, but the exact cause remains unknown. Abnormalities include prolonged sleep apnea, increased frequency of brief inspiratory pauses, excessive periodic breathing, and impaired arousal responsiveness to increased carbon dioxide or decreased oxygen; however, sleep apnea is not the cause of SIDS. Another hypothesis is that SIDS is related to a brainstem abnormality in the neurologic regulation of cardiorespiratory control. The association between the incidence of SIDS and the following hypothesized causes have yet to be clearly demonstrated: prolonged Q-T interval, rebreathing of carbon dioxide by infants in the prone position, impaired ability to achieve full arousal in prone position during sleep, or overheating while sleeping prone. A genetic predisposition to SIDS has been postulated as a cause.

Risk factors associated with SIDS deaths include prone sleeping, maternal smoking during pregnancy, infant bed sharing with an adult or older child on a noninfant bed (cosleeping), infants placed to sleep in a side-lying position, and soft bedding. Supine sleeping, breastfeeding, and pacifier use are associated with a decreased risk for SIDS in some studies.

SIDS is a distinct entity from an **apparent life-threatening event**, formerly referred to as aborted SIDS death or near-miss SIDS, which refers to an event that is sudden and frightening to the observer, in which the infant exhibits a combination of apnea, change in color (pallor, cyanosis, redness), change in muscle tone (usually hypotonia), choking, gagging, or coughing, and which usually involves a significant intervention and even cardiopulmonary resuscitation by the caregiver who witnesses the event.

Clinical Signs and Symptoms
Autopsies reveal consistent pathologic findings such as pulmonary edema and intrathoracic hemorrhages that confirm the diagnosis of SIDS.

Diagnostic Evaluation
There is no diagnostic test for SIDS.

Treatment
The treatment of SIDS is prevention. The Back to Sleep campaign is an educational program aimed at teaching parents and caretakers about placing the infant to sleep on the back and by avoiding other risk factors known to be associated with SIDS.

Nursing Care Management
- Prevention: teaching parents and caretakers about risk factors for SIDS.
- Modeling: serving as role models in health care settings to place infants on their back to sleep

■ Caregiver: providing support and comfort to the parents (family) who experience a SIDS death and discussing options for care of the deceased infant; care for the mother who was breast-feeding to stop milk production, should this be desired; providing resources and follow-up for parents who have experienced a SIDS death through support groups

Patient and Family Teaching
■ Teaching is focused on avoiding prone sleeping position in infants: avoiding risk factors such as cosleeping with an adult, smoking during pregnancy, and soft bedding surfaces; removing bedding items such as stuffed animals or toys; avoiding sleeping on a noninfant bedding surface; and avoiding tobacco smoke exposure.
■ Teach day care and other caretakers to place infant to sleep in supine position.

SYNDROME OF INAPPROPRIATE ANTIDIURETIC HORMONE
Description
The disorder that results from oversecretion of the posterior pituitary hormone, or ADH, is known as SIADH.

Pathophysiology
It is observed with increased frequency in a variety of conditions, especially those involving infections, tumors, or other CNS disease or trauma.

Clinical Signs and Symptoms
■ Signs and symptoms are directly related to fluid retention and hypotonicity.
■ When serum sodium levels are diminished to 120 mEq/L, affected children display anorexia, nausea (and sometimes vomiting), stomach cramps, irritability, and personality changes.
■ With progressive reduction in sodium, other neurologic signs, stupor, and convulsions may occur.

Diagnostic Evaluation
■ Excess ADH causes most of the filtered water to be reabsorbed from the kidneys back into central circulation.

- Serum osmolality is low.
- Urine osmolality is inappropriately elevated.

Treatment
- The immediate management consists of restricting fluids.
- Subsequent management depends on the cause and severity.

Nursing Care Management
- The first goal of nursing management is recognizing the presence of SIADH from symptoms.
- Accurately measure intake and output.
- Weight child daily.
- Observe for signs of fluid overload.
- Implement seizure precautions.

Patient and Family Teaching
- Child and family need education regarding the rationale for fluid restrictions.

SYSTEMIC LUPUS ERYTHEMATOSUS
Description
Systemic lupus erythematosus (SLE) is a chronic, multisystem, autoimmune disease of the connective tissues and blood vessels characterized by inflammation in potentially any body tissue. Its course and symptoms are variable and unpredictable, with mild to life-threatening complications.

Pathophysiology
The cause of SLE is not known. It appears to result from a complex interaction of genetics with an unidentified trigger that causes the disease to activate. Suspected triggers include exposure to ultraviolet light, estrogen, pregnancy, infections, and drugs.

Clinical Signs and Symptoms
- Constitutional: fever, fatigue, weight loss, anorexia
- Cutaneous: erythematosus butterfly rash over bridge of nose and across cheeks, discoid rash, photosensitivity, mucocutaneous ulceration, alopecia, periungual telangiectasias
- Musculoskeletal: arthritis, arthralgia, myositis, myalgia, tenosynovitis

- Neurologic: headache, seizure, forgetfulness, behavior change, change in school performance, psychosis, chorea, stroke, cranial and peripheral neuropathy, pseudotumor cerebri
- Pulmonary and cardiac: pleuritis, basilar pneumonitis, atelectasis, pericarditis, myocarditis, and endocarditis
- Renal: glomerulonephritis, nephrotic syndrome, hypertension
- Gastrointestinal: abdominal pain, nausea, vomiting, blood in stool, abdominal crisis, esophageal dysfunction, colitis
- Hepatic, splenic, and nodal: hepatomegaly, splenomegaly, lymphadenopathy
- Hematologic: anemia, cytopenia
- Ophthalmologic: cotton wool spots, papilledema, retinopathy
- Vascular: Raynaud phenomenon, thrombophlebitis, livedo reticularis

Diagnostic Evaluation

The diagnosis of SLE is established when 4 of the following 11 diagnostic criteria are met:

1. Malar rash: fixed malar erythema
2. Discoid rash: patchy erythematous lesions
3. Photosensitivity: rash with sun exposure
4. Oronasal ulcers: painless ulcers in mouth/nose
5. Arthritis: swelling, tenderness, or effusion in two or more peripheral joints (nonerosive)
6. Serositis: pleuritis/pericarditis
7. Renal disorder: proteinuria/casts
8. Neurologic disorder: psychosis/seizures
9. Hematologic disorder: hemolytic anemia, thrombocytopenia, leukopenia, lymphopenia
10. Immunologic disorder: anti–double-stranded DNA, anti-SM, antiphospholipid antibodies; lupus anticoagulant; false-positive syphilis test (RPR; rapid plasma reagin)
11. Antinuclear antibodies

Treatment

- Supportive therapy
- Medications: corticosteroids to control inflammation
- NSAIDS
- Antimalarial preparations: for rash and arthritis
- Immunosuppressive agents: cyclophosphamide, for renal and central nervous system disease

- Antihypertensives, aspirin, and antibiotics: to treat or avoid complications

Nursing Care Management
- Help child and family recognize subtle signs of disease exacerbation.
- Encourage school involvement and age-appropriate activities as tolerated.
- Assist in dealing with body image issues as a result of rash, corticosteroid therapy.
- Support the child and family.

Patient and Family Teaching
- Recognition of subtle signs of disease exacerbation
- Avoid triggers such as exposure to the sun and UVB light: sunscreens, sun-resistant clothing, and altering outdoor activities.
- Medication administration and potential complications with corticosteroid therapy
- Regular medical follow-up examinations
- Discuss issues related to pregnancy (may exacerbate symptoms).

TETANUS
Description
Tetanus is an acute, preventable, but often fatal disease caused by an exotoxin produced by the anaerobic spore-forming, Gram-positive bacillus *Clostridium tetani*.

Pathophysiology
Tetanus spores are found in soil, dust, and the intestinal tracts of humans and animals, especially herbivorous animals. The organisms are not invasive but enter the body by way of wounds, particularly a puncture wound, burn, or crushed area. In the newborn, infection may occur through the umbilical cord, usually in situations in which infants are delivered in severely contaminated surroundings or the mother is not adequately immunized. The organisms proliferate and form potent exotoxins, one of which is tetanospasmin. Tetanospasmin affects the central nervous system to produce the clinical manifestations of the disease. The ideal conditions for growth of the organisms are devitalized tissues without access to air, such as wounds that have not been washed or

kept clean and those that have crusted over, trapping pus beneath. The exotoxin appears to reach the central nervous system by way of either the neuron axons or the vascular system. The toxin becomes fixed on nerve cells of the anterior horn of the spinal cord and the brainstem. The toxin acts at the myoneural junction to produce muscular stiffness and lower the threshold for reflex excitability. The manner of onset varies, but the initial symptoms are usually a progressive stiffness and tenderness of the muscles in the neck and jaw. Eventually all voluntary muscles are affected.

Clinical Signs and Symptoms
Initial Symptoms
- Progressive stiffness and tenderness of muscles in neck and jaw
- Characteristic difficulty in opening the mouth (trismus)
- Risus sardonicus (sardonic smile) caused by facial muscle spasm

Progressive Involvement
- Opisthotonic positioning
- Boardlike rigidity of abdominal and limb muscles
- Difficulty swallowing
- Extreme sensitivity to external stimuli (slight noise, gentle touch, or bright light)
- Trigger paroxysmal muscular contractions that last seconds to minutes
  - Contractions recur with increased frequency until almost continuous (sustained, tetanic).
- Laryngospasm and tetany of respiratory muscles
  - Accumulated secretions
  - Respiratory arrest
  - Atelectasis
  - Pneumonia

Other Aspects
- Mentation unaffected; patient alert
- Pain, anxiety, and distress are reflected by:
  - Rapid pulse
  - Sweating
  - Anxious facial expression
- Fever usually absent or only mild

Diagnostic Evaluation
- Based on clinical manifestations and the history

Treatment
- Prevention by immunization (DTaP, Td, or Tdap)
- Exposed child: administer tetanus toxoid and tetanus immune globulin (TIG); both are given IM at separate sites and in separate syringes.
- Clean wound thoroughly.
- Acutely ill child with tetanus: supportive care including maintaining adequate airway and fluid and electrolyte balance, pain management, and ensuring adequate caloric intake
- Indwelling oral or nasogastric feedings may be required to maintain adequate fluid and caloric intake; continued laryngospasm may necessitate total parenteral nutrition or gastrostomy feeding.
- Severe or recurrent laryngospasm or excessive secretions may require advanced airway management such as endotracheal intubation.
- Antibiotics to control the proliferation of the vegetative forms of the organism at the site of infection
- Seizures—administer either diazepam or lorazepam.
- For acutely ill child, consider sedation and pain management as muscle spasms are painful.
- Intrathecal baclofen, magnesium sulfate, dantrolene sodium, and midazolam may also be used in the management of tetanus.
- Patients who do not respond to muscle relaxants may require the administration of a neuromuscular blocking agent, such as rocuronium or vecuronium.

Nursing Care Management
- Prevention: administer immunizations, and encourage parents to obtain boosters.
- Acutely ill child: wound cleansing; administration of medications; airway support; nutrition support; emotional support; monitoring neurological signs for progression of symptoms; decrease stimuli; pain management; communication with intubated child; seizure precautions

Patient and Family Teaching

- Encourage support of child in acute phase; communication with child; discuss plan of care with family.
- Encourage immunizations in all children.

TETRALOGY OF FALLOT

Description

The classic form includes four defects: (1) ventricular septal defect (VSD), (2) pulmonic stenosis, (3) overriding aorta, and (4) right ventricular hypertrophy.

Pathophysiology

The alteration in hemodynamics varies widely, depending primarily on the degree of pulmonary stenosis, but also on the size of the VSD and the pulmonary and systemic resistance to flow. Because the VSD is usually large, pressures may be equal in the right and left ventricles. Therefore the shunt direction depends on the difference between pulmonary and systemic vascular resistance. If pulmonary vascular resistance is higher than systemic resistance, the shunt is from right to left. If systemic resistance is higher than pulmonary resistance, the shunt is from left to right. Pulmonic stenosis decreases blood flow to the lungs and, consequently, the amount of oxygenated blood that returns to the left side of the heart. Depending on the position of the aorta, blood from both ventricles may be distributed systemically.

Clinical Signs and Symptoms

Some infants may be acutely cyanotic at birth; others have mild cyanosis that progresses over the first year of life as the pulmonic stenosis worsens. There is a systolic ejection murmur heard at the mid and upper left border that may radiate toward the back. There may be acute episodes of cyanosis and hypoxia, called *blue spells* or *tet spells*. These hypercyanotic spells occur when the infundibular area below the pulmonary valve acutely narrows and increases obstruction of blood flow to the lungs. These spells can occur during crying or after feeding. Squatting is a common posture in toddlers having a hypercyanotic spell. Squatting increases the systemic venous return and systemic vascular resistance forcing blood flow toward the pulmonary circulation. Patients are at risk for emboli, seizures, and loss of consciousness or sudden death following a hypercyanotic spell.

Diagnostic Evaluation
See Tables 3-1 and 3-2.

Treatment
Surgical Treatment
Palliative shunt:—In infants who cannot undergo primary repair, a palliative procedure to increase pulmonary blood flow and increase oxygen saturation may be performed. The preferred procedure is a modified Blalock-Taussig shunt operation, which provides blood flow to the pulmonary arteries from the left or right subclavian artery via a tube graft.

Complete repair:—Elective repair is usually performed in the first year of life. Indications for repair include increasing cyanosis and the development of hypercyanotic spells. Complete repair involves closure of the VSD and resection of the infundibular stenosis, with placement of a pericardial patch to enlarge the right ventricular outflow tract. In some repairs, the patch may extend across the pulmonary valve annulus (transannular patch), making the pulmonary valve incompetent. The procedure requires a median sternotomy and the use of cardiopulmonary bypass.

Nursing Care Management
Assist in Measures to Assess and Improve Cardiac Function
Monitor Cardiac Function
- Vital signs monitoring
- Respiratory assessment
- Cardiac assessment
  - Cardiac output (color, pulses, perfusion, capillary refill, renal function, and neurologic function)
  - Heart sounds
  - Dysrhythmias
- Monitor for any neurologic changes.
- Monitor all intravenous lines for air. No air can be allowed in any IV line.
- Keep accurate record of intake and output.
- Monitor for adequate hydration.

- Weigh child or infant on same scale at same time of day.
- Following shunt placement:
  - Monitor shunt patency by auscultating over the shunt and hearing the "shunt murmur."
  - Monitor for increased cyanosis.
  - Monitor platelets.

Administer Medications
- Review child's history related to cardiac management.
- Administer medications on schedule.
- Assess effectiveness of medications and any side effects noted.
- Be aware of drug-drug and drug-food interactions.
- Follow guidelines for medication administration.

Manage Common Side Effects of Cardiac Defects
- Prevent fatigue during feeding; offer small frequent feedings to infant's or child's tolerance.
- Organize nursing care to allow child/infant uninterrupted rest.
- Promote activities that do not cause fatigue.
- Provide support for the child and family.
- Communicate with the child and family in an appropriate style.
- Provide the child and family with honest answers.
- Provide emotional support.
- Offer age-appropriate interventions.
- Provide information on available resources for support for the child and family.

Patient and Family Teaching
Prepare the Child and Family for Diagnostic and Operative Procedures
- Provide explanation of diagnostic tests and why each test is performed because many of them are invasive procedures.
- Prepare the child prior to the invasive procedure. Remember discussion is dependent upon the child's age and development.
- Use simple words or pictures to describe procedures and answer all questions the child and family may have.
- Postoperative wound care teaching as needed.
- Post-cardiac catheterization wound care teaching as needed.
- Assess and record results of teaching and family's participation in care.

Educate the Child and Family

- Assess child's and family's level of knowledge regarding tetralogy of Fallot.
- Assess child's and family's understanding of what they have heard about tetralogy of Fallot.
- Assess child's and family's understanding of the surgery and/or cardiac catheterization.
- Teach the child and/or family at least four characteristics of congestive heart failure that may occur because of tetralogy of Fallot such as:
  - Fatigue after exertion
  - Fast heart rate
  - Fast breathing, shortness of breath, dyspnea
  - Retractions
  - Nasal flaring
  - Cool extremities
  - Diaphoresis
  - Decreased urine output
  - Puffiness (edema)
  - Fussiness
  - Decreased appetite
- Teach the family signs and symptoms of dehydration.
- Teach the family signs and symptoms of hypercyanotic spells.
- Teach the family how to manage a hypercyanotic spell.
  - "Knee-chest" position
  - Notify the child's physician immediately.
- Educate child and family about care such as medication preparation and administration.
- Assess child's and family's access to appropriate pharmacy for any special preparation medications.
- Educate child and family to notify their physician of any clinical changes.
- Assess and record results and family's participation in care.
- Provide appropriate educational resources, and review materials with them.
- Clarify information presented by the health care team including appointment for follow-up visit.
- Discuss SBE (subacute bacterial endocarditis) prophylaxis with your pediatric cardiologist.

TINEA CORPORIS

Description
The dermatophytoses (ringworm) are infections caused by a group of closely related filamentous fungi that invade primarily the stratum corneum, hair, and nails. Dermatophytoses are designated by the Latin word *tinea*, with further designation related to the area of the body where they are found (e.g., tinea capitis [ringworm of the scalp]).

Pathophysiology
Tinea corporis lives on, not in, the skin. The fungi are confined to the dead keratin layers and are unable to survive in the deeper layers. Because the keratin is desquamated constantly, the fungus must multiply at a rate that equals the rate of keratin production to maintain itself; otherwise, the infection would be shed with the discarded skin cells. Dermatophyte infections are most often transmitted from one person to another or from infected animals to humans.

Clinical Signs and Symptoms
Generally round or oval, erythematous scaling patch that spreads peripherally and clears centrally; usually unilateral; may involve nails (tinea unguium)

Diagnostic Evaluation
- Diagnosis is made from microscopic examination of scrapings taken from the advancing periphery of the lesion.

Treatment
- Oral griseofulvin
- 2% ketoconazole and 1% selenium sulfide shampoos
- Local application of antifungal preparation such as tolnaftate, haloprogin, miconazole, clotrimazole; apply 1 inch beyond periphery of lesion; continual application 1 to 2 weeks after no sign of lesion

Nursing Care Management
- Identify fungal infection.
- Parent and child teaching regarding medication administration, hygiene, and prevention of spread

Patient and Family Teaching
- Affected children should not exchange grooming items, head-gear, scarves, or other articles of apparel that have been in proximity to the infected area with other children.
- Affected children are provided with their own towels and directed to wear a protective cap at night to avoid transmitting the fungus to bedding.
- Household pets should be examined for the presence of the fungus.
- Use of antifungal shampoo which should be applied to the scalp for 5 to 10 minutes at least 3 times per week.
- Medication administration: emphasize compliance with length of treatment; side effects (headache, gastrointestinal upset, fatigue, insomnia, and photosensitivity).

TONSILLITIS
Description
An inflammation of the tonsils that usually occurs in association with an upper respiratory infection. The *palatine*, or *faucial tonsils*, are located on either side of the oropharynx, behind and below the pillars of the fauces (opening from the mouth). The *pharyngeal tonsils*, also known as the *adenoids*, are located above the palatine tonsils on the posterior wall of the nasopharynx. Their proximity to the nares and Eustachian tubes causes difficulties in instances of inflammation. The *lingual tonsils* are located at the base of the tongue.

Pathophysiology
The tonsils are masses of lymphoid tissue located in the pharyngeal cavity. They filter and protect the respiratory and alimentary tracts from invasion by pathogenic organisms and play a role in antibody formation. Tonsillitis often occurs with pharyngitis. The causative agent may be viral or bacterial. Because of the abundant lymphoid tissue and the frequency of URIs, tonsillitis is a common cause of illness in young children.

Clinical Signs and Symptoms
- Enlarged and edematous tonsils
- Difficulty breathing
- Difficulty swallowing
- Mouth breathing when adenoids are swollen

Diagnostic Evaluation
- Inspection of the oral cavity
- Clinical manifestations

Treatment
- GABHS (group A beta hemolytic streptococcus) tonsillitis requires a penicillin regimen.
- Otherwise, supportive treatment: warm saline gargles for throat pain; mild analgesic such as acetaminophen
- Tonsillectomy: surgical removal of tonsils—indications for a tonsillectomy are malignancy, recurrent peritonsilar abscess, and airway obstruction.
- Adenoidectomy: surgical removal of the adenoids; recommended for children who have hypertrophied adenoids that obstruct nasal breathing; recurrent adenoiditis and sinusitis, otitis media with effusion, airway obstruction and subsequent sleep-disordered breathing, and recurrent rhinorrhea

Nursing Care Management
- Detection
- Teaching comfort measures to patient and family
- If surgical intervention required: preoperative preparation; keep parents informed of child's operative and recuperative progress; observe for complications (bleeding, nausea, vomiting, inadequate fluid intake); pain management; monitoring vital signs; discharge teaching.

Patient and Family Teaching
- Comfort measures for tonsillitis.
- If surgery is performed: encourage contact with child; postoperative care; discharge instructions regarding pain management, bleeding, fluid intake.

TRANSPOSITION OF THE GREAT ARTERIES OR TRANSPOSITION OF THE GREAT VESSELS
Description
Also referred to as *D-Transposition of the Great Arteries*. The pulmonary artery arises from the left ventricle, and the aorta arises from the right ventricle. Therefore, oxygenated blood is pumped back to the lungs, and deoxygenated blood is pumped to the body.

There is mixing of oxygenated and deoxygenated blood at the atrial level, but patients present with cyanosis. There may or may not be a ventricular septal defect present. There is typically a patent foramen ovale and a patent ductus arteriosus.

Pathophysiology

Associated defects such as septal defects or patent ductus arteriosus must be present to permit blood to enter the systemic circulation or the pulmonary circulation for mixing of saturated and desaturated blood. The most common defect associated with transposition of the great arteries (TGA) is a patent foramen ovale. Another associated defect may be a ventricular septal defect (VSD). The presence of a VSD increases the risk of congestive heart failure (CHF), because it permits blood to flow from the right to the left ventricle, into the pulmonary artery, and finally to the lungs. However, it also produces high pulmonary blood flow under high pressure, which can result in high pulmonary vascular resistance.

Clinical Signs and Symptoms

Depend on the type and size of the associated defects. Newborns with minimum communication are severely cyanotic and have depressed cardiac function at birth. Those with large septal defects or a patent ductus arteriosus may be less cyanotic but have symptoms of CHF (see Box 3-1). Heart sounds vary according to the type of defect present. Cardiomegaly is usually evident a few weeks after birth.

Diagnostic Evaluation

See Tables 3-1 and 3-2 .

Treatment

(**To provide intracardiac mixing**): The administration of intravenous prostaglandin E_1 may be initiated to keep the ductus arteriosus open to temporarily increase blood mixing and provide an oxygen saturation of 75% or to maintain cardiac output. During cardiac catheterization or under echocardiographic guidance, a balloon atrial septostomy (Rashkind procedure) may also be performed to increase mixing by opening the atrial septum.

Surgical Treatment

An arterial switch procedure is the procedure of choice performed in the first weeks of life. It involves transecting the great arteries and anastomosing the main pulmonary artery to the proximal aorta (just above the aortic valve) and anastomosing the ascending aorta to the proximal pulmonary artery. The coronary arteries are removed as buttons from the proximal aorta and reimplanted to the proximal pulmonary artery (neoaorta). Reimplantation of the coronary arteries is critical to the infant's survival, and they must be reattached without torsion or kinking to provide the heart with its supply of oxygen. The advantage of the arterial switch procedure is the reestablishment of normal circulation, with the left ventricle acting as the systemic pump. Potential complications of the arterial switch include narrowing at the great artery anastomoses and coronary artery insufficiency.

Rastelli procedure: This procedure is the operative choice in infants with TGA, VSD, and severe pulmonic stenosis. It involves closure of the VSD with a baffle, so that left ventricular blood is directed through the VSD into the aorta. The pulmonic valve is then closed, and a conduit is placed from the right ventricle to the pulmonary artery to create a physiologically normal circulation. Unfortunately, this procedure requires multiple conduit replacements as the child grows.

Nursing Care Management
Assist in Measures to Assess and Improve Cardiac Function
Monitor Cardiac Function
- Vital signs monitoring
- Respiratory assessment
- Cardiac assessment
  - Cardiac output (color, pulses, perfusion, capillary refill, renal function, and neurologic function)
  - Heart sounds
  - Dysrhythmias
- Keep accurate record of intake and output.
- Weigh child or infant on same scale at same time of day.

Administer Medications
- Review child's history related to cardiac management.
- Administer medications on schedule.

- Assess effectiveness of medications and any side effects noted.
- Be aware of drug-drug and drug-food interactions.
- Follow guidelines for medication administration.

Manage Common Side Effects of Cardiac Defects
- Prevent fatigue during feeding; offer small frequent feedings to infant's or child's tolerance.
- Organize nursing care to allow child/infant uninterrupted rest.
- Promote activities that do not cause fatigue.

Provide Support for the Child and Family
- Communicate with the child and family in an appropriate style.
- Provide the child and family with honest answers.
- Provide emotional support.
- Offer age-appropriate interventions.
- Provide information on available resources for support for the child and family.

Patient and Family Teaching
Prepare the Child and Family for Diagnostic and Operative Procedures
- Provide explanation of diagnostic tests and why each test is performed because many of them are invasive procedures.
- Prepare the child prior to the invasive procedure. Remember that discussion is dependent upon the child's age and development.
- Use simple words or pictures to describe procedures, and answer all questions the child and family may have.
- Postoperative wound care teaching as needed
- Post-cardiac catheterization wound care teaching as needed
- Assess and record results of teaching and family's participation in care.

Educate the Child and Family
- Assess child's and family's level of knowledge regarding the transposition of the great arteries.
- Assess child's and family's understanding of what they have heard about transposition of the great arteries.
- Assess child's and family's understanding of the surgery and/or cardiac catheterization.

- Teach the child and/or family at least four characteristics of congestive heart failure that may occur because of the transposition of the great arteries such as:
  - Fatigue after exertion
  - Fast heart rate
  - Fast breathing, shortness of breath, dyspnea
  - Retractions
  - Nasal flaring
  - Cool extremities
  - Diaphoresis
  - Decreased urinary output
  - Puffiness (edema)
  - Fussiness
  - Decreased appetite
- Educate child and family about care such as medication preparation and administration.
- Assess child's and family's access to appropriate pharmacy for any special preparation medications.
- Educate child and family about when to notify their physician of any clinical changes.
- Assess and record results and family's participation in care.
- Provide appropriate educational resources and review materials with them.
- Clarify information presented by the health care team including appointment for follow-up visit.
- Discuss SBE (subacute bacterial endocarditis) prophylaxis with your pediatric cardiologist.

TRICUSPID ATRESIA
Description
The tricuspid valve fails to develop; consequently there is no communication from the right atrium to the right ventricle. Blood flows through an atrial septal defect (ASD) or a patent foramen ovale to the left side of the heart and through a VSD to the right ventricle and out to the lungs. Patients with tricuspid atresia may have pulmonic stenosis and transposition of the great arteries. There is complete mixing of unoxygenated and oxygenated blood in the left side of the heart, which results in systemic desaturation.

Pathophysiology

At birth, the presence of a patent foramen ovale (or other atrial septal opening) is required to permit blood flow across the septum into the left atrium; the patent ductus arteriosus allows blood flow to the pulmonary artery into the lungs for oxygenation. A VSD allows a modest amount of blood to enter the right ventricle and pulmonary artery for oxygenation. Pulmonary blood flow usually is diminished.

Clinical Signs and Symptoms

Cyanosis is usually seen in the newborn. There may be tachycardia and dyspnea. A low-frequency holosystolic murmur may be present. In patients with pulmonary stenosis, there may be a systolic crescendo-decrescendo murmur. Older children have signs of chronic hypoxemia with clubbing.

Diagnostic Evaluation

See Tables 3-1 and 3-2.

Treatment

For the neonate whose pulmonary blood flow depends on the patency of the ductus arteriosus, a continuous infusion of prostaglandin E_1 is started at 0.05-0.1 mcg/kg of body weight per minute until surgical intervention can be arranged.

Surgical Treatment

Some children have increased pulmonary blood flow and require pulmonary artery banding to lessen the volume of blood to the lungs. Other children are cyanotic and require staged palliation. The first stage is the placement of a systemic-to-pulmonary artery shunt to increase blood flow to the lungs. If the ASD is small, an atrial septostomy is performed during cardiac catheterization. The second stage is often a bidirectional Glenn shunt procedure or a hemi-Fontan operation. Both involve anastomosing the superior vena cava to the right pulmonary artery so superior vena cava flow bypasses the right atrium and flows directly to the lungs. The procedure is usually done at 3 to 6 months of age to relieve cyanosis and reduce the volume load on the right ventricle. The final repair is a modified Fontan procedure.

Modified Fontan procedure: Systemic venous return from the inferior vena cava is directed to the lungs through a conduit using the lateral tunnel or extracardiac technique. A fenestration (opening) is sometimes made in the conduit to relieve pressure. The patient must have normal ventricular function and a low pulmonary vascular resistance for the procedure to be successful. The modified Fontan procedure separates oxygenated and unoxygenated blood inside the heart and eliminates the excess volume load on the ventricle but does not restore normal anatomy or hemodynamics. This operation is also the final stage in the correction of many complex defects with a functional single ventricle, including HLHS.

Nursing Care Management
Assist in Measures to Assess and Improve Cardiac Function
Monitor Cardiac Function
- Vital signs monitoring
- Respiratory assessment
- Monitor oxygen saturation. Patients with shunts will not have normal oxygen saturations after the first and second stage surgeries. SpO_2 should be 75-80% after the first- and second-stage surgeries. Following the Fontan, the saturations will be close to normal.
- Following shunt placement:
  - Monitor shunt patency by auscultating over the shunt and hearing the "shunt murmur."
  - Monitor for increased cyanosis.
  - Monitor platelets.
- Following the Glenn, facilitate drainage from the SVC to the lungs by keeping the head of the bed elevated.
- Following the Fontan, monitor for signs and symptoms of pleural effusions.
- Monitor cardiac output (color, pulses, perfusion, capillary refill, renal function, and neurologic function).
- Monitor for dysrhythmias.
- Monitor for excessive sweating.
- Monitor for neurologic changes.
- Monitor for fussiness or inconsolability.
- Keep accurate record of intake and output (including chest-tube output following surgery).
- Weigh child or infant on same scale at same time of day.

Administer Medications
- Review child's history related to cardiac management.
- Administer medications on schedule.
- Assess effectiveness of medications and any side effects noted.
- Be aware of drug-drug interactions and drug-food interactions.
- Follow guidelines for medication administration.

Manage Common Side Effects of Cardiac Defects
- Prevent fatigue during feeding; offer small frequent feedings to infant's or child's tolerance.
- Organize nursing care to allow child/infant uninterrupted rest.
- Promote activities that do not cause fatigue.

Provide Support for the Child and Family
- Communicate with the child and family in an appropriate style.
- Provide the child and family with honest answers.
- Provide emotional support.
- Offer age-appropriate interventions.
- Provide information on available resources for support for the child and family.

Patient and Family Teaching
Prepare the Child and Family for Diagnostic and Operative Procedures
- Provide explanation of diagnostic tests and why each test is performed because many of them are invasive procedures.
- Prepare the child prior to the invasive procedure. Remember that discussion is dependent upon the child's age and development.
- Use simple words to describe procedures, and answer all questions the child and family may have.

Educate the Child and Family
- Assess child's and family's level of knowledge regarding tricuspid atresia.
- Assess child's and family's understanding of what they have heard about tricuspid atresia.
- Assess child's and family's understanding of the surgery.

- Teach the child and/or family at least four characteristics of heart failure that may occur because of tricuspid atresia such as:
  - Fatigue after exertion
  - Fast heart rate
  - Fast breathing, shortness of breath, dyspnea
  - Retractions
  - Nasal flaring
  - Cool extremities
  - Diaphoresis
  - Decreased urinary output
  - Puffiness (edema)
  - Fussiness
  - Decreased appetite
- Educate child and family about medication administration.
- Provide appropriate educational resources, and review materials with them.
- Clarify information presented by the health care team.
- Postoperative wound care teaching as needed
- Post-cardiac catheterization wound care teaching as needed
- Assess and record results of teaching and family's participation in care.

TUBERCULOSIS
Description
Tuberculosis (TB) is an infectious disease that primarily affects the lungs; extrapulmonary TB may be manifested as superior lymphadenitis, meningitis, or osteoarthritis and may appear in the middle ear and mastoid and on the skin. TB is caused by *Mycobacterium tuberculosis,* an acid-fast bacillus not readily decolorized by acids after staining. The source of tuberculosis infection in children is usually an infected member of the household or a frequent visitor to the home such as a babysitter or domestic worker.

Definitions
TST: tuberculin skin test—intradermal injection of purified protein derivative on volar aspect of the arm; ***positive reaction*** indicates that the individual has been infected and has developed sensitivity to the tubercle bacillus. It does not, however, confirm the presence of active disease. Once an individual reacts positively, he will always react positively.

Latent tuberculosis infection (LTBI):—infection in a person who has a positive TST, no physical findings of disease, and normal chest radiograph findings; there may be evidence of a healed infection.

Tuberculosis disease:—disease in a child who has clinical symptoms or radiographic manifestations caused by the *M. tuberculosis* organism; the child may have pulmonary infection, extrapulmonary, or both.

DOT: direct observation therapy—medication is provided directly to affected person by a trained third party or health care worker.

Pathophysiology

The lung is the usual portal of entry for *M. tuberculosis*. The organism is airborne, and transmission occurs by inhalation of the droplet cells from an infected (contagious) person. In the lungs, a proliferation of epithelial cells surround and encapsulate the multiplying bacilli in an attempt to wall it off, thus forming the typical tubercle. Extension of the primary lesion at the original site causes progressive tissue destruction as it spreads within the lung, discharges material from foci to other areas of the lungs (e.g., bronchi, pleura), or produces pneumonia. Erosion of blood vessels by the primary lesion can cause widespread dissemination of the tubercle bacillus to near and distant sites (miliary tuberculosis).

Clinical Signs and Symptoms

- May be asymptomatic or produce a broad range of symptoms
  - Fever
  - Malaise
  - Anorexia
  - Weight loss
  - Cough may or may not be present (progresses slowly over weeks to months).
  - Aching pain and tightness in the chest
  - Hemoptysis (rare)
- With progression
  - Respiratory rate increases.
  - Poor expansion of lung on the affected side
  - Diminished breath sounds and crackles
  - Dullness to percussion

- Fever persists.
- Generalized symptoms are manifested.
- Pallor, anemia, weakness, and weight loss

Diagnostic Evaluation
- Physical examination and history
- TST
- Chest radiograph
- Isolation and identification of *M. tuberculosis* from sputum or in small children, from gastric washing (i.e., aspiration of lavaged contents from the fasting stomach)

Treatment
Pharmacotherapy
- For LTBI: INH (isoniazid) daily for 9 months
- For active TB: combinations of isoniazid (INH), rifampin, and pyrazinamide (PZA)

Prevention
- Identification of persons with disease, and treatment of those in close contact
- High-risk screening
- Prevention of disease among persons with immunodeficiency who are most likely to acquire disease (e.g. , person with HIV infection)
- Prevention of spread and contraction of antibiotic-resistant TB

Surgery
- Surgical removal of infected tissue
- Nutrition support of person with active disease

Nursing Care Management
- Administer and interpret of TST.
- Perform high-risk screening for TB.
- Assist with diagnostic procedures such as sputum collection, gastric lavage.
- Help the family understand the rationale for diagnostic procedures.
- Prevent spread from infected person to others; standard precautions in asymptomatic child.

- Airborne precautions and a negative-pressure room for children who are contagious and hospitalized with active tuberculosis disease
- Infection control for hospital personnel in contagious cases should include the use of a personally fitted air-purifying N95 or N100 respirator (PAPR) for all patient contacts.

Patient and Family Teaching
- Diagnostic testing
- Primary prevention in household with infected person; handwashing; cover mouth and nose when sneezing, coughing; food preparation.
- Importance of drug therapy

TUMORS, BRAIN
Description
Brain tumors occur as primary tumors that arise in the regions of the brain. They may be benign or malignant.

Pathophysiology
Because the neoplasms can arise from any cell within the cranium, it is possible to have tumors originating from the glial cells, nerve cells, neuroepithelium, cranial nerves, blood vessels, pineal gland, and hypophysis. Within each of these structures, specific cells may be involved to provide a histologic classification of the major tumors found in children. Astrocytes, cells that form most of the supportive tissue for the neurons, may form astrocytomas, the most common glial tumor.

Clinical Signs and Symptoms
- Signs and symptoms of brain tumors are directly related to their anatomic location and size and to some extent the age of the child.
- In infants, whose sutures are still open, virtually no early detectable symptoms develop. It is not until spinal fluid obstruction causes markedly increased head size that a lesion may be suspected. Head circumference allows for detection of increased head size. Even in older children, clinical manifestations are nonspecific. See Table 3-10.

▌ TABLE 3-10

Brain Tumor Signs and Symptoms in Children

SIGNS AND SYMPTOMS	ASSESSMENT
HEADACHE Recurrent and progressive In frontal or occipital areas Usually dull and throbbing Worse on arising, less during day Intensified by lowering head and straining, such as during bowel movement, coughing, sneezing	Record description of pain, location, severity, and duration. Use pain rating scale to assess severity of pain. Note changes in relation to time of day and activity. Observe changes in behavior in infants (persistent irritability, crying, head rolling).
VOMITING With or without nausea or feeding Progressively more projectile More severe in morning Relieved by moving about and changing position	Record time, amount and relationship to feeding
NEUROMUSCULAR CHANGES Incoordination or clumsiness Loss of balance (use of wide-based stance, falling, tripping, banging into objects) Poor fine-motor control Weakness Hyporelexia or hyperreflexia Positive Babinski sign Spasticity Paralysis	Test muscle strength, gait, coordination, and reflexes.
BEHAVIORAL CHANGES Irritability Decreased appetite Failure to thrive Fatigue (frequent naps) Lethargy Coma Bizarre behavior (staring, automatic movements)	Observe behavior regularly. Compare observations with parental reports of normal behavioral patterns. Monitor growth and food intake. Monitor activity and sleep.

TABLE 3-10—cont'd	
Brain Tumor Signs and Symptoms in Children	
SIGNS AND SYMPTOMS	ASSESSMENT

CRANIAL NERVE NEUROPATHY
Cranial nerve involvement varies according to tumor location.
Most common signs:
    Head tilt
    Visual defects (nystagmus, diplopia, strabismus, episodic "graying out" of vision, visual field defect)
	Assess cranial nerves, especially VII (facial), IX (glossopharyngeal), X (vagus), V (trigeminal, sensory roots), and VI (abducens).
	Assess visual acuity, binocularity, and peripheral vision.

VITAL SIGN DISTURBANCES Decreased pulse and respiration Increased blood pressure Decreased pulse pressure Hypothermia or hyperthermia	Measure vital signs frequently. Monitor pulse and respirations for 1 full minute. Record pulse pressure (difference between systolic and diastolic blood pressure).
OTHER SIGNS Seizures Cranial enlargement Tense, bulging fontanel at rest Nuchal rigidity Papilledema (edema of optic nerve)	Record seizure activity. Measure head circumference daily (infant and young child). Perform funduscopic examination if skilled in procedure.

Diagnostic Evaluation

- The gold standard diagnostic procedure is MRI, which permits early diagnosis of brain tumors as well as assessment of tumor growth during or following treatment.
- Magnetic resonance (MR) angiography can be performed during the same session as MRI to determine the vascularity of the tumor.
- A CT scan permits direct visualization of the brain parenchyma, ventricles, and surrounding subarachnoid space. Through the IV injection of radiographic contrast agents, intracranial blood vasculature can be demonstrated. When a positive CT scan is obtained, angiography may be done to

provide information about the tumor's blood supply and degree of vascularity, which may assist the surgeon in planning the operative approach.

■ Other tests (e.g., electroencephalography, tomographies, lumbar puncture, or ventriculography) may be performed.

■ Lumbar puncture is dangerous in the presence of increased ICP because of possible brainstem herniation following sudden release of pressure.

■ Definitive diagnosis is based on tissue specimens obtained during surgery. Occasionally, special techniques are required for determining the cell type.

Treatment

Treatment may involve the use of surgery, radiotherapy, and chemotherapy. All three may or may not be used, depending on the type of tumor. The treatment of choice is total removal of the tumor without residual neurologic damage. Patients with the most complete tumor removal have the greatest chance of survival. Several surgical advances have allowed the biopsy and removal of tumors in areas previously considered too dangerous for traditional operative techniques. Stereotactic surgery involves the use of CT and MRI in conjunction with other special computer techniques to reconstruct the tumor in three dimensions. With computer-assisted instruments, removal is sometimes possible. Stereotactic biopsy is performed with CT or MRI computer guidance for inserting the biopsy needle. Other procedures include the use of lasers to vaporize tumor tissue and brain mapping to determine the precise location of critical brain areas that are avoided during surgery.

Radiotherapy is used to treat most tumors and to shrink the size of the tumor before attempting surgical removal. The use of chemotherapy has emerged in the past decades with an increasingly important role, either in combination with irradiation or alone.

Nursing Care Management

A child admitted to the hospital with neurologic dysfunction is often suspected of having a brain tumor, although the actual diagnosis is as yet unconfirmed. Establishing a baseline of data on which to compare preoperative and postoperative changes is an essential step toward planning physical care and preventing complications.

Nursing care for the child with a brain tumor involves:
▪ Preparing the child and family for diagnostic and operative procedures
▪ Administering therapy
▪ Managing treatment side effects
▪ Monitoring to prevent complications related to the brain tumor and treatment
▪ Educating the child and family
▪ Providing child and family support

Prepare the Child and Family for Diagnostic and Operative Procedures

▪ The suspected diagnosis of a brain tumor is always a crisis event. The physician can rarely give definitive answers regarding the prognosis until after surgery. Parents and older children require emotional support to face the diagnostic procedures and a craniotomy.
▪ The hair is usually shaved in the operating room just before surgery, or sometimes in the child's room, usually the night before surgery. Children are also told about the size of the dressing. Usually the entire scalp is covered to maintain a tight wound closure, even if a small incision is made. Infratentorial head dressings may be attached to the upper back and extend forward to the neck in order to maintain slight extension and alignment as a precaution against wound rupture.

Provide Postoperative Nursing Care

▪ Vital signs are taken as frequently as every 15 to 30 minutes until stable. Temperature measurement is particularly important because of hyperthermia resulting from surgical intervention in the hypothalamus or brainstem and from some types of general anesthesia. To prepare for this reaction, a cooling blanket may be placed on the bed before the child returns to the unit, or it may be used when needed.
▪ Once the younger child is alert, the arms may need to be restrained to preserve the dressing. Even a child who has been cooperative before surgery must be closely supervised during the initial stages of regaining consciousness, when disorientation and restlessness are common. Elbow restraints are satisfactory to prevent the hands from reaching the head, although

additional restraint may be necessary to preserve an infusion line and maintain a specific position.

▪ Correct positioning after surgery is critical to prevent pressure against the operative site, reduce intracranial pressure, and avoid the danger of aspiration. If a large tumor was removed, the child is not placed on the operative side, because the brain may suddenly shift to that cavity, causing trauma to the blood vessels, linings, and the brain itself. The nurse confers with the surgeon to be certain of the correct position, including the degree of neck flexion. The first 24 to 48 hours after brain surgery are critical.

▪ The child with an infratentorial procedure is usually positioned flat and on either side. Pillows should be placed against the child's back, not head, to maintain the desired position. Ordinarily the head and neck are kept in midline with the body and slightly extended. In a supratentorial craniotomy, the head is usually elevated above the heart to facilitate cerebrospinal fluid drainage and decrease excessive blood flow to the brain to prevent hemorrhage.

▪ With an infratentorial craniotomy, the child is allowed nothing by mouth for at least 24 hours and longer if the gag and swallowing reflexes are depressed or the child is comatose. With a supratentorial procedure, feeding may be resumed soon after the child is alert, sometimes within 24 hours. Clear water is always started first because of the danger of aspiration. If the child vomits, oral liquids are stopped. Vomiting not only predisposes the child to aspiration, but also increases ICP and the risk for incisional rupture.

▪ IV fluids are continued until fluids are well tolerated. Because of the cerebral edema postoperatively and the danger of increased ICP, fluids are carefully monitored and usually infused at one half the maintenance rate. If drugs, such as prophylactic antibiotics, are given intravenously, the medication amount is calculated as part of the IV fluid. A hypertonic solution such as mannitol or dextrose may be necessary to remove excess fluid. These drugs cause rapid diuresis. After surgery, the child may have a Foley catheter in place. Urinary output is monitored after administration of these drugs to evaluate their effectiveness.

▪ Headache may be severe and is largely the result of cerebral edema. Measures to relieve some of the discomfort include providing a quiet, dimly lit environment, restricting visitors to a minimum, preventing any sudden jarring movement, such as banging into the bed, and preventing an increase in ICP. The last is most effectively achieved by proper positioning and prevention of straining, such as during coughing, vomiting, or defecating. The use of opioids, such as morphine, to relieve pain is controversial because it is thought that they may mask signs of altered consciousness or depress respirations. However, they can be given safely because naloxone can be used to reverse opioid effects, such as sedation or respiratory depression.

▪ Bowel movements are monitored to prevent constipation. Stool softeners may be given as soon as liquids are tolerated to facilitate easy passage of stool. Placing an ice bag on the forehead may also provide some headache relief, especially if facial edema is severe.

▪ Brain edema may severely depress the gag reflex, necessitating suctioning of oral secretions. Facial edema may also be present, necessitating eye care if the lids remain partially open. Ice compresses applied to the eyes for short periods help in relieving the edema. A depressed blink reflex also predisposes the corneas to ulceration. Irrigating the eyes with saline drops and covering them with eye dressings are important steps in preventing this complication.

Administer Therapy

▪ Once surgery is completed and the child has recovered, many children with brain tumors receive chemotherapy and/or radiation therapy. The nurse plays a major role in chemotherapy administration.

▪ Review child's history related to previous tolerance to therapy.

▪ Determine appropriate medications to manage side effects.

▪ Be aware of drug-specific interactions.

▪ Assess the child's laboratory findings prior to therapy administration.

▪ Ensure that the chemotherapy doses are correct by checking orders according to the institution's policies and procedures.

▪ Follow the guidelines for chemotherapy administration.

▪ If the treatment is given intravenously, observe the IV site for signs of irritation or infiltration.

▪ Follow the institution's policy for safe handling chemotherapy wastes, including the patient's bodily fluids.
▪ Observe the child for signs of reaction during and following treatment.

Manage Common Side Effects of Cancer Treatment
▪ Assess for toxicities specific to the cancer treatment.
▪ Monitor for signs of infection, and obtain cultures and initiate antibiotics if indicated.
▪ Monitor nutrition and weight changes and alternative methods of nutrition if appropriate.
▪ Monitor fluid and electrolytes.
▪ Evaluate child's response to treatment.
▪ Manage central line care.

Monitor for Complications Related to the Brain Tumor and Treatment
▪ Assess for symptoms related to the brain tumor and treatment.
▪ Review laboratory findings.
▪ Obtain a complete history evaluating the incidence and duration of symptoms.
▪ Perform a complete physical examination; assess for signs similar to the child's presenting signs and symptoms as well as for pain, fatigue, weakness, developmental delay, morning vomiting, headache, seizures, ataxia, and signs of infection.

Patient and Family Teaching
Educate the Child and Family
▪ Assess child's and family's level of knowledge regarding the brain tumor and treatment.
▪ Assess child's and family's understanding of what they have heard about brain tumor and treatment.
▪ Explain that chemotherapeutic reactions vary with the specific drug regimen. Explain that the most common side effects from chemotherapy include nausea and vomiting, body image changes, neuropathy, and mucosal ulceration.
▪ If the child is to receive radiation therapy, review the common side effects associated with radiation therapy and precautions that should be followed during treatment. High-dose radiotherapy often causes a skin reaction of dry or moist desquamation

followed by hyperpigmentation. Because of increased sensitivity, the area is protected from sunlight and sudden changes in temperature, such as from heating pads or ice packs.
- Educate the family regarding neutropenia, anemia, and thrombocytopenia, the signs and symptoms of infection, and fever precautions.
- Provide appropriate educational resources, and review materials with them.
- Clarify information presented by the health care team.

Provide Support for the Child and Family
- Communicate with the child and family in an appropriate style.
- Provide the child and family with honest answers.
- Provide emotional support.
- Offer age-appropriate interventions.
- Provide information on available resources for support for the child and family.

URINARY TRACT INFECTION
Description
Urinary tract infection refers to the presence of a significant number of microorganisms in the urinary system; this may involve the urethra and bladder, or the ureters, renal pelvis, calyces, and renal parenchyma. The distal third of the urinary tract is usually colonized with bacteria, so it is not included. Females have a higher incidence of UTI, and the peak incidence is between 2 and 6 years of age. Organisms associated with UTI include *E. coli, Proteus, Pseudomonas, Klebsiella, Staphylococcus aureus, Haemophilus,* and coagulase-negative *Staphylococcus.*

Pathophysiology
Urinary stasis is a major factor influencing the development of UTI. Urine is usually sterile, but at 37 °C (98.6° F) it provides an excellent medium for bacteria when it remains in the bladder. Incomplete bladder emptying may occur as a result of reflux, anatomic abnormalities, dysfunction of the voiding mechanism, or extrinsic ureteral or bladder compression caused by constipation. The short urethra in females may contribute to bacterial colonization.

Clinical Signs and Symptoms
Neonatal Period (Birth to 1 Month)
- Poor feeding
- Vomiting
- Failure to gain weight
- Rapid respiration (acidosis)
- Respiratory distress
- Spontaneous pneumothorax or pneumomediastinum
- Frequent urination
- Screaming on urination
- Poor urine stream
- Jaundice
- Seizures
- Dehydration
- Enlarged kidneys or bladder
- May be afebrile

Infancy (1 to 24 Months)
- Poor feeding
- Vomiting
- Failure to gain weight
- Excessive thirst
- Frequent urination
- Straining or screaming on urination
- Foul-smelling urine
- Pallor
- Fever
- Persistent diaper rash
- Seizures (with or without fever)
- Dehydration
- Enlarged kidneys or bladder

Childhood (2 to 14 Years)
- Poor appetite
- Vomiting
- Growth failure
- Excessive thirst
- Enuresis, incontinence, frequent urination
- Painful urination
- Swelling of face
- Seizures

- Pallor
- Fatigue
- Blood in urine
- Abdominal or back pain
- Edema
- Hypertension
- Tetany

Diagnostic Evaluation
- Based in part on clinical manifestations
- Detection of bacteria in a urine culture
- A positive urine dipstick for leukocyte esterase or nitrite may be used as a screening tool to determine need for urine culture (must be a clean catch or catheterized specimen).
- Ultrasonography, VCUG (voiding cystourethrogram), IVP (intravenous pyelogram), and DSMA (dimercaptosuccinic acid scan) may be performed to localize anatomic abnormality contributing to recurrent infections.

Treatment
- Identification of the causative pathogen
- Antibiotic therapy
- Identification of anatomical structural defect contributing to UTI, with subsequent surgical correction
- Follow-up evaluation to ensure permanent damage is not caused by recurring UTIs

Nursing Care Management
- Recognize signs and symptoms of UTI in children.
- Obtain urine specimen for urinalysis and culture.
- Assist with diagnostic procedures.
- Medication administration
- Postoperative care for child undergoing surgery; monitoring vital signs; pain management; assessment of renal function

Patient and Family Teaching
- Prevention: urethral cleansing after voiding—wipe front to back (females); additional fluid intake; types of oral fluid; avoiding holding urine for prolonged periods; sexually active females should void after intercourse.
- Medication administration: complete course of antibiotics

■ Follow up with practitioner to evaluate effectiveness of antibiotic therapy.

VENTRICULAR SEPTAL DEFECT
Description
Abnormal opening between the right and left ventricles. May be classified according to location: membranous (accounting for 80%) or muscular. May vary in size from a small pinhole to absence of the septum, which results in a common ventricle. Ventricular septal defects (VSDs) are frequently associated with other defects, such as pulmonary stenosis, transposition of the great vessels, patent ductus arteriosus, atrial defects, and coarctation of the aorta. Many VSDs (20% to 60%) will close spontaneously. Spontaneous closure is most likely to occur during the first year of life in children having small or moderate defects. A left-to-right shunt is caused by the flow of blood from the higher-pressure left ventricle to the lower-pressure right ventricle. Defects left unrepaired will most likely cause pulmonary vascular disease.

Pathophysiology
Because of the higher pressure within the left ventricle and because the systemic arterial circulation offers more resistance than the pulmonary circulation, blood flows through the defect into the pulmonary artery. The increased blood volume is pumped into the lungs, which may eventually result in increased pulmonary vascular resistance. Increased pressure in the right ventricle as a result of left-to-right shunting and pulmonary resistance causes the muscle to hypertrophy. If the right ventricle is unable to accommodate the increased workload, the right atrium may also enlarge as it attempts to overcome the resistance offered by incomplete right ventricular emptying. Defects left unrepaired will most likely cause pulmonary vascular disease. If the resistance in the pulmonary bed becomes higher than systemic resistance, blood flow through the shunt reverses and becomes right to left. This is called *Eisenmenger's syndrome*.

Clinical Signs and Symptoms
CHF is common (see Box 3-1). Slow weight gain, feeding difficulties, duskiness, and dyspnea may occur. There is a characteristic holosystolic murmur (blowing sound) heard loudest at the fourth

intercostal space. A thrill may or may not be present. S$_2$ heart sound is loud and widely split. Patients are at risk for bacterial endocarditis and pulmonary vascular obstructive disease.

Diagnostic Evaluation
See Tables 3-1 and 3-2.

Treatment
Surgical Treatment
Palliative: Pulmonary artery banding (placement of a band around the main pulmonary artery to decrease pulmonary blood flow) may be done in infants with multiple muscular VSDs or complex anatomy. Improvements in surgical techniques and postoperative care make complete repair in infancy the preferred approach.

Complete repair (procedure of choice)*:* Small defects are repaired with sutures. Large defects usually require that a knitted Dacron or pericardial patch be sewn over the opening. Cardiopulmonary bypass is used for both procedures. The approach for the repair is generally through the right atrium and the tricuspid valve. Postoperative complications include residual VSD and conduction disturbances.

Nonsurgical Treatment
Device closure during cardiac catheterization is being performed in some centers under investigational protocols. One device has been approved for closure of muscular defects and another is in clinical trials. Early results are encouraging, with successful defect closure and few complications.

Nursing Care Management
Assist in Measures to Assess and Improve Cardiac Function
Monitor Cardiac Function
- Vital signs monitoring
- Respiratory assessment
- Cardiac assessment
  - Cardiac output (color, pulses, perfusion, capillary refill, renal function, and neurologic function)
  - Heart sounds
  - Dysrhythmias

- Keep accurate record of intake and output.
- Weigh child or infant on same scale at same time of day.

Administer Medications
- Review child's history related to cardiac management.
- Administer medications on schedule.
- Assess effectiveness of medications and any side effects noted.
- Be aware of drug-drug and drug-food interactions.
- Follow guidelines for medication administration.

Manage Common Side Effects of Cardiac Defects
- Prevent fatigue during feeding; offer small frequent feedings to infant's or child's tolerance.
- Organize nursing care to allow child/infant uninterrupted rest.
- Promote activities that do not cause fatigue.

Provide Support for the Child and Family
- Communicate with the child and family in an appropriate style.
- Provide the child and family with honest answers.
- Provide emotional support.
- Offer age-appropriate interventions.
- Provide information on available resources for support for the child and family.

Patient and Family Teaching
Prepare the Child and Family for Diagnostic and Operative Procedures
- Provide explanation of diagnostic tests and why each test is performed because many of them are invasive procedures.
- Prepare the child prior to the invasive procedure. Remember that discussion is dependent upon the child's age and development.
- Use simple words or pictures to describe procedures, and answer all questions the child and family may have.
- Postoperative wound care teaching as needed
- Post-cardiac catheterization wound care teaching as needed
- Assess and record results of teaching and family's participation in care.

Educate the Child and Family
- Assess child's and family's level of knowledge regarding the VSD.
- Assess child's and family's understanding of what they have heard about VSD.
- Assess child's and family's understanding of the surgery and/or cardiac catheterization.
- Teach the child and/or family at least four characteristics of congestive heart failure that may occur because of the VSD such as:
    - Fatigue after exertion
    - Fast heart rate
    - Fast breathing, shortness of breath, dyspnea
    - Retractions
    - Nasal flaring
    - Cool extremities
    - Diaphoresis
    - Decreased urinary output
    - Puffiness (edema)
    - Fussiness
    - Decreased appetite
- Educate child and family about care such as medication preparation and administration.
- Assess child's and family's access to appropriate pharmacy for any special preparation medications.
- Educate child and family about when to notify their physician of any clinical changes.
- Assess and record results and family's participation in care.
- Provide appropriate educational resources, and review materials with them.
- Clarify information presented by the health care team including appointment for follow-up visit.
- Discuss SBE (subacute bacterial endocarditis) prophylaxis with your pediatric cardiologist.

VESICOURETERAL REFLUX
Description
Vesicoureteral reflux (VUR) refers to the abnormal retrograde flow of bladder urine into the ureters.

Pathophysiology

During voiding, urine is swept up the ureters and then flows back into the empty bladder, where it acts as a reservoir for bacterial growth until the next void. *Primary reflux* results from congenitally abnormal insertion of ureters into the bladder; *secondary reflux* occurs as a result of an acquired condition. Reflux is more likely to be associated with recurring kidney infections rather than simple bladder infections (cystitis).

Clinical Signs and Symptoms

■ In the presence of reflux, infected urine (bacteria) from the bladder has access to the kidney, resulting in kidney infections (pyelonephritis). These children are usually very symptomatic with high fevers, vomiting, and chills.

Diagnostic Evaluation

■ Voiding cystourethrogram
■ Urinalysis and urine culture
■ Renal ultrasound may be performed.

Treatment

■ The goal for treatment of VUR is to prevent any kidney damage from occurring.
■ VUR is managed conservatively with daily low-dose antibiotic therapy.
■ A urine culture should be done every 2 to 3 months and any time the child has a fever.
■ An annual voiding cystourethrogram is done to assess the status of the reflux.

Nursing Care Management

■ Nurses should instruct parents to observe regularly for clues suggesting UTI.
  ■ A careful history regarding voiding habits, stooling pattern, and episodes of unexplained irritability may assist in detecting less obvious cases of UTI.

Patient and Family Teaching

■ Advise parents of proper antibiotic dosage and administration.
■ Parents should be aware that many children will outgrow the reflux over a period of years.

WILMS TUMOR
Description
Wilms tumor, or nephroblastoma, is the most common intraabdominal and kidney tumor of childhood.

Pathophysiology
Wilms tumor is one of the childhood cancers that show an increased incidence among siblings and identical twins, reflecting evidence of genetic inheritance. The mode of inheritance in familial cases, which account for less than 2% of all Wilms tumors, is autosomal dominant with variable penetrance and expressivity. Wilms tumor is heritable in about 15% to 20% of all cases, including some unilateral sporadic cases. Unfortunately, there is no method of identification of gene carriers.

Wilms tumor is also associated with several congenital anomalies; the most common are aniridia, hemihypertrophy, genitourinary anomalies (such as hypospadias, cryptorchidism, ambiguous genitalia), and Beckwith-Wiedemann syndrome. Other, less common anomalies are microcephaly, pigmented and vascular nevi, pinna deformities, and mental and growth retardation.

Clinical Signs and Symptoms
- Swelling or mass within the abdomen. The mass is characteristically firm, nontender, confined to one side, and deep within the flank. If it is on the right side, it may be difficult to distinguish from the liver, although, unlike that organ, it does not move with respiration. Parents usually discover the mass during routine bathing or dressing of the child.
- Other clinical signs and symptoms are the result of compression from the tumor mass, metabolic alterations secondary to the tumor, or metastasis.
- Hematuria occurs in less than one fourth of children with Wilms tumor.
- Anemia, usually secondary to hemorrhage within the tumor, results in pallor, anorexia, and lethargy.
- Hypertension, probably caused by secretion of excess amounts of renin by the tumor, occurs occasionally.
- Other effects of malignancy include weight loss and fever.

- If metastasis has occurred, symptoms of lung involvement, such as dyspnea, cough, shortness of breath, and pain in the chest, may be evident.

Diagnostic Evaluation

- History and physical examination for the presence of congenital anomalies; a family history of cancer; and signs of malignancy, such as weight loss, size of the liver and spleen, indications of anemia, and lymphadenopathy
- Specific tests include radiographic studies, including abdominal ultrasound, CT, MRI, hematologic studies (polycythemia is sometimes present if the tumor secretes excess erythropoietin).
- Biochemical studies and urinalysis
- Studies to demonstrate the relationship of the tumor to the ipsilateral kidney and the presence of a normally functioning kidney on the contralateral side are essential. If a large tumor is present, an inferior venacavogram is necessary to demonstrate possible tumor involvement adjacent to the vena cava.
- The histology of the tumor cells is also identified and classified according to two groups: favorable histology (FH) and unfavorable histology (UH). Only about 12% of Wilms tumors demonstrate UH, which is associated with a poorer prognosis and demands a more aggressive treatment protocol, regardless of the clinical stage. Survival rates for Wilms tumor are one of the highest among all childhood cancers.

Treatment

Combined treatment of surgery and chemotherapy with or without irradiation is based on the clinical stage and histologic pattern. In unilateral disease, a large transabdominal incision is performed for optimum visualization of the abdominal cavity; the tumor, affected kidney, and adjacent adrenal gland are removed. Great care is taken to keep the encapsulated tumor intact because rupture can seed cancer cells throughout the abdomen, lymph channel, and bloodstream. The contralateral kidney is carefully inspected for evidence of disease or dysfunction. Regional lymph nodes are inspected, and a biopsy is performed when indicated. Any involved structures, such as part of the colon, diaphragm, or vena cava, are removed. Metal clips are placed around the tumor site for exact marking during radiotherapy.

If both kidneys are involved, the child may be treated with radiotherapy or chemotherapy preoperatively to shrink the tumor, allowing more conservative therapy. In some cases, a partial nephrectomy is performed on the less affected kidney, with a total nephrectomy performed on the opposite side. When a transplant is feasible, such as from a twin, sibling, or parent, bilateral nephrectomy is considered as a last resort. Postoperative radiotherapy is indicated for children with large tumors, metastasis, residual disease at the primary tumor site, UH, or recurrence. Chemotherapy is indicated for all stages.

Nursing Care Management
Nursing care for the child with Wilms tumor involves:
- Preparing the child and family for diagnostic and operative procedures
- Administering therapy
- Managing treatment side-effects
- Monitoring to prevent complications related to leukemia and treatment
- Educating the child and family
- Providing child and family support

Prepare the Child and Family for Diagnostic and Operative Procedures
- As with many of the other cancers, the diagnosis of Wilms tumor is a shock. Frequently the child has no physical indication of the seriousness of the disorder other than a palpable abdominal mass. Because it is the parents who usually discover the mass, the nurse needs to take into account their feelings regarding the diagnosis. Whereas some parents are grateful for their detection of the tumor, others feel guilty for not finding it sooner or anger toward the practitioner for missing it on earlier examinations.
- The preoperative period is one of swift diagnosis. Typically, surgery is scheduled within 24 to 48 hours of admission. The nurse is faced with the challenge of preparing the child and parents for all laboratory and operative procedures. Because of the little time available, explanations should be kept simple and repeated often with attention to what the child will experience. Besides usual preoperative observations, blood pressure

is monitored, because hypertension from excess renin production is a possibility.

■ There are several special preoperative concerns, the most important of which is that the tumor is not palpated unless absolutely necessary because manipulation of the mass may cause dissemination of cancer cells to adjacent and distant sites.

■ Because radiotherapy and chemotherapy are usually begun immediately after surgery, parents need an explanation of what to expect, such as major benefits and side effects, although the timing of the information should be considered to avoid overwhelming the family.

Provide Postoperative Nursing Care

■ Despite the extensive surgical intervention necessary in many children with Wilms tumor, the recovery period is usually rapid. Because these children are at risk for intestinal obstruction from vincristine-induced adynamic ileus, radiation-induced edema, and postsurgical adhesion formation, gastrointestinal activity, such as bowel movements, bowel sounds, distention, and vomiting, is monitored. Other considerations are frequent evaluation of blood pressure and observation for signs of infection. Because of the myelosuppression from the drugs, pulmonary hygiene measures are instituted in the immediate postoperative period to prevent complications.

Administer Therapy

■ Review child's history related to previous tolerance to therapy.
■ Determine appropriate premedication prior to therapy.
■ Be aware of drug-specific interactions.
■ Assess the child's laboratory findings prior to therapy administration.
■ Ensure that the chemotherapy doses are correct by checking orders according to the institution's policies and procedures.
■ Follow the guidelines for chemotherapy administration.
■ If the treatment is given intravenously, observe the IV site for signs of irritation or infiltration.
■ Follow the institution's policy for safe handling chemotherapy wastes, including the patient's bodily fluids.
■ Observe the child for signs of reaction during and following treatment.

Manage Common Side Effects of Cancer Treatment
- Assess for toxicities specific to the cancer treatment.
- Monitor for signs of infection and obtain cultures and initiate antibiotics if indicated.
- Monitor nutrition and weight changes and alternative methods of nutrition if appropriate.
- Monitor fluid and electrolytes.
- Evaluate child's response to treatment.
- Manage central line care.

Monitor for Complications Related to Wilms Tumor and Treatment
- Assess for symptoms related to Wilms tumor and treatment.
- Review laboratory findings.
- Obtain a complete history evaluating the incidence and duration of symptoms.
- Perform a complete physical examination; assess for fever, night sweats, weight loss, pallor, signs of infection, lymphadenopathy.

Patient and Family Teaching
Educate the Child and Family
- Assess child's and family's level of knowledge regarding Wilms tumor and treatment.
- Assess child's and family's understanding of what they have heard about Wilms tumor and treatment.
- Explain that chemotherapeutic reactions vary with the specific drug regimen. Explain the most common side effects from chemotherapy include nausea and vomiting, body image changes, neuropathy, and mucosal ulceration.
- If the child is to receive radiation therapy, review the common side effects associated with radiation therapy and precautions that should be followed during treatment: High-dose radiotherapy often causes a skin reaction of dry or moist desquamation followed by hyperpigmentation. The child should wear loose-fitting clothes over the irradiated area to minimize additional skin irritation. Because of increased sensitivity, the area is protected from sunlight and sudden changes in temperature, such as from heating pads or ice packs. The child is encouraged to use the extremity as tolerated. Occasionally an active exercise

program may be planned by the physical therapist to preserve maximum function.

▪ Educate the family regarding neutropenia, anemia, and thrombocytopenia, the signs and symptoms of infection and fever precautions.

▪ Because the child is left with only one kidney, certain precautions, such as avoiding contact sports or any other activity that has a high-risk potential, are recommended to prevent injury to the organ. Urinary tract infections should be prevented with good hygiene, especially in girls. Prompt detection and treatment of any genitourinary signs or symptoms is mandatory.

Provide Support for the Child and Family
▪ Communicate with the child and family in an appropriate style.
▪ Provide the child and family with honest answers.
▪ Provide emotional support.
▪ Offer age-appropriate interventions.
▪ Provide information on available resources for support for the child and family.

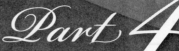

Common Diagnostic and Laboratory Tests

ARTERIAL BLOOD GAS ANALYSIS

Arterial blood gas (ABG) analysis results are rapidly available and provide a baseline to determine a patient's current respiratory and metabolic status and needs.

Blood gas interpretation is based on assessing the arterial serum levels of the following variables:

TABLE 4-1

Arterial Blood Gas Values

ABG COMPONENT	NORMAL LEVELS
pH	7.35-7.45
$PaCO_2$	35-45 mmHg
HCO_3	22-26 mEq/liter
PaO_2	90-110 mmHg

Consistent Approach Is Key

In order to make an interpretation based on the individual ABG values, a consistent sequence of steps should be followed:

1. Evaluate pH to determine the presence of acidosis or alkalosis. The lungs and kidneys regulate the hydrogen ion status within the plasma. Alterations in these systems affect the acid-base balance, causing pH changes that affect multiple body systems.

Within normal limits (WNL) indicates normal or compensated state.

Outside normal limits

<7.35: Acidosis—Acidosis may cause pulmonary vasoconstriction leading to decreased pulmonary blood flow. Acidosis may also cause vasoconstriction to cerebral blood vessels.

>7.45: Alkalosis—Alkalosis may diminish cellular metabolism, depress myocardial function, and dilate pulmonary blood vessels.

2. Evaluate $PaCO_2$ to assess the alveolar ventilation status. In an uncompensated acidosis or alkalosis, an abnormal $PaCO_2$ level will generally indicate that the origin of the pH imbalance is respiratory rather than metabolic.

Within normal limits—adequate ventilation

Outside normal limits

>**45:** Hypercarbia—Hypoventilation leads to an increase in $PaCO_2$, which in turn lowers the pH, resulting in a respiratory acidosis.

<**30:** Hypocarbia—Hyperventilation leads to decreased $PaCO_2$, which in turn raises the pH, resulting in a respiratory alkalosis.

3. Evaluate HCO_3 to assess the effectiveness of renal regulation of blood pH. In an uncompensated acidosis or alkalosis, an abnormal HCO_3 level will generally indicate that the origin of the pH imbalance is metabolic rather than respiratory.

Within normal limits—normal renal function

Outside normal limits

<**22:** Decreased bicarbonate—Renal mechanisms lead to increased excretion of bicarbonate and a lower serum bicarbonate level. Owing to the absence of normal levels of bicarbonate to buffer serum H^+ (acid), the pH lowers and metabolic acidosis is the result.

>**29:** Increased bicarbonate—Renal mechanisms lead to increased retention of bicarbonate. Owing to the higher levels of bicarbonate, more serum H^+ (acid) is buffered, the pH increases, and metabolic alkalosis is the result.

4. Look for signs of compensation—With prolonged abnormalities in pH, the body tries to return the pH to normal through respiratory compensation (adjusting $PaCO_2$ levels)

or metabolic compensation (adjusting HCO_3 levels). In compensated acidosis or alkalosis, the pH will be normal, but the $PaCO_2$ and HCO_3 will both be abnormal in the same "direction" (increased or decreased).

The following table may be used to assist with differentiation of respiratory versus metabolic acid-base imbalances, including presence of compensation:

TABLE 4-2			
ABG Interpretation			
INTERPRETATION	**pH**	**PaCO₂**	**HCO₃**
ACIDOSIS			
Respiratory	<7.35	>45	WNL
Compensated respiratory	WNL	>45	>29
Metabolic	<7.35	WNL	<22
Compensated metabolic	WNL	<30	<22
Alkalosis			
Respiratory	>7.45	<30	WNL
Compensated respiratory	WNL	<30	<22
Metabolic	>7.45	WNL	>29
Compensated metabolic	WNL	>45	>29

WNL, Within normal limits.

5. Evaluate PaO_2 to assess the oxygenation status. It is important to be aware of a patient's specific "normal" values. Patients with certain cardiac or pulmonary conditions may have "acceptable" PaO_2 that is below normal limits. Assess each patient's unique needs, and treat accordingly.

Within normal limits—adequate oxygenation

Outside normal limits

    55-85: Mild hypoxemia

    40-55: Moderate hypoxemia

    <40: Severe hypoxemia

BONE MARROW ASPIRATION AND BIOPSY

Insertion of a needle into the bone marrow to obtain (by aspiration) either (1) bone marrow, or (2) piece of bone (biopsy) for evaluation of cells and bone tissue, respectively. Procedure is performed with child under sedation and with local anesthetic used for dermal penetration. Child should be prepared beforehand. Care after procedure: A small pressure dressing may be used; child may be sore and require analgesic for 24 hours. May be performed on an outpatient basis, and the child may go home once he or she is fully awake and alert. No activity restrictions are required for the test.

BRONCHOSCOPY

BOX 4-1

Bronchoscopy

Bronchoscopy is the direct observation of tracheobronchial tree via bronchoscope.
> Localizes abnormalities in major airways
> Provides access to (1) remove aspirated foreign bodies from major airways, (2) remove obstructive mucous plugs, (3) perform bronchial lavage, (4) directly observe and assess anatomic structures of airway for any pathology.
> Procedure requires sedation and monitoring of vital signs during and after procedure until child is awake and alert.

CARDIAC CATHETERIZATION AND COMMON CARDIOLOGY TESTS

TABLE 4-3

Cardiac Catheterization and Common Cardiology Tests

PROCEDURE	DESCRIPTIVE
Chest radiograph (X-ray)	Produces images of internal structures of chest, including air-filled lungs, airways, vascular markings, heart, and great vessels; shows heart size
Electrocardiography (ECG)	Graphic measure of electrical activity of heart
Holter monitor	24-hour continuous ECG recording used to assess dysrhythmias
Echocardiography	Use of high-frequency sound waves obtained by a transducer to produce an image of cardiac structures
Transthoracic	Performed with transducer on chest
M-mode	One-dimensional graphic view used to estimate ventricular size and function
Two-dimensional (2-D)	Real-time, cross-sectional views of heart used to identify cardiac structures and cardiac anatomy
Doppler	Identifies blood flow patterns and pressure gradients across structures
Fetal	Imaging fetal heart in utero
Transesophageal (TEE)	Transducer placed in esophagus behind heart to obtain images of posterior heart structures or in patients with poor images from chest approach
Cardiac catheterization	Imaging study using radiopaque catheters placed in a peripheral blood vessel and advanced into heart to measure pressures and oxygen levels in heart chambers and visualize heart structures and blood flow patterns

Continued

TABLE 4-3—cont'd

Cardiac Catheterization and Common Cardiology Tests

PROCEDURE	DESCRIPTIVE
Hemodynamics	Measures pressures and oxygen saturations in heart chambers
Angiography	Use of contrast material to illuminate heart structures and blood flow patterns
Biopsy	Use of special catheter to remove tiny samples of heart muscle for microscopic evaluation; used in assessing infection, inflammation, or muscle dysfunction disorders; also used to evaluate for rejection after heart transplant
Electrophysiology (EPS)	Special catheters with electrodes employed to record electrical activity from within heart; used to diagnose rhythm disturbances
Exercise stress test	Monitoring of heart rate, blood pressure, electrocardiogram (ECG), and oxygen consumption at rest and during progressive exercise on a treadmill or bicycle
Cardiac magnetic resonance imaging (MRI)	Noninvasive imaging technique; used in evaluation of vascular anatomy outside of heart (e.g., coarctation of the aorta, vascular rings), estimates of ventricular mass and volume; uses for MRI are expanding

LABS

COMPLETE BLOOD CELL COUNT

TABLE 4-4	
Complete Blood Cell Count	
TEST (AVERAGE VALUE)	**DESCRIPTION/COMMENTS**
Red blood cell (RBC) count (4.5-5.5 million/mm³)	Number of RBCs/mm³ of blood Indirectly estimates Hgb content of blood Reflects function of bone marrow
Hemoglobin (Hgb) determination (11.5-15.5 g/dl)*	Amount of Hgb (g)/dl of whole blood Total blood Hgb primarily depends on number of circulating RBCs but also on amount of Hgb in each cell
Hematocrit (Hct) (35%-45%)	Percent volume of packed RBCs in whole blood Indirectly measures Hgb content Is approximately three times Hgb content
RBC indexes	
Mean corpuscular volume (MCV) (77-95 fl)	Average or mean volume (size) of a single RBC MCV values are expressed as femtoliters (fl) or cubic microns (μm³)
Mean corpuscular hemoglobin (MCH) (25-33 pg/cell)	Average or mean quantity (weight) of Hgb in a single RBC MCH values are expressed as picograms (pg) or micromicrograms (μmcg) MCV and MCH depend on accurate counts of RBCs, whereas MCHC does not; therefore, MCHC is often more reliable. All indexes depend on average cell measurements and do not show individual RBC variations (anisocytosis).
Mean corpuscular hemoglobin concentration (MCHC) (31%-37% Hgb [g]/dl RBC)	Average concentration of Hgb in a single RBC MCHC values are expressed as percent Hgb (g)/cell or Hgb (g)/dl RBC.

Continued

TABLE 4-4—cont'd

Complete Blood Cell Count

TEST (AVERAGE VALUE)	DESCRIPTION/COMMENTS
RBC volume distribution width (RDW) (13.4% ± 1.2%)	Average size of RBCs Differentiates some types of anemia
Reticulocyte count (0.5%-1.5% erythrocytes)	Percent reticulocytes in RBCs Index of production of mature RBCs by bone marrow Decreased count indicates depressed bone marrow function. Increased count indicates erythrogenesis in response to some stimulus. When reticulocyte count is extremely high, other forms of immature RBCs (normoblasts, even erythroblasts) may be present. Indirectly estimates hypochromic anemia Usually elevated in patients with chronic hemolytic anemia
White blood cell (WBC) count (4.5-13.5×10^3 cells/mm³)	Number of WBCs/mm³ of blood Total number of WBCs less important than differential count
Differential WBC count	Inspection and quantification of WBC types present in peripheral blood Values are expressed as percentages; to obtain the absolute number of any type of WBC, multiply its respective percentage by total number of WBCs.
Neutrophils (polys) (54%-62%) (3-5.8×10^3 cells/mm³)	Primary defense in bacterial infection; capable of phagocytizing and killing bacteria
Bands (3%-5%) (0.15-0.4×10^3 cells/mm³)	Immature neutrophil Increased numbers in bacterial infection Also capable of phagocytosis and killing bacteria

TABLE 4-4—cont'd

Complete Blood Cell Count

TEST (AVERAGE VALUE)	DESCRIPTION/COMMENTS
Eosinophils (1%-3%) (0.05-0.25 × 10^3 cells/mm³)	Named for their staining characteristics with eosin dye Increased in allergic disorders, parasitic diseases, certain neoplasms, and other diseases
Basophils (0.075%) (0.015-0.030 × 10 cubed cells/mm³)	Named for their characteristic basophilic stippling Contain histamine, heparin, and serotonin; believed to cause increased blood flow to injured tissues while preventing excessive clotting
Lymphocytes (25%-33%) (1.5-3.0 × 10^3 cells/mm³)	Involved in development of antibody and delayed hypersensitivity
Monocytes (3%-7%)	Large phagocytic cells that are involved in early stage of inflammatory reaction
Absolute neutrophil count (ANC) (>1000)	Percent neutrophils/bands times WBC count Indicates body's capability to handle bacterial infections
Platelet count (150-400 × 10³/mm³)	Number of platelets/mm³ of blood Cellular fragments that are necessary for clotting to occur
Stained peripheral blood smear	Visual estimation of amount of Hgb in RBCs and overall size, shape, and structure of RBCs Various staining properties of RBC structures may be evidence of immature forms of erythrocytes Shows variation in size and shape of RBCs: microcytic, macrocytic, poikilocytic (variable shapes)

*Hemoglobin values may vary according to the child's age and gender.

COMMON NEUROLOGIC TESTS

TABLE 4-5

Common Neurologic Tests

TEST	DESCRIPTION	PURPOSE
Lumbar puncture (LP)	Spinal needle is inserted between L3-L4 or L4-L5 vertebral spaces into subarachnoid space; cerebrospinal fluid (CSF) pressure is measured, and sample is collected for examination.	Diagnostic—measures spinal fluid pressure, obtains CSF for laboratory analysis; monitors for presence of bacteria (meningitis) Therapeutic—injection of medication (intrathecal)
Subdural tap	Needle is inserted into anterior fontanel or coronal suture (midline to pupil).	Helps rule out subdural effusions Removes CSF to relieve pressure
Ventricular puncture	Needle is inserted into lateral ventricle via coronal suture (midline to pupil).	Removes CSF to relieve pressure
Electroencephalography (EEG)	EEG records changes in electric potential of brain. Electrodes are placed at various points to assess electrical function in a particular area. Impulses are recorded by electromagnetic pen or digitally.	Detects spikes, or bursts of electrical activity that indicate the potential for seizures Used to determine brain death
Nuclear brain scan	Radioisotope is injected intravenously, and then counted and recorded after fixed time intervals. Radioisotope accumulates in areas where blood-brain barrier is defective.	Identifies focal brain lesions (e.g., tumors, abscesses) Positive uptake of material with encephalitis and subdural hematoma Visualizes CSF pathways

Endocephalography	Pulses of ultrasonic waves are beamed through head; echoes from reflecting surfaces are recorded graphically.	Identifies shifts in midline structures from their normal positions as a result of intracranial lesions May show ventricular dilation
Real-time ultrasonography (RTUS)	RTUS is similar to CT but uses ultrasound instead of ionizing radiation.	Allows high-resolution anatomic visualization in variety of imaging planes
Radiography	Skull films are taken from different views—lateral, posterolateral, axial (submentoventricular), and half-axial.	Shows fractures, dislocations, spreading suture lines, craniostenosis Shows degenerative changes, bone erosion, calcifications
Computed tomography (CT) scan	Pinpoint X-ray beam is directed on horizontal or vertical plane to provide series of images that are fed into computer and assembled in image displayed on video screen. CT uses ionizing radiation.	Visualizes horizontal and vertical cross section of brain in three planes (axial, coronal, and sagittal) Distinguishes density of various intracranial tissues and structures—congenital abnormalities, hemorrhage, tumors, demyelinating and inflammatory processes, calcification
Magnetic resonance imaging (MRI)	MRI produces radiofrequency emissions from elements (e.g., hydrogen, phosphorus), which are converted to visual images by computer.	Permits visualization of morphologic feature of target structures Permits tissue discrimination unavailable with many techniques

Continued

TABLE 4-5—cont'd

Common Neurologic Tests

TEST	DESCRIPTION	PURPOSE
Positron emission tomography (PET)	PET involves IV injection of positron-emitting radionucleotide; local concentrations are detected and transformed into visual display by computer.	Detects and measures blood volume and flow in brain, metabolic activity, biochemical changes within tissue
Digital subtraction angiography (DSA)	Contrast dye is injected intravenously; computer "subtracts" all tissues without contrast medium, leaving clear image of contrast medium in vessels studied.	Visualizes vasculature of target tissue Visualizes finite vascular abnormalities
Single-photon emission computed tomography (SPECT)	SPECT involves IV injection of photon-emitting radionuclide; radionuclides are absorbed by healthy tissue at a different rate than diseased or necrotic tissue; data are transferred to computer that converts image to film.	Provides information regarding blood flow to tissues; analyzing blood flow to organ may help determine how well it is functioning.

PULMONARY FUNCTION TESTS

TABLE 4-6

Pulmonary Function Tests

TEST	MEASUREMENT	SIGNIFICANCE
Forced vital capacity (FVC) (peak flow)	Maximum amount of air that can be expired after maximum inspiration	Reduced in obesity Reduced in obstructive airway disease Normal in restrictive disease
Forced expiratory volume in 1 second (FEV$_1$) or 3 seconds (FEV$_3$)	Amount of air that can be forced from lungs after maximum inspiration in 1 and 3 seconds	Normally 80% of FVC in 1 second Reduced in obstructive disease Is the single best measure of airway function
Tidal volume (TV or V$_T$)	Amount of air inhaled and exhaled during any respiratory cycle	Multiplied by respiratory rate to provide minute volume Information needed to determine rate and depth of artificial ventilation
Functional residual volume (FRV); functional residual capacity (FRC)	Volume of air remaining in lungs after passive expiration	Allows for aeration of alveoli Increased in hyperinflated lungs of obstructive lung disease

Continued

TABLE 4-6—cont'd

Pulmonary Function Tests

TEST	MEASUREMENT	SIGNIFICANCE
Dynamic compliance	Relationship between change in volume and pressure difference	Reflects elastic recoil of lung Normal volume but decreased airflow in obstructive disease (e.g., asthma) Normal flow but decreased volume in restrictive disease (e.g., pulmonary fibrosis)
Pulmonary resistance	Changes in pressure with changes in flow on inspiration and expiration	
Work of breathing	Total work expended moving lung and chest	
Respiratory time constancy	Time for proximal and alveolar airway pressure to equilibrate	
Capnography	Measures CO_2 during inhalation and exhalation cycle and produces a graph of CO_2 concentration over time	Provides end-tidal CO_2 levels to determine trends and identify shunts
FEV_1 or FEV_3/FVC	Percentage of maximum inspiration that is expired in 1 or 3 seconds	Normally 95% of FVC in 3 seconds Reduced in obstructive disease

RADIOLOGIC EXAMS

▌ TABLE 4-7

Radiologic Exams

TEST	DESCRIPTION	PURPOSE
Radiography	Pictures obtained by passing X-rays through the body and recording them on sensitized film	Produces images of internal structures of chest, including air-filled lungs, airways, vascular markings, heart, and great vessels
Fluoroscopy	Projection of electronically intensified image on viewing screen	Used primarily to study diaphragmatic excursion and respiratory motion of lungs Examination of barium-filled esophagus to outline mediastinal abnormalities
Bronchography	Contrast medium instilled directly into bronchial tree through opaque catheter inserted via orotracheal tube	Valuable to demonstrate and inspect bronchiectasis Detects distal bronchial obstruction Detects malformations
Barium swallow (or other contrast agent)	Esophagus outlined when barium solution or colloid is swallowed	Esophageal displacement defining mediastinal masses Detects swallowing disorders and malformations (e.g., tracheoesophageal fistula)
Angiography	Injection of dye to produce image of pulmonary vasculature	Investigation of pulmonary vascular anomalies and pulmonary hypertension

Continued

TABLE 4-7—cont'd

Radiologic Exams

TEST	DESCRIPTION	PURPOSE
Computed tomography (CT)	Sequence of X-rays, each representing a cross section or "cut" through lung tissue at different depth	Useful in identifying presence of calcium or cavity within a lesion, hilar adenopathy, mediastinal masses, or abnormalities
KUB	Flat plate roentgenogram of abdomen and pelvis for kidney, ureters, and bladder (KUB); intestine also included in child	Visualizes gastrointestinal outline for air, masses, stool; problems such as intestinal obstruction
Magnetic resonance imaging (MRI)	Use of large magnet and radio waves to produce 2- or 3-dimensional image	Clearly identifies soft tissues
Radioisotope scanning	Intravenous injection of albumin labeled with radioisotopes or inhalation of radioactive aerosols or xenon gas followed by radiation scanning	Delineates defects in pulmonary arterial perfusion and diseased areas of lungs. Detects location of aspirated foreign body
Ultrasonography	Transmission of sound waves through chest	Identifies opacification, internal structures, masses

UROLOGIC DIAGNOSTIC TESTS

TABLE 4-8		
Urologic Diagnostic Tests		
TEST	**PROCEDURE**	**PURPOSE**
Renal/bladder ultrasound	Transmission of ultrasonic waves through renal parenchyma, along ureteral course, and over bladder	Allows visualization of renal parenchyma, renal pelvis without exposure to external beam radiation or radioactive isotopes Visualization of dilated ureters and bladder wall also possible
Testicular (scrotal) ultrasound	Transmission of ultrasonic waves through scrotal contents and testis	Allows visualization of scrotal contents, including testis Testicular ultrasound is used to identify masses, and Doppler-enhanced ultrasound is used to differentiate hyperemia of epididymo-orchitis from ischemia or torsion.
Scout film, (KUB)	Flat plate roentgenogram of abdomen and pelvis for kidney, ureters, and bladder (KUB)	Detects and establishes renal outlines, presence of calculi, or opaque foreign bodies in bladder
Voiding cystourethrography	Contrast medium injected into bladder through urethral catheter until bladder is full; films taken before, during, and after voiding	Visualizes bladder outline and urethra, reveals reflux of urine into ureters, and shows complications of bladder emptying

Continued

TABLE 4-8—cont'd

Urologic Diagnostic Tests

TEST	PROCEDURE	PURPOSE
Radionuclide (nuclear) cystogram	Radionuclide-containing fluid injected through urethral catheter until bladder is full; images generated before, during, and after voiding	Alternative to voiding cystourethrography in children with allergy to intravesical contrast material Allows evaluation of reflux, although visualization of anatomic details is relatively poor
Radioisotope imaging studies	Contrast medium injected intravenously; computer analysis to measure uptake or washout (excretion) for analysis of organ function	DTPA radioisotope used to measure glomerular filtration rate; estimate of differential renal function and renal washout to determine presence and location of upper urinary tract obstruction DMSA radioisotope allows visualization of renal scars and differential renal function; ureters and bladder are not visualized. MAG 3 radioisotope combines features of DTPA (evaluation of upper urinary tract obstruction) with features of DMSA radioisotope (differential renal function).

TABLE 4-8—cont'd

Urologic Diagnostic Tests

TEST	PROCEDURE	PURPOSE
Intravenous pyelography (IVP) (intravenous urogram; excretory urogram)	Intravenous injection of a contrast medium Medium secreted and concentrated by tubules X-ray films made 5, 10, and 15 minutes after injection; delayed films (30, 60 minutes, and so on), are obtained if obstruction is suspected.	Defines urinary tract Provides information about integrity of kidneys, ureters, and bladder Visualizes retroperitoneal masses when they shift position of ureters
Computed tomography (CT)	Narrow-beam x-rays and computer analysis provide precise reconstruction of area.	Visualizes vertical or horizontal cross section of kidney Especially valuable to distinguish tumors and cysts
Cystoscopy	Direct visualization of bladder and lower urinary tract through small scope inserted via urethra	Investigation of bladder and lower tract lesions; visualizes ureteral openings, bladder wall, trigone, and urethra
Retrograde pyelography	Contrast medium injected through ureteral catheter	Visualizes pelvic calyces, ureters, and bladder
Renal angiography	Contrast medium injected directly into renal artery via catheter placed in femoral artery (or umbilical artery in newborn) and advanced to renal artery	Visualizes renal vascular system, especially for renal arterial stenosis

Continued

TABLE 4-8—cont'd
Urologic Diagnostic Tests

TEST	PROCEDURE	PURPOSE
Whitaker perfusion test	Injection of contrast material through renal pelvis and ureters Pressures are measured in renal pelvis and urinary bladder.	Determine presence of obstruction causing upper urinary tract dilation
Renal biopsy	Removal of kidney tissue by open or percutaneous technique for study by light, electron, or immunofluorescent microscopy	Yields histologic and microscopic information about glomeruli and tubules; helps to distinguish between types of nephritic syndromes Distinguishes other renal disorders
Urodynamics	Set of tests designed to measure bladder filling, storage, and evacuation functions Uroflowmetry is a test to determine efficiency of urination. Cystometrogram is a graphic comparison of bladder pressure as a function of volume. Voiding pressure study is a comparison of detrusor contraction pressure, sphincter electromyelogram, and urinary flow.	Determines characteristic of voiding dysfunction Used to identify type (cause) of incontinence or urinary retention Especially valuable for voiding dysfunction complicated by urinary infection, urinary retention, or neurogenic bladder dysfunction

TABLE 4-9

Lumbar Puncture†

CELL COUNT	CELLS/MM3
Preterm	0-25 mononuclear 0-10 polymorphonuclear 0-1000 RBC
Newborn	0-20 mononuclear 0-10 polymorphonuclear 0-800 RBC
Neonate	0-5 mononuclear 0-10 polymorphonuclear 0-50 RBC
Thereafter	0-5 mononuclear
LEUKOCYTE DIFFERENTIAL COUNT	**PERCENT (%)**
Lymphocytes	62±34
Monocytes	36±20
Neutrophils	2 ± -5
Eosinophils	0-rare
Glucose	40-70 mg/dL* (adult values)
Protein	8-32 mg/dL

†Obtain CSF for analysis: cell count, protein, glucose, culture and sensitivity, Gram stain
*Approximately 75% of serum glucose

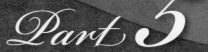

Part 5

Common Nursing Care Procedures

MEDICATION ADMINISTRATION
Safety Precautions
1. Take a drug allergy history.
2. Check the following five *R*s for correctness:
   - Right drug
   - Right dosage
   - Right time
   - Right route
   - Right child (Always check identification band.)
3. Double-check drug and dosage with another nurse.
4. Always double-check the following:
   - Digoxin
   - Insulin
   - Heparin
   - Blood
   - Chemotherapy
   - Cardiotoxic drugs
5. May also double-check the following:
   - Epinephrine
   - Opioids (narcotics)
   - Sedatives
6. Be aware of drug-drug or drug-food interactions.
7. Document all drugs administered.

Oral Administration
1. Follow Safety Precautions for identification and administration.

2. Select appropriate vehicle, for example, calibrated cup, oral medication syringe, dropper, measuring spoon, or nipple.
3. Prepare medication:
   ■ Measure into appropriate vehicle.
   ■ Crush tablets (except when contraindicated, e.g., time-released or enteric-coated preparations) for children who will have difficulty swallowing; mix with syrup, apple sauce, juice, and so on.
4. Avoid mixing medications with essential food items, such as milk and formula.

Infants
Hold in semi-reclining position.
Place oral syringe, measuring spoon, or dropper in mouth well back on the tongue or to the side of the tongue.
Administer slowly to reduce likelihood of choking or aspiration.
Allow infant to suck liquid medication placed in a nipple.

Older Infant or Toddler
Offer medication in a cup or spoon.
Administer with oral syringe, measuring spoon, or dropper (as with infants).
Use mild or partial restraint with reluctant children.
Do not force actively resistive children because of danger of aspiration; postpone 20 to 30 minutes, and offer medication again.

Preschool Children
Use straightforward approach.
For reluctant children, use the following:
   ■ Simple persuasion
   ■ Innovative containers
   ■ Reinforcement, such as stars, stickers, or other tangible rewards for compliance

Intramuscular Administration
Obtain necessary equipment.
Explain procedure to child as developmentally appropriate, and provide atraumatic care.
Follow Safety Precautions for administration of medications (see p. 411).

Select needle and syringe appropriate to the following:

- Amount of fluid to be administered (syringe size)
- Viscosity of fluid to be administered (needle gauge)
- Amount of tissue to be penetrated (needle length)

If withdrawing medication from an ampule, use a needle equipped with a filter that removes glass particles; then use a new, nonfilter needle for injection. Replace needle after withdrawing medication from a vial.

Maintain aseptic technique, and follow Standard Precautions.

Provide for sufficient help in restraining the child; children are often uncooperative, and their behavior is usually unpredictable.

Determine the site of injection (see pp. 418-421); make certain that muscle is large enough to accommodate volume and type of medication.

- Older children—Select site as with the adult patient; allow child some choice of site, if feasible.
- Following are acceptable sites for infants and small or debilitated children:
  - Vastus lateralis muscle
  - Ventrogluteal muscle

Prepare area for puncture with antiseptic agent, and allow to dry completely.

Administer the medication:

- Expose injection area for unobstructed view of landmarks.
- Select a site where the skin is free of irritation and danger of infection; palpate for and avoid sensitive or hardened areas. With multiple injections, rotate sites.
- Place the child in a lying or sitting position; the child is not allowed to stand for the following reasons:
  - Landmarks are more difficult to assess.
  - Restraint is more difficult.
  - The child may faint and fall.
  - Grasp the muscle firmly between the thumb and fingers to isolate and stabilize the muscle for deposition of the drug in its deepest part; in obese children, spread the skin with the thumb and index finger to displace subcutaneous tissue and grasp the muscle deeply on each side.
- Insert needle quickly using a dartlike motion.
- Avoid tracking any medication through superficial tissues.
  - Use the Z track and/or air-bubble technique as indicated.

■ Avoid any depression of the plunger during insertion of the needle.

Aspirate for blood.

■ If blood is found, remove syringe from site, change needle, and reinsert into new location.

■ If no blood is found, inject into a relaxed muscle.

■ Inject medication slowly over several seconds.

Remove needle quickly; hold gauze firmly against skin near needle when removing it to avoid pulling on tissue.

Apply firm pressure with dry gauze to the site after injection; massage the site to hasten absorption unless contraindicated (e.g., with iron, dextran).

Clean area of prepping agent with water to decrease absorption of agent in neonate.

PRAISE CHILD FOR COOPERATION.

Discard syringe and needle in puncture-resistant container near site of use. Do not recap needle.

Record the date, time, dose, drug, and site of injection.

Subcutaneous and Intradermal Administration

Obtain necessary equipment.

Explain procedure to child as developmentally appropriate, and provide atraumatic care.

Maintain aseptic technique, and follow Standard Precautions.

Follow Safety Precautions for administration of medications (see p. 411).

Any site may be used where there are relatively few sensory nerve endings and large blood vessels and bones are relatively deep.

Suggested sites:

■ Center third of lateral aspect of upper arm

■ Abdomen

■ Center third of anterior thigh

■ Avoid the medial side of arm or leg, where skin is more sensitive.

Needle Size and Insertion

Use 26- to 30-gauge needle; change needle before skin puncture if it pierced a rubber stopper on a vial.

Prepare area for puncture with antiseptic agent. Inject small volumes (up to 0.5 ml).

Text continued on p. 417

TABLE 5-1

Intramuscular Administration: Location, Needle Length, Gauge, and Fluid Administration Amount

	LOCATION OF INJECTION	NEEDLE LENGTH	NEEDLE GAUGE (G)	SUGGESTED MAXIMUM AMOUNT (ML)
Preterm newborn	Anterolateral thigh	⅝ inch	23-25 ga	¼-½ ml[†]
Term newborn	Anterolateral thigh	⅝ inch	23-25 ga	½-1 ml[†]
Infant (1-12 months)	Anterolateral thigh	⅝-1 inch	22-25 ga	1 ml[†]
Toddler (13-36 months)	Deltoid	⅝-1 inch	22-25 ga	½-1 ml[†]
	Anterolateral thigh or ventrogluteal	⅝-1 inch* 1-1¼inches[‡]	22-25 ga	1-2 ml[†]
Preschool and older children	Deltoid	⅝-1 inch	22-25 ga	½-1 ml[†]
	Anterolateral thigh or ventrogluteal	1-1¼ inches[‡]	22-25 ga	2-3 ml[†]

Continued

TABLE 5-1—cont'd

Intramuscular Administration: Location, Needle Length, Gauge, and Fluid Administration Amount

	LOCATION OF INJECTION	NEEDLE LENGTH	NEEDLE GAUGE (G)	SUGGESTED MAXIMUM AMOUNT (ML)
Adolescent	Deltoid	5/8-1 inch 1-1½ inches* 1-1¼ inches‡	22-25 ga	1-1½ ml† 2 ml‡
	Anterolateral thigh or ven-trogluteal	1-1¼ inches‡ 1-1½ inches*	22-25 ga**	2-3 ml† 2-5 ml‡

Modified from Becton-Dickinson Media Center: *A guide for managing the pediatric patient: reducing the anxiety and pain of injections,* Franklin Lakes, NJ, 1998, Becton-Dickinson; Centers for Disease Control and Prevention: General recommendations on immunization: recommendations of the Advisory Committee on Immunization Practices (ACIP), *MMWR* 55(RR-15):16-18, 2006; American Academy of Pediatrics; *Red Book, 2006 Report of the Committee on Infectious Diseases,* ed. 27, Elk Grove Village, IL, American Academy of Pediatrics, 2006, pp. 19-21; and Nicoll LH, Hesby A: Intramuscular injection: an integrative research review and guideline for evidence-based practice, *Appl Nurs Res* 16(2): 149-162, 2002.
*Evaluate size of muscle mass before administration.
*Centers for Disease Control and Prevention, 2006.
‡American Academy of Pediatrics, 2006.
**Nicoll and Hesby, 2002.

Subcutaneous and Intradermal Administration (cont'd.)
Subcutaneous Administration
Pinch tissue fold with thumb and index finger.

Using a dartlike motion, insert needle at a 90-degree angle. (Some practitioners use a 45-degree angle on children with little subcutaneous tissue or those who are dehydrated. However, the benefit of using the 45-degree angle rather than the 90-degree angle remains controversial.)

Aspirate for blood. (Some practitioners believe it is not necessary to aspirate before injecting subcutaneously; however, this is not universally accepted. Automatic injector devices do not aspirate before injecting.)

Inject medication slowly without tracking through tissues.

Intradermal Administration
Spread skin site with thumb and index finger if needed for easier penetration.

Insert needle with bevel up and parallel to skin.

Aspirate for blood.

Inject medication slowly.

After injection:
- Clean area of prepping agent with water to decrease absorption of agent in neonate.
- Praise child for cooperation.
- Discard syringe and uncapped, uncut needle in puncture-resistant container near site of use.
- Record date, time, dose, drug, and site of injection.

Use of Insuflon for Subcutaneous Administration of Insulin
Small indwelling catheter placed in the subcutaneous tissues

The average indwelling time is 3 to 5 days.

The catheter is most often inserted in the abdomen, but the buttocks and other areas can also be used. Topical anesthetic cream is recommended before insertion.

Use needles that are 10 mm (0.39 inches) or shorter for injecting to avoid penetration of the tubing of the catheter.

Using indwelling catheters for up to 4 to 5 days does not affect the absorption of insulin.

The long-term (measured by HbA1c) and short-term glucose control (measured by blood glucose profiles and insulin levels) is not altered.

TABLE 5-2

Intramuscular Injection Sites in Children

SITE VASTUS LATERALIS

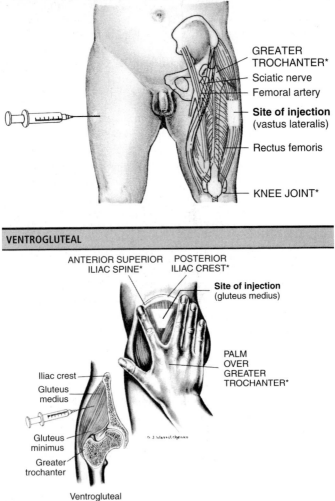

GREATER TROCHANTER*
Sciatic nerve
Femoral artery
Site of injection (vastus lateralis)
Rectus femoris
KNEE JOINT*

VENTROGLUTEAL

ANTERIOR SUPERIOR ILIAC SPINE*   POSTERIOR ILIAC CREST*
Site of injection (gluteus medius)
PALM OVER GREATER TROCHANTER*

Iliac crest
Gluteus medius
Gluteus minimus
Greater trochanter

Ventrogluteal site of injection

▌ TABLE 5-2—cont'd

Intramuscular Injection Sites in Children

DISCUSSION LOCATION*

Palpate to find greater trochanter and knee joints; divide vertical distance between these two landmarks into thirds; inject into middle one third.

NEEDLE INSERTION AND SIZE
Insert needle at 90-degree angle between syringe and upper thigh in infants and in young children
22-25 gauge, ⅝-1 inch

ADVANTAGES
Large, well-developed muscle that can tolerate larger quantities of fluid (0.5 ml [infant] to 2 ml [child])
Easily accessible if child is supine, side lying, or sitting

DISADVANTAGES
Thrombosis of femoral artery from injection in midthigh area (rectus femoris muscle)
Sciatic nerve damage from long needle injected posteriorly and medially into small extremity
More painful than deltoid or gluteal sites

LOCATION*

Palpate to locate greater trochanter, anterior superior iliac tubercle (found by flexing thigh at hip and measuring up to 1-2 cm above crease formed in groin), and posterior iliac crest; place palm of hand over greater trochanter, index finger over anterior superior iliac tubercle, and middle finger along crest of ilium posteriorly as far as possible; inject into center of V formed by fingers.

NEEDLE INSERTION AND SIZE
Insert needle perpendicular to site, but angled slightly toward greater trochanter.
22-25 gauge, ½-1 inch

ADVANTAGES
Free of important nerves and vascular structures
Easily identified by prominent bony landmarks
Thinner layer of subcutaneous tissue than in dorsogluteal site, thus less chance of depositing drug subcutaneously rather than intramuscularly
Can accommodate larger quantities of fluid (0.5 ml [infant] to 2 ml [child])
Easily accessible if child is supine, prone, or side lying
Less painful than vastus lateralis

DISADVANTAGES
Health professionals' unfamiliarity with site

*Locations of landmarks are indicated by asterisks on illustrations.

Continued

TABLE 5-2—cont'd

Intramuscular Injection Sites in Children

DELTOID

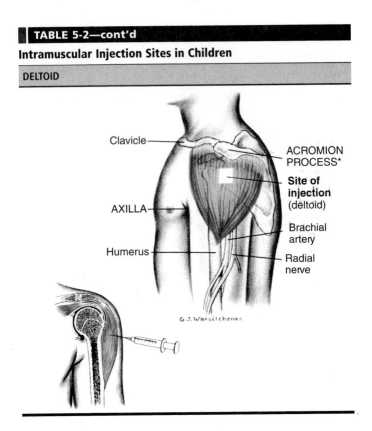

Clavicle

ACROMION PROCESS*

Site of injection (deltoid)

AXILLA

Brachial artery

Humerus

Radial nerve

G.J.Wassilchenko

Use of Insuflon for Subcutaneous Administration of Insulin (cont'd.)

The dead space of the catheter is about 0.5 unit of U100, so it may be necessary to give 0.5 units extra with the first dose after insertion if the child uses small doses.

Intravenous Administration

Obtain necessary equipment.

Explain procedure to the child as developmentally appropriate, and provide atraumatic care.

Use pain prevention interventions before procedure.

TABLE 5-2—cont'd

Intramuscular Injection Sites in Children

LOCATIONS*

Locate acromion process; inject only into upper third of muscle that begins about two finger-breadths below acromion but is above axilla.

NEEDLE INSERTION AND SIZE
Insert needle perpendicular to site, but angled slightly toward greate trochanter.
22-25 gauge, ½-1 inch

ADVANTAGES
Faster absorption rates than gluteal sites
Easily accessible with minimum removal of clothing
Less pain and fewer local side effects from vaccines as compared with vastus lateralis

DISADVANTAGES
Small muscle mass; only limited amounts of drug can be injected (0.5-1 ml).
Small margin of safety with possible damage to radial nerve and axillary nerve (not shown, lies under deltoid at head of humerus)

*Locations of landmarks are indicated by asterisks on illustrations.

Maintain aseptic technique, and follow Standard Precautions.

Follow Safety Precautions for administration of medications. (See p. 411.)

Assess the status of IV infusion to determine that it is functioning properly.

Inspect injection site to make certain the catheter or needle is secure.

Dilute the drug in an amount of solution according to the following:

- Compatibility with infusion fluids or other IV drugs child is receiving
- Size of the child
- Size of the vein being used for infusion

- Length of time over which the drug is to be administered (e.g., 30 minutes, 1 hour, 2 hours)
- Rate at which the drug is to be infused
- Strength of the drug or the degree to which it is toxic to subcutaneous tissues
- Need for fluid restriction

Monitor until medication has been infused. Medication is not completely administered until solution in tubing has infused also (amount of solution depends on tubing length).

Praise child for cooperation.

Discard syringe or bag.

Record date, time, dose, drug, and site of injection.

Procedure for Inserting and Taping a Peripheral Intravenous Catheter

Obtain necessary equipment.

Explain procedure to child as developmentally appropriate, and provide atraumatic care.

Verify order and confirm patient identity.

Follow manufacturer's directions for all devices used.

Wash hands, and observe aseptic technique throughout procedure.

Choose catheter insertion site and an alternative site in case the initial attempt is unsuccessful.

Sites are as follows:

- Superficial veins of the upper extremities are preferred, then the foot.
- Scalp veins (infants)
- A site is chosen that restricts the child's movements as little as possible (e.g., avoid a site over a joint).

For extremity veins, start with the most distal site, especially if irritating or sclerosing agents are to be used.

Apply a topical analgesic such as EMLA or LMX 4 to two sites.

Prepare insertion site by applying with friction an antiseptic solution.

Allow solution to dry completely, but do not blow, blot dry, or fan the area.

Don gloves.

Apply tourniquet when site is ready for catheter insertion.

Stretch the skin taut downward below the point of insertion, upward above the site of insertion, or from underneath level with the point of insertion. This technique helps stabilize veins that roll or move away from the catheter as attempts are made to enter the vein.

Inspect catheter, looking for damage (e.g., bent stylet, shavings on the catheter, frayed catheter tip [follow employer's policy for reporting defective devices]).

Insert catheter through the skin, bevel up, at a 15- to 30-degree angle, and enter the vein. This direct approach is best for large veins and allows the skin and vein to be entered in one step. The indirect approach for smaller veins enables the catheter to enter the vein from the side at an angle. It is sometimes helpful with short veins to start the catheter below the intended site and advance through the superficial layers of skin so that the advancement of the catheter in the vein is a shorter distance. In infants or children with very small veins, insert the catheter bevel down, which prevents the needle from puncturing the back wall of the vein and provides an earlier flashback of blood as the vein is entered.

Watch for blood return in the flashback chamber. Some 24-gauge catheters provide visualization of the flashback within the catheter, so immediate vein entrance is recognized before the needle punctures the back of the vessel or goes through the other side of the vessel.

Once the flashback is seen, lower the angle between the skin and catheter to 15 degrees. Advance the catheter another ¹⁄₁₆ to ⅛ inch to ensure that both the metal stylet and the catheter are inside the vein. Look closely at the IV catheter before inserting it, and note that the stylet tip is slightly longer than the catheter. It is necessary to have both pieces inside the vein before the catheter is advanced. Holding the stylet steady, push the catheter off the stylet and into the vein until the catheter hub is situated against the skin at the insertion site. Activate safety mechanism if necessary (some safety catheters are passive and activate automatically), remove the stylet, and discard into sharps container. Apply pressure to catheter within the vein to prevent backflow of blood before attachment of tubing.

Collect blood if ordered. Remove the tourniquet. Flush the IV line with NS to check for patency (ease of flushing fluid, lack of resistance while flushing), complaints of pain, or swelling at the site. If line flushes easily, proceed to secure the catheter to the skin.

Connect the T-connector, J-connector, injection cap, or tubing, and reinforce connection with a junction securement device (e.g., Luer-Lok, clasping device, threaded device) to prevent accidental disconnection and subsequent air embolism or blood loss.

Place transparent dressing across catheter hub, up to but not including the junction securement device, and surrounding skin.

Further secure the catheter to the skin using tape or adhesive securement devices (e.g., StatLock). Follow manufacturer's directions for adhesive anchors.

Place a ¼ to ½-inch strip of clear tape across the width of the transparent dressing and the catheter hub, but avoid the insertion site. This will serve as an anchor tape strip, and all other tape will be affixed to this strip (tape-on-tape method). This strip will not compromise the transparent dressing properties or interfere with visual inspection of the catheter-skin insertion site.

To stabilize the catheter and junction securement device, attach 1 to 1½ inches of clear tape that is ¼ to ½ inch wide, adhesive side up, to the underneath side of the catheter hub and junction securement device at their connection. Wrap the ends of the tape around the connections, and meet on top to form a *V* shape (sometimes referred to as a *chevron*); secure the overlapping ends onto the anchor tape strip.

Loop the IV tubing away from the catheter hub and toward the IV fluid source. Secure the looped tubing with a piece of tape on the anchor tape strip. Be certain fingers or toes are visible whenever extremity is used.

Consider use of a commercial protective device (e.g., I.V. House) over the catheter hub and looped tubing. Bending one corner of the tape over and onto itself provides a free tab to lift the tape easily for site visualization.

Nasogastric, Orogastric, or Gastrotomy Tube Administration

Use elixir or suspension preparations of medication (rather than tablets) whenever possible.

Dilute viscous medication or syrup with a small amount of water if possible.

Avoid oily medications because they tend to cling to the sides of the tube.

If administering tablets, crush them to a very fine powder and dissolve drug in a small amount of warm water.

Never crush enteric-coated or sustained-release tablets or capsules.

Do not mix medication with enteral formula unless fluid is restricted. If adding a drug:
- Check with pharmacist for compatibility.
- Shake formula well, and observe for any physical reaction (e.g., separation, precipitation).
- Label formula container with name of medication, dosage, date, and time infusion started.
- Have medication at room temperature.
- Measure medication in calibrated cup or syringe.

Check for correct placement of nasogastric (NG) or orogastric tube. *Place 5 ml of air in the syringe. Connect the syringe to the tube.
- Place the stethoscope over the child's stomach area.
- Inject the air quickly into the tube while listening for the sound of gurgling through the stethoscope.
- Remove the air by gently pulling the plunger back to the 5-ml mark.
- If stomach contents appear in the tube as you pull the plunger back, the tube is assumed to be in the correct place.
- If you are unable to see stomach contents in the tube, place the child on the left side or advance the tube a short distance. Pull plunger back again to check for stomach contents.

If more than one fourth of the last feeding is still present, return the food to the stomach and wait 30 to 60 minutes. When there is less than one fourth of the amount of food, return the stomach contents and feed the child.

Attach syringe (with adaptable tip but without plunger) to tube.

Pour medication into syringe.

Unclamp tube, and allow medication to flow by gravity.

Adjust height of container to achieve desired flow rate (e.g., increase height for faster flow).

As soon as syringe is empty, pour 10 ml of water to flush tubing.
- Amount of water depends on length and gauge of tubing.
- Determine amount before administering any medication by using a syringe to completely fill an unused NG or

---

* To test the stomach contents' pH (acidity), as well as listening with a stethoscope to confirm placement, follow directions for pH testing. At the time of this writing, a pH greater than or equal to 5 obtained on stomach aspirate is confirmation of adequate placement in children. Confirmation of feeding tube placement by X-ray is the only method with 100% accuracy. Ellett MLC, Croffie JMB, Cohen MD, Perkins SM: Gastric tube placement in young children, *Clin Nurs Res* 14(3): 238-252, 2005.

orogastric tube with water. The amount of flush solution is
usually 1½ times this volume.
- With certain drug preparations (e.g., suspensions), more
fluid may be needed.

If administering more than one drug at the same time, flush the
tube between each medication with clear water.

Clamp tube after flushing, unless tube is left open or replace cap on
G-tube.

Procedure: Placement of a Nasogastric or Orogastric Tube

1. Place the child supine with the head slightly hyperflexed or in a
   sniffing position (nose pointed toward ceiling).
2. Measure the tube for approximate length of insertion, and mark
   the point with a small piece of tape. Two standard methods of
   measuring length are as follows:
   - Measuring from the nose to the earlobe, then to the distal
     end of the xiphoid process
   - Measuring from the nose to the earlobe, then to a point mid-
     way between the xiphoid process and umbilicus
3. Lubricate the tube with sterile water or water-soluble lubricant,
   and insert through one of the nares or the mouth to the prede-
   termined mark. In older infants and children, the tube is passed
   through the nose and the position alternated between nostrils.
   An indwelling tube is almost always placed through the nose.
   Because most young infants are obligatory nose breathers, insertion through the mouth may be used for intermittent gavage
   feedings because it causes less distress.
   - When using the nose, slip the tube along the base of the nose
     and direct it straight back toward the occiput.
   - When entering through the mouth, direct the tube toward
     the back of the throat.
   - If the child is able to swallow on command, synchronize
     passing the tube with swallowing.
4. Confirm placement by X-ray if available. Document pH and color
   of aspirate with initial placement and ongoing placement checks.*

---

* To test the stomach contents' pH (acidity), as well as listening with a stethoscope to
confirm placement, follow directions for pH testing. At the time of this writing, a pH
greater than or equal to 5 obtained on stomach aspirate is confirmation of adequate
placement in children. Confirmation of feeding tube placement by X-ray is the only
method with 100% accuracy. Ellett MLC, Croffie JMB, Cohen MD, Perkins SM: Gastric
tube placement in young children, *Clin Nurs Res* 14(3): 238-252, 2005.

5. Stabilize the tube by holding or taping it to the cheek, not to the forehead because of possible damage to the nostril. To assist in maintaining correct placement, measure and record the amount of tubing extending from the nose or mouth to the distal port when the tube is first positioned. Recheck position before each feeding. A hydrocolloid barrier (DuoDerm or Coloplast) may be placed on the cheeks to protect the skin from tape irritation.

Procedure: NG TUBE Feeding

1. Whenever possible, hold the infant or young child during the feeding to associate the comfort of physical contact with the procedure. When this is not possible, place the infant or child supine or slightly toward the right side with head and chest slightly elevated.
   - Use a folded blanket under the head and shoulders for infants and a pillow for small children.
   - Raise the head of the bed for larger children.
   - If possible, allow infant to suck on a pacifier during feeding for association of suck and satiation (feeling satisfied).
2. Warm the formula to room temperature. Do not microwave.
3. For feedings delivered by mechanical pump, pour formula into bag or syringe, and prime tubing. Connect to patient and set desired rate.
4. For gravity feedings via syringe, pour formula into the barrel of the syringe attached to the feeding tube. To start the flow, give a gentle push with the plunger, but then remove the plunger and allow the fluid to flow into the stomach by gravity. To prevent nausea and regurgitation, the rate of flow should not exceed 5 ml every 5 to 10 minutes in preterm and very small infants and 10 ml/min in older infants and children. The rate is determined by the diameter of the tubing and the height of the reservoir containing the feeding. The rate is regulated by adjusting the height of the syringe. A typical feeding may take 15 to 30 minutes to complete.
5. Flush the tube with sterile water: 1 or 2 ml for small tubes; 5 to 15 ml or more for large ones.
6. Cap or clamp indwelling tubes to prevent loss of feeding. If the tube is to be removed, first pinch it firmly to prevent escape of fluid as the tube is withdrawn, then withdraw the tube quickly.

7. Position the child with the head elevated about 30 degrees and on the right side for at least 1 hour in the same manner as following any infant feeding to minimize the possibility of regurgitation and aspiration. If the child's condition permits, bubble the child after the feeding.

8. Record the feeding, including the type and amount of residual, the type and amount of formula, and the manner in which it was tolerated. For most infant feedings, any amount of residual fluid aspirated from the stomach is refed to prevent electrolyte imbalance. The amount is subtracted from the prescribed amount of feeding. For example, if the infant or child is to receive 30 ml, and 10 ml is aspirated from the stomach before the feeding, the 10 ml of aspirated stomach contents are refed, plus 20 ml of feeding. Another method in children is that if residual is more than one fourth of the last feeding, the aspirate is returned and rechecked in 30 to 60 minutes. When residual is less than one fourth of last feeding, give scheduled feeding. If high aspirates persist and the child is due for another feeding, notify the practitioner.

9. Between feedings, give infant pacifier to satisfy oral needs.

Procedure: Gastrostomy Tube Feeding

Equipment
    Liquid food at room temperature in pour container
    Water to rinse tube
    Syringe

Instructions

1. Gather equipment.
2. Wash hands.
3. Tell the child (even if infant) what you will be doing.
4. Place the child on your lap or reclining in an infant seat. The older child can sit in a chair or on a bed.
5. Use a pacifier for the infant to enjoy sucking during the feeding.
6. Attach the feeding syringe to the gastrostomy tube.
7. Unclamp the tube.
8. Pull back gently on the plunger to see the amount of food left in the child's stomach.
9. If more than ¼ of the last feeding is still present, return the food to the stomach and wait 30 to 60 minutes. When there is less than ¼ of the amount of food, feed the child.

10. Remove the plunger from the syringe. Hold syringe and tubing below stomach level when filling syringe to prevent excess air getting into stomach.
11. Fill syringe with the right amount of liquid food.
12. A gentle push with the plunger of the syringe may be necessary to start the flow of food; then remove the plunger and allow the food to flow by itself. Do not forcefully push on plunger to speed up the feeding. If the feeding is pushed back into the feeding syringe instead of flowing by gravity, leave the plunger in the barrel of the syringe until the feeding is completed.
13. Do not hold the bottom of the syringe higher than the child's chin.
14. Continue adding food to the syringe until you have finished the right amount. Do not let the syringe become empty.
15. When the food is at the bottom of the syringe add water (1 to 2 teaspoons [5 to 10 ml] or more depending on the child's size and the size of the gastrostomy tube) to rinse the tube and keep it from clogging.
16. Clamp the tube and remove the syringe.
17. Gently pull the tube to allow the balloon to rest against the inside of the stomach at the opening.
18. Tape the tube to the skin to prevent it from advancing or allowing stomach contents to leak on the skin.
19. Hold and cuddle child after the feeding.
20. PRAISE THE CHILD FOR HELPING.

Wash the syringe in soap and warm water using a bottle brush. Rinse the inside well with clear water. Dry the syringe and plunger. Put plunger in syringe when dry, and store in a clean dry container between feedings (e.g., plastic bag).

Procedure: Skin-Level Device Feeding
Equipment
    Liquid food at room temperature in pour container
    Feeding tube with adapter.
    Clamp (usually on the feeding tube)
    Water to rinse tube
    Syringe

Instructions
1. Gather equipment.
2. Wash hands with soap and water.
3. Tell the child (even if infant) what you will be doing.
4. Place the child on your lap or reclining in an infant seat. The older child can sit on a chair or bed.
5. Use a pacifier for the infant to enjoy sucking during the feeding.
6. Align the black line on the feeding tube adapter with the black line on the skin-level device.
7. Turn the feeding tube adapter to the right (clockwise) to lock the feeding tube in place and prevent accidental disconnection and leaking.
8. Attach syringe to the tubing.
9. If the stomach seems full and gassy, air can be removed by putting the feeding tube adapter into the skin-level device and opening the safety plug on the skin-level device. If more than one-fourth of the previous feeding comes out, wait 30 minutes before feeding, and try again.
   (Note: Most skin level gastrostomy buttons have an anti-leak valve so air and fluid does not escape under pressure when the safety plug is open; however, in many cases this feature becomes sticky with the constant presence of formula and gastrointestinal fluid and the valve remains open, thus permitting back flow of air and gastric contents.)
10. Place the desired amount of formula or liquid food in the syringe. This keeps too much air from going into the stomach.
11. A gentle push with the syringe plunger may be necessary to start the flow of food; then remove the plunger and allow the food to flow by itself. Do not forcefully push on plunger to speed up the feeding. If the feeding is pushed back into the feeding syringe instead of flowing by gravity, leave the plunger in the barrel of the syringe until the feeding is completed.
12. Avoid holding the bottom of the syringe higher than the child's chin.
13. Continue adding formula or food to the syringe until you have finished the right amount. Do not let the syringe become empty.
14. When the formula is at the bottom of the syringe, add 1 to 2 teaspoons (5 to 10 ml) of water to rinse the tube.

15. Remove the tube from the device by unlocking (turn counterclockwise) the adapter and feeding tube.
19. Replace the safety plug on the device.
20. Hold and cuddle the child after the feeding.
21. PRAISE THE CHILD FOR HELPING.

Rinse the tubing and syringe with water after each feeding. Place in a clean container.

Care of the Skin-Level Device (G-Button)

Clean around the site each day with mild soap and water. Clean the button with a cotton-tip applicator to remove encrusted formula.

Turn the button around in a complete circle to make sure it is completely cleaned. Dry the area and leave it exposed to air for about 20 minutes so it can dry completely.

If the device is leaking, refer to the Troubleshooting section that follows. A small amount of leakage (less than 1 teaspoon) may occur on occasion, but more than that may lead to problems with the skin around the stoma.

Check the device at least once a week (or more if leakage is noted) by placing a 6-ml syringe on the side port and withdrawing the water from the balloon to make sure it is properly inflated. Keep your hand on the device to prevent it from coming out while the balloon is deflated; it may be necessary to have a helper keep pressure on the button device while doing this. Most skin-level devices have a balloon that requires 5 ml (1 teaspoon) of water; proper inflation maintains the seal and prevents leaking.

Medications can plug the device. Medicines in tablet form should be crushed well and mixed with water or food before putting them in the feeding syringe. Thick liquids can be mixed with warm water to make them thinner. The medicine should be given before the feeding, to make sure the medicine goes into the stomach. If it is not time for a feeding, rinse the tubing with 1 to 2 teaspoons (5 to 10 ml) of water after giving the medicine.

If the child is on continuous feedings, flush the device and tubing with water (1 to 2 teaspoons [5 to 10 ml]) to rinse the tube and keep it from clogging.

Troubleshooting the Skin-Level Device

Once the tube tract has formed (usually in 6 to 12 weeks), the surgeon will approve of changing the tube if it comes out. If the device accidentally comes out, it is not an emergency. Do not throw the device away, and follow these directions.

Examine the device carefully; if the balloon has completely deflated or is partially empty, attach a 6-ml syringe to the port on the side of the button device and try to inflate the balloon.

If the balloon will not inflate and appears to be ruptured, apply a small amount of water-soluble lubricant to the tip of the tube, replace the tube into the stomach hole, and tape it in place.

If the balloon has simply discharged some or all of its water but still inflates, withdraw all the water from the balloon with the 6-ml syringe, apply a small amount of water-soluble lubricant to the tip of the tube, and insert the tube into the stomach hole. Then reinflate the balloon by pushing 5-ml of water into the side port with the 6-ml syringe. The balloon will inflate and hold the tube in place. Remove the syringe after balloon inflation.

If the device comes out and you cannot replace the tube into the stomach hole, place a gastrostomy tube into the opening. Inflate the gastrostomy tube balloon with sterile water (usually the amount is 5 mls), and contact the practitioner in charge of the child's care.

Skin Care

Keep the skin around the gastrostomy tube or skin-level device clean and dry. A bandage does not have to be put over the area. A cloth diaper or cotton cloth can be wrapped around the child's abdomen and secured with tape. This will keep the child from playing with the tube. Other ways to keep the tube out of reach are to use one-piece outfits, tube tops, the tops of panty hose, or children's tights with the legs cut off.

Zinc oxide ointment, Duoderm-CGF (a thin dressing that can be kept on the skin for 7 days), Pro Shield Plus Skin Protectant, or Cavilon No Sting Barrier Film (spray or foam); or any other skin barrier can be used on the skin around the gastrostomy tube or skin-level device.

A single layer 2 × 2 gauze pad may also be placed around the tube or device. It should be changed at least daily or when soiled. These measures will provide protection for the skin in case there is a small leakage of gastric fluid. If the area becomes red or sore, or if drainage continues to be a problem after every feeding, contact the practitioner or an enterostomal therapist for further evaluation.

OXYGEN THERAPY

Methods include use of a mask, hood, nasal cannula, face tent, or oxygen tent.

Method is selected on the basis of the following:

- Concentration of inspired oxygen needed
- Ability of the child to cooperate in its use

Oxygen is a drug and is administered only in prescribed dose.

Concentration is regulated according to the needs of the child (usually 40% to 50%, or 4- to 6-L flow).

Oxygen is dry; therefore it must be humidified.

Use the following precautions with an oxygen hood:

- Do not allow oxygen to blow directly on the infant's face.
- Position hood to avoid rubbing against the infant's neck, chin, or shoulders.

Use the following precautions with an oxygen tent:

- Plan nursing activities so that tent is opened as little as possible.
- Tuck open edges of tent carefully to reduce oxygen loss (oxygen is heavier than air).
- Check temperature inside tent frequently.
- Keep child warm and dry.
- Make certain cooling mechanism is functioning.
- Examine bedding and clothing periodically, and change as needed.
- Inspect any toys placed in the tent for safety and suitability.
- Note that any source of sparks (e.g., from mechanical or electrical toys) is a potential fire hazard.
- Monitor child's color, respirations, and O_2 saturation.
- Periodically analyze oxygen concentration at a point near the child's head, and adjust oxygen flow rate to maintain desired concentration.
- Provide comfort and reassurance to the child. Make sure the child is able to see someone nearby.

Pulse Oximetry

Measures arterial hemoglobin oxygen saturation (SaO_2) by passage of two different wavelengths of light through blood-perfused tissues to a photodetector. SaO_2 and heart rate are displayed on digital readout.

Attach sensor to earlobe, finger, or toe; make certain light source and photodetector are in opposition.

Avoid sites with restricted blood flow (e.g., distal to a blood pressure cuff or indwelling arterial catheter).

Secure sensor cord self-adhering wrap or tape to avoid interference by patient movement. Shield sensor from bright light. Keep extremity warm (e.g., use a sock over foot or hand if extremity is cool).

Avoid IV dyes; green, purple, or black nail polish; nonopaque synthetic nails; and possibly footprint ink, which may cause erroneous readings.

Change placement of sensor every 4 to 8 hours. Inspect skin at sensor site in children with compromised circulation and oxygenation, and change sensor more frequently if needed to prevent pressure necrosis.

Advantages:

- Noninvasive technique
- No complicated preparation or calibration of sensor
- No special skin care needed
- Convenient sites can be used.

Disadvantages:

- Requires peripheral arterial pulsation
- Limited use in hypotension or with vasoconstricting drugs
- Sensor affected by movement (Safety Alert)
- SaO_2 is related to PO_2, but the values are not the same. As a rule of thumb, an SaO_2 of:
  - **98%** = PO_2 of 100 mmHg or greater
  - **90%** = PO_2 of 60 mmHg
  - **80%** = PO_2 of 45 mmHg
  - **60%** = PO_2 of 30 mmHg

In general, normal range is 95% to 99%, except in preterm infant. A consistent SaO_2 less than 95% should be investigated, and an SaO_2 of 90% signifies developing hypoxia.

Aerosol Therapy

The purpose is the inhalation of a solution in droplet (particle) form for direct deposition in the tracheobronchial tree.

Aerosols consist of liquid medications (e.g., bronchodilators, steroids, mucolytics, decongestants, antibiotics, antiviral agents) suspended in a particulate form in air.

Aerosol generators propelled by air or air-oxygen mixtures generally fall into three categories:
- Small-volume jet nebulizers or handheld nebulizers
- Ultrasonic nebulizers for sterile water or saline aerosol only
- Metered-dose inhalers (MDIs) (sometimes with a "spacer" device that acts as a reservoir and simplifies use of the inhaler; devices such as the Rotohaler or Turbuhaler eliminate the need for a spacer device and are easier for young children to use.)

Deposition of aerosol is maximized by instructing the child to breathe through the mouth with slow, deep inhalations, followed by holding the breath for 5 to 10 seconds, then slow exhalations while in an upright position. A small face mask is more effective for aerosol delivery to the infant and toddler. The medication chamber must be held upright for the aerosol to be nebuziled effectively.

Using an incentive spirometer can help a cooperative child learn this ventilatory pattern.

For infants and young children, activities to produce deep breathing and coughing include feet tapping, tactile stimulation, and crying.

Assessment of breath sounds and work of breathing is performed before and after treatments.

Tracheostomy Care
Tracheostomy is a surgical opening in the trachea between the second and fourth tracheal rings. Pediatric tracheostomy tubes are usually made of plastic or Silastic.

Tracheostomy Suctioning
The practice of instilling sterile saline in the tracheostomy tube before suctioning is not supported by research and is no longer recommended by many institutions. Suctioning should require no more than 5 seconds. Counting 1, one thousand, 2, one thousand, 3, one thousand, and so on while suctioning is a simple means for monitoring the time. Without a safeguard, the airway may be obstructed for too long. Hyperventilating the child with 100% O_2 before and after suctioning (using a bag-valve-mask or increasing the FiO_2 ventilator setting) is also performed to prevent hypoxia. Closed tracheal suctioning systems that allow for uninterrupted O_2 delivery may also be used. In a closed suction system, a suction catheter is directly

attached to the ventilator tubing. This system has several advantages. First, there is no need to disconnect the patient from the ventilator, which allows for better oxygenation. Second, the suction catheter is enclosed in a plastic sheath, which reduces the risk of exposure to the patient's secretions.

Suctioning, Catheter Length, and Saline

Traditional technique for suctioning ET or tracheostomy tubes recommends advancing a suction catheter into the tube until it meets resistance, then withdrawing it slightly and applying suction. However, studies indicate that this approach causes trauma to the tracheobronchial wall. This trauma can be avoided by inserting the catheter and advancing it to the premeasured depth of just to the tip (especially in infants) or no more than 0.5 cm beyond the tube (Kleiber, Krutzfield, and Rose, 1988).[*]

Calibrated catheters are easier to use for premeasured suctioning technique, but unmarked catheters can also be used. To measure the length for catheter insertion, place the catheter near a sample ET or tracheostomy tube (same size as child's tube) with the end of the catheter at the correct position. Grasp the catheter with a sterile-gloved hand to mark the length, and insert the catheter until the hand reaches the stoma.

It has been common practice to instill a bolus of NS into the tube before suctioning. However, this technique may contribute to lower airway colonization and nosocomial pneumonia through repeated washing of organisms from the tube's surface into the lower airway (Hagler and Traver, 1994).[†] The use of saline has been shown to have an adverse effect on SaO_2, and it should not be used routinely in patients receiving mechanical ventilation who have a pulmonary infection (Ackerman, 1998).[‡] Although the pediatric research is scarce, routine use of NS with ET tube suctioning should be avoided (Curley and Moloney-Harmon, 2001).[§]

---

[*]Kleiber C, Krutzfield N, Rose EF: Acute histologic changes in tracheobronchial tree associated with different suction catheter insertion techniques, *Heart Lung* 17:10-14, 1988.
[†]Hagler DA, Traver GA: Endotracheal saline and suction catheters: sources of lower airway contamination, *Am J Crit Care* 3(6):444-447, 1994.
[‡]Ackerman MH: Instillation of normal saline before suctioning in patients with pulmonary infections: a prospective randomized controlled trial, *Am J Crit Care* 7(4): 261-266, 1998.
[§]Curley MAQ, Moloney-Harmon PA: *Critical care nursing of infants and children*, ed 2, Philadelphia, 2001, Saunders.

TABLE 5-3

Fluid Management

Estimates of Daily Caloric Expenditure (Under Normal Conditions)

HOLLIDAY-SEGAR METHOD*

BODY WEIGHT	Water ML/KG/DAY	Water ML/KG/HR		ELECTROLYTES (MEQ/100 ML H$_2$O)
First 10 kg	100	÷ 24 hr/day ≈4	Na$^+$	3
Second 10 kg	50	÷ 24 hr/day ≈2	Cl$^-$	2
Each additional kg	20	÷ 24 hr/day ≈1	K$^+$	2

EXAMPLE: 8-YEAR-OLD WEIGHING 25 kg

ml/kg/day

100 (for first 10 kg)	× 10 kg	= 1000 ml/day	
50 (for second 10 kg)	× 10 kg	= 500 ml/day	
20 (per additional kg)	× 5 kg	= 100 ml/day	
	25 kg	1600 ml/day	

ml/kg/hr

4 (for first 10 kg)	× 10 kg	= 40 ml/hr	
2 (for second 10 kg)	× 10 kg	= 20 ml/hr	
1 (per additional kg)	× 5 kg	= 5 ml/hr	
	25 kg	65 ml/hr	

From Robertson J, Shilkofski N: *The Harriet Lane handbook*, ed 17, St Louis, 2005, Elsevier.
*Not suitable for neonates <14 days old.

Positioning for Procedures
Extremity Venipuncture or Injection
Place child on parent's (or assistant's) lap, with the child facing toward the parent and in the straddle position.

For venipuncture, place child's arm on a firm surface such as the treatment table (for support) and on top of a soft cloth or towel.

Have parent or assistant immobilize child's arm for venipuncture.

Have parent hug the child around the back to hold the child's free arm, or place child on parent's lap, with the child facing away from the parent.

To hold the child's legs still, place them between the parent's legs. This position is appropriate for an injection into the thigh; for an injection into the arm, place child in parent's lap, with the child facing sideward.

Place the child's arm closest to the parent under the parent's arm, and wrap toward the back.

Have the parent hold the arm receiving the injection against the child's body.

Femoral Venipuncture
Place infant supine with legs in frog position to provide extensive exposure of the groin.

Restrain legs in frog position with hands while controlling the child's arm and body movements with downward and inward pressure of forearms.

Cover genitalia to protect the operator and the venipuncture site from contamination if the child urinates during the procedure.

Site is not advisable for long-term venous access in mobile child because of risk of infection and trauma to flexion area.

Subdural Puncture (through Fontanel or Bur Holes)
Place active infant in mummy restraint.

Position supine with head accessible to examiner.

Control head movement with firm hold on each side of the head.

Nose and/or Throat Access
Position supine with face accessible to examiner.

Control head and arms by holding child's extended arms over and close to the head, thus immobilizing both head and arms.

Ear Access

Place child in parent's (or assistant's) lap with the child's body sideways and the ear to be examined away from the parent.

Place the child's arm closest to the parent under the parent's arm and wrap toward the back.

Have the parent hold the other arm against the child's body and use the free arm to hold the head against the parent's chest.

To hold the child's legs still, place them between the parent's legs.

Lumbar Puncture

Infant

Place infant in sitting position with buttocks extended over the edge of the table and head flexed on chest.

In neonates, use side-lying position with modified head extension to decrease respiratory distress during procedure. Pulse oxime try and heart rate monitoring are advisable.

Immobilize arms and legs with nurse's hands.

Observe child for difficulty in breathing.

Child

Place child on side with back close to or extended over the edge of examining table, head flexed, and knees drawn up toward the chest.

Reach over the top of the child, and place one arm behind child's neck and the other behind the knees.

Stabilize this position by clasping own hands in front of the child's abdomen.

Take care that excessive pressure does not compromise circulation or breathing and that the nose and mouth are not covered by the restrainer's body.

Bone Marrow Examination

For posterior iliac site:

- Position child prone.
- Place a small pillow or folded towel under the hips to raise them slightly.
- Apply restraint at upper body and lower extremities, preferably with two persons.

For anterior iliac site or tibia:

- Position child supine.

- Apply restraint at upper body and lower extremities, preferably with two persons.

Urinary Catheterization

Have the parent sit in a chair or on an examining table with a back support. Place the child leaning back in the parent's lap with the parent's arms hugging the child's upper body.

Place the child's legs in the froglike position, with the parent's legs over the child's to stabilize them. In this comfortable position, the perineum is exposed for the procedure.

Place the child supine in bed with legs in the froglike position. Raise head of bed as much as possible while still allowing good visualization of the perineum. A semi-upright position is less stressful to a child.

COLLECTION OF SPECIMENS
Urine
Non–Toilet-Trained Child
Equipment
    Antiseptic cleanser
    Urine collection bag for small child

Use a pediatric urine collection bag. The bag is not sterile, therefore usually only a clean –catch specimen may be obtained.

Cleanse the infant's genitalia with an approved antiseptic before applying the urine bag.

Have your helper hold the child's legs apart while you apply the bag.

Hold the urine collector with the bag portion downward.

Remove the bottom half of the adhesive protector.

For Girls

Spread the labia and buttocks, keeping the skin tight.

Begin with the bottom of the adhesive. Place the sticky portion of the bag as flat as possible against the skin.

Smooth the plastic to avoid any wrinkles.

Remove the top half of the adhesive protector, and smooth it also on the labia.

For Boys

Place the boy's penis and scrotum into the bag if possible. If only the penis fits in the bag, put the sticky part of the bag on the scrotum.

Smooth the sticky portion of the bag on the skin, taking care to avoid making any wrinkles.

Remove the top half of the adhesive protector, and smooth the top part on the skin to remove any wrinkles.

Cut a small slit in the diaper, and pull the bag through to allow room for urine to collect and to facilitate checking the contents. To obtain small amounts of urine, use a syringe without a needle to aspirate urine directly from the diaper; if diapers with absorbent gelling material that traps urine are used, place a small gauze dressing, some cotton balls, or a urine collection device inside the diaper to collect urine, and then aspirate the urine with a syringe.

Check the bag frequently, and remove as soon as specimen is available.

Wash the child's genitalia with warm water after removing the urine collection device.

Urine collected for culture should be tested within 30 minutes, refrigerated, or placed in a sterile container with a preservative.

Toilet-Trained Young Child
Instructions for the Toilet-Trained Child
Equipment
  Urine specimen cup
  Potty chair, potty hat, or toilet
  Antiseptic cleanser
  Washcloth and warm water
Clean-catch urine sample (boys and girls)
  ▪ Tell the child that you need to get some urine.
  ▪ If the child is able to obtain the sample of urine, have the child wash his or her hands.
  ▪ Wash your hands.
  ▪ Gather the equipment needed.
For boy: Cleanse the tip of the penis with an antiseptic (or instruct parent assisting to cleanse penis). If the child is uncircumcised, pull back the foreskin only as far as it will easily go, then cleanse the tip of the penis with antiseptic. Rinse well after procedure. Make sure the foreskin is pushed back toward the tip after cleaning.
For girl: Spread the child's labia (lips) with your fingers (or instruct parent assisting to cleanse labia). Cleanse the area with antiseptic.

Wipe from front to back (top to bottom). Rinse area with washcloth after completing urine collection.

Open the urine container, being careful not to touch the inside of
the cup or lid.

Have the child begin to urinate in the potty chair or toilet.

Tell child to stop.

If child cannot stop the flow of urine, place the urine cup so that
you can catch some of the urine.

Have child urinate directly into the cup (or potty hat if more convenient for female).

Replace the lid on the cup.

Label the cup with the child's first and last name.

Rinse antiseptic off penis or labia with a warm washcloth and water after the child has voided (or instruct child or assistant to
cleanse area).

PRAISE THE CHILD FOR HELPING.

Bladder Catheterization

Bladder catheterization is employed for the following reasons:

- Collection of a urine specimen
- Diagnostic testing
- Continuous urinary drainage
- Intravesical instillation of medications or chemotherapeutic
  agents

Materials needed:

- Sterile gloves
- Sterile catheter—either a straight catheter (in and out) or in-
  dwelling Foley catheter
- Antiseptic solution and sterile gauze pad or cotton (or ap-
  plicator)
- Sterile drape
- Sterile urine container
- Sterile lubricant
- Sterile water to fill balloon (for Foley) and a syringe to insert
  water into balloon

Catheter

Select a catheter based on the purpose of the procedure, the age and
gender of the child, and any history of prior urologic surgery.

When collecting a urine specimen or completing a diagnostic test
requiring catheterization for a brief period, use:

- A 4-5, or 8 French straight catheter for an infant

- A 5-8 French catheter for a toddler or young school-aged child
- An 8-12 French straight catheter for an adolescent girl
- An 8-12 French, straight-tipped or coudé-tipped catheter for an older school-aged or adolescent boy

When placing an indwelling catheter, use:

- A 5, 6-8 French Foley catheter with a 3-ml retention balloon for an infant
- A 6-8 French Foley catheter with a 3-5-ml retention balloon for a toddler or school-aged child
- An 8-12 French Foley catheter with a 5-ml retention balloon for an adolescent girl
- An 8-16 French Foley catheter with a 5-ml retention balloon for an adolescent boy
- Larger French sizes (14 to 16) are reserved for older adolescents with more fully developed prostates. A coudé-tipped catheter is selected for the adolescent boy with a history of urologic surgery.

Procedure

1. Assemble necessary equipment.
2. Explain procedure to child and parents.
   - Give a careful and thorough explanation of the procedure, according to the developmental level of the child, before preparation of the perineum. Include an explanation of the purpose of the catheterization, and reassure child that it is not punishment.
   - Reassure parents that catheterization will not harm their child or damage the urethra or hymen.
   - Reassure child that insertion of the catheter will not feel like having a sharp object inserted but will produce a feeling of pressure and desire to urinate.
3. Give instruction on pelvic muscle relaxation whenever possible.
   - Young child is taught to blow (using a pinwheel is helpful) and to press the hips against the bed or procedure table during catheterization in order to relax the pelvic and periurethral muscles.
   - Older child or adolescent is taught to contract and relax the pelvic muscles, and the relaxation procedure is repeated during catheter insertion. If the youngster vigorously contracts the pelvic muscles when the catheter reaches the striated

sphincter (proximal urethra in boys and midurethra in girls), catheter insertion is temporarily stopped. The catheter is neither removed nor advanced; instead the child is assisted to press the hips against the bed or examining table and relax the pelvic muscles. The catheter is then gently advanced into the bladder.

4. Place the infant or child in a supine position with the perineum adequately exposed. Girls may bend the knees and abduct the legs in a froglike position; boys should lie with the penis lying above the upper thighs. For a young child, have the parent sit on the bed or examining table with a back support. Place the child leaning back in the parent's lap with the parent's arms hugging the child's upper body. When the child's legs are in the frog position, the parent's legs can be placed over the child's to stabilize them. In this comfortable position, the perineum is exposed for the procedure and the child is helped to lie still.

5. Put on a pair of sterile gloves.

6. Place a sterile drape over the perineum of girls, ensuring that the vagina, labia, and urethral meatus remain exposed. Most catheter insertion kits provide a sterile drape with a diamond-shaped hole in the middle to assist with this. For boys, the sterile drape is placed over the upper aspect of the thighs.

7. Place 5 ml of sterile lubricating jelly on the sterile drape. During catheterization of an adolescent or child accustomed to the procedure, the catheter may be placed on the sterile drape laid over the perineum. When an anxious child is being catheterized, the catheter should remain on a sterile field that will not be contaminated should the child move during the procedure.

8. Cleanse the perineum of girls, including the labia, vaginal introitus, and urethral meatus. Use a new cotton ball for each wipe, moving in a front-to-back motion along each side of the labia minora, along the sides of the urinary meatus, and finally straight down over the urethral opening. For boys, the entire glans penis is cleansed, in an outward circular fashion, using one cotton ball for each wipe. The foreskin is retracted in the uncircumcised boy to ensure adequate exposure. If the foreskin cannot be easily retracted, particular care is taken to ensure that the glans penis is adequately cleaned before catheter insertion.

9. Wipe the cleanser from the skin using sterile cotton balls.

10. Girls: Spread the labia (if necessary) using one hand in order to clearly visualize the urethral meatus. With the other hand, grasp the catheter and apply a small amount of sterile lubricant from the sterile field onto the tip of the catheter. (It is rarely necessary to spread the labia in infants; instead, locate the urethra, which often appears as a dimple above the hymen.) Gently insert the catheter until urine return is seen. If inserting an indwelling catheter, advance the catheter an additional 1-2 inches before attempting to fill the retention balloon.

11. Boys: Hold the penile shaft just under the glans to prevent the foreskin from contaminating the area. Grasp the catheter with the other hand, and apply a small amount of sterile lubricant from sterile field onto the tip of the catheter. Insert the catheter while gently stretching the penis and lifting it to a 90-degree angle to the body. Resistance may occur when the catheter meets the urethral sphincter. Ask the patient to inhale deeply and advance the catheter at that time. Insert the catheter until urine return occurs; this may take several seconds longer because of the additional lubricant present in the urethra. If inserting an indwelling catheter, advance until urine return is noted, then advance to the bifurcation of the filling port before filling the retention balloon.

12. When catheterizing for specimen collection, allow 15 to 30 ml for urinalysis and urine culture. Drain bladder, and record postvoid urinary volume if collected soon after urination. Cap the specimen, label it, and send it to the laboratory.

13. When inserting an indwelling catheter, inject the recommended amount of sterile water into the side port injection site to fill the balloon.

14. When inserting an indwelling catheter, gently pull the catheter back until resistance is met; this ensures that the retention balloon lies just above the bladder neck. Tape tubing to the leg to avoid pulling, or use a commercially available catheter securement device. Hang drainage apparatus to bed frame (avoid bed rails to prevent pulling on catheter).

Blood
Heel or Finger
Heel lancing has been shown to be more painful than venipuncture; consider venipuncture when the amount of blood from the heel would require much squeezing (e.g., genetic tests).

Puncture should be no deeper than 2 mm. Use of an automatic lancing device is recommended, as this prevents too deep a puncture.

- Obtain necessary equipment, including appropriate specimen container(s).
- Explain procedure to child as developmentally appropriate, and provide atraumatic care.
- Maintain aseptic technique, and follow Standard Precautions.
- To increase blood flow, warm heel by using a commercial heel warmer for 3 minutes before puncture; may hold finger under warm water for a few seconds before puncture.
- Prepare area for puncture with antiseptic agent.
- Provide comfort for neonate (e.g., swaddling, holding in containment, allowing sucking on pacifier, using a 24% concentrated sucrose [2 ml] during procedure).
- Perform puncture on heel or finger in proper location with an automatic lancet device:
    - Usual site for heel puncture is outer aspects of heel. Boundaries can be marked by an imaginary line extending posteriorly from a point between the fourth and fifth toes and running parallel to the lateral aspect of the heel and another line extending posteriorly from the middle of the great toe and running parallel to the medial aspect of the heel.
    - Usual site for finger puncture is just to the side of the finger pad, which has more blood vessels and fewer nerve endings. Avoid the tip of the finger just below the nail. Avoid steadying the finger against a hard surface.
- Collect blood sample in appropriate specimen container.
- Apply pressure to puncture site with a dry, sterile gauze pad until bleeding stops.
- Clean area of prepping agent with water to avoid absorption in neonate.
- PRAISE CHILD FOR COOPERATION.
- Discard puncture device in puncture-resistant container near site of use.
- Document site and amount of blood withdrawn as well as type of test performed.

Respiratory (Nasal) Secretions

To obtain nasal secretions using a nasal washing:

- Place child supine if maximal restraint is needed; an upright or semi-reclining position allows the child more control and causes less anxiety.
- Instill 1 to 3 ml sterile NS with a sterile syringe (without needle or with 2 inches of 18- or 20-gauge tubing) into one nostril.
- Allow child to blow nose into the specimen cup; if child is unable to blow nose, aspirate contents with a small sterile bulb syringe, or a wall suction (or suction machine) attached to a DeLee mucus trap with sterile specimen cup.
- A BBG Nasal Aspirator connected to wall suction and DeLee mucus trap is adequate for neonates and small infants (less trauma to nasal passages than a catheter).
- Place specimen in sterile container.

VEIN (VENIPUNCTURE)

Obtain necessary equipment, including appropriate specimen container(s).

Explain procedure to child as developmentally appropriate, and provide atraumatic care.

Maintain aseptic technique, and use Standard Precautions.

Restrain child only as needed to prevent injury.

Prepare area for puncture with antiseptic agent. Allow skin to dry.

Apply tourniquet; alternative tourniquet for neonate is a rubber band.

Visualize or palpate vein.

Insert needle with bevel up; a slight pop may be felt when entering a child's vein; in small and preterm infants, this may not occur.

Withdraw required amount of blood, and place in appropriate container.

Release tourniquet.

Withdraw needle from site, and apply dry, sterile gauze or cotton ball to site with firm pressure until bleeding stops. If antecubital site is used, keep arm extended to reduce bruising.

Clean area of prepping agent with water to decrease absorption in neonate.

PRAISE CHILD FOR COOPERATION.

Discard syringe and needle in puncture-resistant container near site of use. Document site and amount of blood withdrawn as well as type of test obtained.

Caring for a Central Venous Catheter
Changing the Injection Cap
If the cap is changed at the time of rinsing, the heparin or saline is given (flushed) through the new injection cap.

Equipment
  Antiseptic swab
  Injection cap

Procedure
1. Gather the equipment you will need.
2. Wash your hands with soap and water.
3. Clamp the tube midway between the skin and the end of the tube or on the reinforced clamping sleeve that is on some catheters; do not clamp a Groshong catheter.
4. With the swab, clean around the tip of the tube below the injection cap.
5. Open the new injection cap package.
6. Remove the used injection cap from the tube, and attach the new injection cap.
7. Remove the clamp from the catheter (not needed with Groshong).

Dressing Change
  Equipment
■ Adhesive remover pad
■ Transparent dressing
■ Antiseptic swabs
■ Bag for disposing of used supplies and dressing
■ Tape

Instructions
1. Gather the equipment on a clean, dry surface.
2. Wash hands.
3. Gently peel off the edges of the old dressing, using adhesive remover if necessary. Peel off one edge at a time. Another way to remove the dressing is to grasp opposite corners of the plastic film and pull them away from each other to stretch and loosen the film. After the film begins to loosen, grasp the other two corners of the film and pull. This method is easier and more comfortable than pulling the dressing up and off the skin.

CAUTION: Avoid using scissors around a central line dressing.
PICC Line Dressing removal—The PICC line is often held in place by one or two sutures. During dressing removal, locate the entrance point of the PICC line and place a gloved finger over the catheter at the insertion point while loosening the dressing edges to avoid pulling or dislodging the PICC line.

4. Carefully look at the skin around the tube for redness or drainage.
5. Using each antiseptic swab only once, clean the skin where the tube enters the body. Use a circular motion starting at the tube and moving out about 3 inches from the tube.
6. Loop the tube around the entry site, leaving the injection cap below the dressing.
7. Carefully place the dressing on the child's skin. Hold the dressing in both hands. When the top of the dressing is on the skin, slowly bring the dressing toward the bottom of the window frame, making sure that it attaches to the skin.
8. Secure the end of the tube with tape to keep it from dangling.
9. Discard all used items in an appropriate container.
10. PRAISE THE CHILD FOR HELPING.

Appendix A

Vital Signs for Infants and Children

Normal Ranges of Heart Rates for Children

AGE	Rate (Beats/Minute)		
	RESTING (AWAKE)	RESTING (SLEEPING)	EXERCISE (FEVER)
Newborn	100-180	80-160	Up to 220
1 week to 3 months	100-220	80-180	Up to 220
3 months to 2 years	80-150	70-120	Up to 200
2 -10 years	70-110	60-100	Up to 180
10 years to adult	55-90	50-90	Up to 180

Modified from Gillette PC: Dysrhythmias. In Adams FH, Emmanouilides GC, Riemenschneider TA, eds: *Moss' heart disease in infants, children, and adolescents,* ed 4, Baltimore, 1989, Williams & Wilkins.

Normal Respiratory Rates for Children

AGE	RATE (BREATHS/MINUTE)
Newborn	35
1-11 months	30
2 years	25
4 years	23
6 years	21
8 years	20
10 years	19
12 years	19
14 years	18
16 years	17
18 years	16-18

Normal Temperatures in Children

	Temperature	
AGE	°F	°C
3 months	99.4	37.5
6 months	99.5	37.5
1 year	99.7	37.7
3 years	99.0	37.2
5 years	98.6	37.0
7 years	98.3	36.8
9 years	98.1	36.7
11 years	98.0	36.7
13 years	97.8	36.6

Modified from Lowery GH: *Growth and development of children,* ed 8, St Louis, 1986, Mosby.

Appendix B

Centigrade to Fahrenheit Temperature Conversions

°C	°F	°C	°F	°C	°F
35.0	95.0	37.0	98.6	39.0	102.2
35.2	95.4	37.2	99.0	39.2	102.6
35.4	95.7	37.4	99.3	39.4	102.9
35.6	96.1	37.6	99.7	39.6	103.3
35.8	96.4	37.8	100.0	39.8	103.6
36.0	96.8	38.0	100.4	40.0	104.0
36.2	97.2	38.2	100.8	40.2	104.4
36.4	97.5	38.4	101.1	40.4	104.7
36.6	97.9	38.6	101.5	40.6	105.1
36.8	98.2	38.8	101.8	40.8	105.4
				41.0	105.8

Conversion Formulas
$°F = (°C \times 9/5) + 32$ or $(°C \times 1.8) + 32$
$°C = (°F - 32) \times 5/9$ or $(°F - 32) \times 0.55$

DOSE CALC

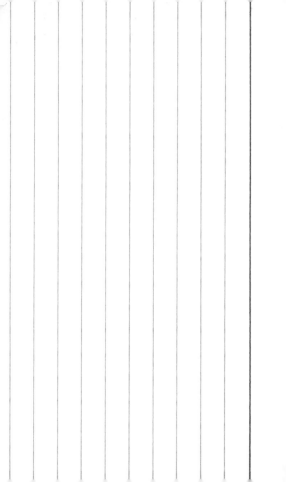

Appendix C

Dosage Calculations

There are 3 basic formulas which can be used for calculating medication dosages.

D/H METHOD

$$\frac{\text{Dosage desired (ordered)}}{\text{Drug Available}} \times \text{Quantity on hand} = x$$

Quantity on hand for pills and tablets will always be equal to 1, whereas for liquids it will vary.

Example: Ordered: Amoxicillin susp 365 mg p.o. BID
Available: Amoxicillin 250 mg/5 ml

$$\frac{365\,\text{mg}}{250\,\text{mg}} \times 5\,\text{ml} = 7.3\,\text{ml}$$

RATIO: PROPORTION

Left side is "known"; right side is desired dose and amount to administer.

On Hand : Unit Measure = Desired : x
Example: Ordered: Amoxicillin susp 365 mg p.o. BID
Available: Amoxicillin susp 250 mg/5ml
$250 : 5 = 365 : x$
$50x = 365$
$x = 7.3$ ml

INTRAVENOUS FLOW RATE

$$\frac{\text{Amount of fluid} \times \text{drops/mL (drip factor)}}{\text{Hours to administer} \times \text{minutes/hour}} = \text{drops/minute}$$

Example:

$$\frac{500\,\text{ml} \times 15\,\text{gtts/ml}}{6\,\text{hours} \times 60} =$$

$$\frac{7500}{360} = 20.8\,\text{gtts/min}$$

REFERENCES

Attia J: Measurement of postoperative pain and narcotic administration in infants using a new clinical scoring system, *Anesthesiology* 67(3A):A532, 1987.

Beyer JE, Denyes MJ, Villarruel AM: The creation, validation and continuing development of the Oucher: a measure of pain intensity in children, *J Pediatr Nurs* 7(5):335-346, 1992. www.oucher.org.

Blauer T, Gerstmann D: A simultaneous comparison of three neonatal pain scales during common NICU procedures, *Clin J Pain* 14(1):39-47, 1998.

Brazzelli M, Griffiths P: Behavioral and cognitive interventions with or without other treatments for the management of faecal incontinence in children (Review), *Cochrane Collaboration 2*: 2007.

Burns CE, Dunn AM, Brady MA and others: *Pediatric Primary Care*, ed 3, Philadelphia, 2004, WB Saunders.

Cline ME, Herman J, Shaw ER and others: Standardization of the visual analogue scale, *Nurs Res* 41(6):378-380, 1992.

Eland JA, Banner W: Analgesia, sedation, and neuromuscular blockage in pediatric critical care. In Hazinski MF, editor: *Manual of pediatric critical care*, St Louis, 1999, Mosby.

Finberg L, Kleinman RE: *Saunders manual of pediatric practice*, ed 2, Philadelphia, 2002, WB Saunders.

Hannallah RS, Broadman LM, Belman AB, et al: Comparison of caudal and ilioinguinal/iliohypogastric nerve blocks for control of post-orchiopexy pain in pediatric ambulatory surgery, *Anesthesiology* 66:832-834, 1987.

Hester NO, Foster RL, Jordan-Mash M, et al: Putting pain measurement into clinical practice. In Finley GA, McGrath PJ, editors: *Measurement of pain in infants and children*, vol 10, Seattle, 1998, International Association for the Study of Pain Press.

Hodgkinson K, Bear M, Thorn J, et al: Measuring pain in neonates: Evaluating an instrument and developing a common language, *Austral J Adv Nurs* 12(1):17-22, 1994.

Jordan-Marsh M, Yoder L, Hall D, et al: Alternate Oucher form testing: gender ethnicity, and age variations, *Res Nurs Health* 17:111-118, 1994.

Joyce BA, Schade JG, Keck JF and others: Reliability and validity of preverbal pain assessment tools, *Issues Comp Pediatr Nurs* 17:121-135, 1994.

Kliegman RM, Behrman RE, Jenson HTB, Stanton BF, editors: *Nelson textbook of pediatrics*, ed 18, Philadelphia, 2007, WB Saunders.

Krechel SW, Bildner J: CRIES: *A* new neonatal postoperative pain measurement score: Initial testing of validity and reliability, *Pediatr Anaesth* 5:53-61, 1995.

Lawrence J, Alcock D, McGrath P, et al: The development of a tool to assess neonatal pain, *Neonat Netw* 12(6):59-66, 1993.

Luffy R, Grove SK: Examining the validity, reliability, and preference of three pediatric pain measurement tools in African-American children, *Pediatr Nurs* 29(1):54-60, 2003.

McGrath PJ, Johnson G, Goodman JT, et al: The CHEOPS: A behavioral scale to measure postoperative pain in children. In Fields H, Dubner R, Cervero F, editors: *Advances in pain research and therapy*, New York: Raven Press, 1985.

Merkel SI, Voepel-Lewis T, Shayevitz JR, et al: The FLACC: A behavioral scale for scoring postoperative pain in young children, *Pediatr Nurs 23*(3):293-297, 1997.

Pickering LK, Baker CJ, Long SS, McMillan JA, editors. *Red book: 2006. Report of the Committee on Infectious Diseases*, ed 27, Elk Grove Village, IL, American Academy of Pediatrics, 2006.

Puchalski M, Hummel P: The reality of neonatal pain, *Adv Neonatal Care 2*(5):233-44, 2002.

Robieux I, Kumar R, Radhakrishnan S, et al: Assessing pain and analgesia with a lidocaine-prilocaine emulsion in infants and toddlers during venipuncture, *J Pediatr 118*(6):971-973, 1991.

Schade JG, Joyce BA, Gerkensmeyer J, et al: Comparison of three preverbal scales for postoperative pain assessment in a diverse pediatric sample, *J Pain Symptom Manage 12*(6):348-359, 1996.

Stevens B, Johnston C, Petryshen P, et al: Premature Infant Pain Profile: development and initial validation, *Clin J Pain 12*:13-22, 1996.

Stevens B: Development and testing of a pediatric pain management sheet, *Pediatr Nurs 16*(6):543-548, 1990.

Taddio A, Nulman I, Koren BS, et al: A revised measure of acute pain in infants, *J Pain Symptom Manage 10*(6):456-463, 1995.

Tesler MD, Savedra MC, Holzemer WL, et al: The word-graphic rating scale as a measure of children's and adolescents' pain intensity, *Res Nurs Health 14*:361-371, 1991.

Villarruel AM, Denyes MJ: Pain assessment in children: Theoretical and empirical validity, *Adv Nurs Sci 14*(2):32-41, 1991.

Wong DL, Baker CM: Pain in children: Comparison of assessment scales, *Pediatr Nurs 14*(1):9-17, 1988.

INDEX

A

Abdominal assessment, 16-17
Abdominal pain
  paroxysmal, 124-126
  recurrent, 306-308
Abdominal reflex, 17
Abducens nerve, 22t
ABG analysis. See Arterial blood gas analysis.
Absence seizures, 167
Absolute neutrophil count, 397t
Accessory nerve, 23t
Acetaminophen, 56t, 57t
  analgesic drugs with, 60t
  hydrocodone with, 59t
Acetylsalicylic acid, 57t. See also Aspirin.
Achilles reflex, 19
Acholic stool, 101
Acid-base balance, 389-391, 389t, 391t
Acidosis
  arterial blood gas values in, 390
  compensated, 391
  in diabetes mellitus, 147-149
  interpretation of, 391t
Acoustic nerve, 22t
Acrocyanosis, 9
Actiq. See Fentanyl.
Activities of daily living, 4
Acute chest syndrome, 336
Acute lymphocytic leukemia, 243-246
  favorable prognostic factors for, 244t
Acute myelogenous leukemia, 243-246
Acute respiratory distress syndrome, 65-67
Adenoidectomy, 357
Adenoids, 355
ADH. See Antidiuretic hormone.

ADHD. See Attention deficit hyperactivity disorder.
Adolescent goiter, 248-249
Adolescents
  intramuscular injections for, 416t
  pain response in, 40
  vital signs in, 451-452t
Adolescent scoliosis, 329
Adrenalectomy, 134-135
Adrenal hyperplasia, congenital, 67-69
Adventitious breath sounds, 14
Advil. See Ibuprofen.
Aerosol therapy, 434-435
Agammaglobulinemia, Swiss-type or X-linked lymphopenic, 333
Agonal respiration, 14t
Akinetic seizures, 167
Alkalosis
  arterial blood gas values in, 390
  compensated, 391
  interpretation of, 391t
ALL. See Acute lymphocytic leukemia.
Allergic conjunctivitis, 127
Allergic rhinitis, 69-71
Allergies, history of, 3
Alveolar ventilation status, 390
Ambiguous genitalia, 68
5-Aminosalicylates, 229
AML. See Acute myelogenous leukemia.
Amplatzer septal occluder, 79t
Amputation, limb, 280-281, 282
Analgesic drugs
  administration routes and methods for, 49-55
  side effects of, 55, 61-64t
  types of, 56-60t
Anal reflex, 18
Anemia
  aplastic, 82-84
  Cooley, 108-110
  iron-deficiency, 71-73
  sickle cell, 335-338, 335b

Note: Page numbers followed by an italic *t* indicate tables and *b* boxes.